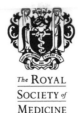

The ROYAL
SOCIETY *of*
MEDICINE
PRESS *Limited*

Type 2 Diabetes

SECOND EDITION

in Practice

Andrew J Krentz

Consultant Physician, Southampton
University Hospitals, UK

Clifford J Bailey

Head of Diabetes Research at Aston
University, UK

2005 Royal Society of Medicine Press Ltd
2001 First edition
Reprinted and updated 2001
2005 Second edition

by the Royal Society of Medicine Press Ltd
Wimpole Street, London W1G 0AE, UK
Tel: +44 (0) 20 7290 2921
Fax: +44 (0) 20 7290 2929
Email: publishing@rsm.ac.uk
Website: www.rsmpress.co.uk

British Library Cataloguing in Publication Data
A catalogue record for this book is available from the British Library

ISBN 1 85315 635 3
ISSN 1473 6845

Distribution in Europe and Rest of World:
Marston Book Services Ltd
PO Box 269
Abingdon
Oxon OX14 4YN, UK
Tel: +44 (0) 1235 465500
Fax: +44 (0) 1235 465555
Email: direct.order@marston.co.uk

Distribution in the USA and Canada:
Royal Society of Medicine Press Ltd
c/o Jamco Distribution Inc.
1401 Lakeway Drive
Lewisville TX 75057, USA
Tel: +1 800 538 1287
Fax: +1 972 353 1303
Email: jamco@majors.com

Distribution in Australia and New Zealand:
Elsevier Australia
30–52 Smidmore Street
Marrickville NSW 2204
Australia
Tel: + 61 2 9517 8999
Fax: + 61 2 9517 2249
Email: service@elsevier.com.au

Typeset by Phoenix Photosetting, Chatham, Kent
Printed and bound by Krips b.v., Meppel, The Netherlands

Dedication

To our families

Foreword to first edition

Type 2 diabetes is a modern-age epidemic estimated to affect 150 million people worldwide. In most occidental societies, 3–7% of adults develop type 2 diabetes and, in certain ethnic groups, the prevalence is much higher. The complications of type 2 diabetes are formidable: microvascular morbidity is the leading cause of adult blindness, amputations and end-stage renal failure, while premature macrovascular disease reduces average life expectancy by almost 10 years. Management of type 2 diabetes is rarely straightforward. It requires rigorous control of blood glucose and special attention to a syndrome of associated vascular risk factors including hypertension, dyslipidaemia and abdominal obesity. There is no place for mediocrity in the treatment of type 2 diabetes; it must be comprehensive, initiated promptly, delivered as intensively as possible and individually tailored.

This book confronts type 2 diabetes with an analysis of its complex aetiology, pathogenesis and natural history. Against this background, the authors provide a clear practical guide to the early diagnosis, organization and optimization of diabetes care. They show how currently available medications can be used effectively to achieve treatment targets that will minimize the complications. With due diligence, they address the awkward day-to-day problems of type 2 diabetes and suggest a rational framework for good clinical practice and informed decision-making.

We must not flinch from the challenge of type 2 diabetes, and this book provides a valuable resource to assist our endeavours.

Professor Sir George Alberti

President of the Royal College of Physicians, London

President of the International Diabetes Federation

About the authors

Andrew J Krentz is a Consultant Physician at Southampton University Hospitals, UK. His clinical and research interests include type 2 diabetes and the metabolic syndrome.

Clifford J Bailey is Head of Diabetes Research at Aston University, UK. He has served as Secretary of the medical and scientific section of Diabetes UK (formerly the British Diabetic Association), held editorial positions with several journals, and is presently editor of The British Journal of Diabetes and Vascular Disease. He has acted as an expert witness to drug licensing authorities. His research involves mainly the development of new antidiabetic therapies.

Preface to second edition

For the second edition of *Type 2 Diabetes in Practice* we have updated the guidelines and targets, noting relevant new information from the latest trials. The key messages, however, remain the same – appreciate who is at high risk and consider pre-emptive advice for prevention, or make an early diagnosis. One should treat as intensively as is practicable for the individual patient, being cognizant of the need to delay the onset and reduce the severity of complications through effective management of glycaemia and all accompanying vascular risk factors.

We thank Peter Altman and Natalie Baderman at the RSM Press.

We hope the additions and revisions made to this book will help you in your management of patients with type 2 diabetes.

Andrew J Krentz
Clifford J Bailey

Preface to first edition

The prevalence of type 2 diabetes is growing inordinately, with numbers projected to exceed 300 million by the year 2025. The condition is also emerging earlier in life, magnifying the prospect of long-term complications and the inexorable havoc they bring. Recent research has provided unequivocal evidence that improved control of blood glucose and vascular risk factors will delay the onset and reduce the severity of diabetic complications. Recognized guidelines are now in place which encourage a new philosophy for the management of type 2 diabetes: that of treating to targets. The targets are based on substantial evidence for the reduced risk of complications. Those responsible for the care of patients with type 2 diabetes are strongly urged to adopt an intensive approach to their management programme to achieve these targets whenever possible.

Intensive treatment requires considerable extra commitment, understanding, resources and, above all, the optimal use of those resources. In this book we attempt to lay the foundations and provide the wherewithal to accomplish the task of effective management of type 2 diabetes. We have tried to provide information in a clear and concise format, with easy references, highlighted key facts and practical advice.

We pay tribute to those whose lessons we have heeded carefully: George Bray, Ian Campbell, Michael Fitzgerald, Peter Flatt, Angus MacCuish, Allen Matty, Malcolm Nattrass, Gerry Reaven, David Schade, Ken Taylor, Alex Wright and Tony Zalin. Thank you.

We also acknowledge with grateful thanks those involved in the preparation of this book. Janet Allen in Birmingham, Sandra Messiou in Southampton, and Peter Altman, Tanya Thomas and Sarah Bayer at the RSM.

We hope you enjoy this book, find it useful, and gain something that will improve the management of your patients with type 2 diabetes.

Andrew J Krentz
Clifford J Bailey

Contents

1. The burden of type 2 diabetes

Epidemiology
Mortality
Morbidity
Prediction and prevention

The term diabetes mellitus refers to a group of metabolic disorders characterized by chronic hyperglycaemia. These disorders usually result from defects in insulin secretion, insulin action or both. Sustained hyperglycaemia is associated with complications in the macrovasculature, microvasculature and nerves, causing protracted morbidity and premature mortality. Macrovascular complications, particularly coronary artery disease and stroke, are increased two- to four-fold, and diabetic patients have a higher prevalence of peripheral vascular disease. Microvascular complications such as retinopathy and nephropathy, and peripheral and autonomic neuropathy, are also common.

Two main categories of diabetes are distinguished. Type 1 – formerly known as insulin-dependent diabetes mellitus (IDDM) or juvenile-onset diabetes – usually manifests before adulthood and accounts for about 5% of all cases. Type 1 diabetes arises mainly through autoimmune destruction of pancreatic β-cells, which leaves the patient with severe insulinopenia and extreme hyperglycaemia. If untreated, insulin deficiency culminates in fatal ketoacidotic coma. Hence, type 1 diabetic patients are dependent on exogenous insulin administration for survival.

Type 2 diabetes – formerly known as non-insulin dependent diabetes mellitus (NIDDM) or maturity-onset diabetes – usually manifests in later adult life and accounts for about 95% of all

cases. This type of diabetes develops mostly through a combination of insulin resistance and defective β-cell function. This causes less severe hyperglycaemia that is not usually life threatening. However, the catalogue of chronic complications of type 2 diabetes represents a serious clinical burden, eroding quality of life and reducing life expectancy. The progressive and heterogeneous nature of type 2 diabetes adds to the complexity of treatment, which usually requires one or more oral antidiabetic agents and may also necessitate the use of insulin.

In most Western societies, the prevalence of all types of diabetes is 3–7%, and it is the fourth or fifth leading cause of death. Its direct costs are currently estimated at 9% in the UK and 14% in the US of total healthcare budgets. The continuing rise in prevalence of type 2 diabetes makes this condition a major focus for every general medical practice. One in three people born in the USA in 2000 are projected to develop diabetes some time in their lifetime.

Epidemiology

Type 2 diabetes is by far the most common form of diabetes on a global scale (~95% of all cases). During the past few decades, type 2 diabetes has reached epidemic proportions in many parts of the world; the increase is closely associated with the development of obesity. The World Health Organization (WHO) has predicted that the global prevalence of all diabetes will increase from ~194 million in 2003 to ~330 million in 2025 and that this increase will affect both industrialized and developing countries. The impact on less-developed countries will be disproportionately high. Some of the countries expecting the greatest increases, such as India (up 38 million to 73 million), China (up 22 million to 46 million), Pakistan, Indonesia and Mexico, are also some of the poorest. The public health implications are formidable. In the US, for example, the age-adjusted death rate for diabetes has increased 30% over the past two decades while death rates for other major multifactorial diseases have declined (Figure 1.1).

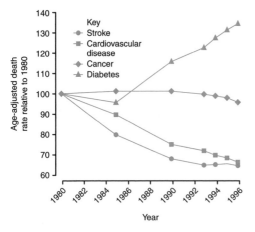

Figure 1.1
The increasing mortality associated with diabetes in the US between 1980 and 1996, contrasting with the declining associations with cardiovascular disease and stroke. Sourced from the National Centre for Health Statistics, 1998 and reproduced with permission from McKinaly J, Marceau L. *Lancet* 2000; **356**: 757-61.

Table 1.1
Ethnic variation in type 2 diabetes prevalence in individuals aged 30–64 years. Sourced from the World Health Organization.

	Prevalence (%)	Risk ratio
Pima Indians (Arizona, USA)	50	12
Nauruans (South Pacific)	40	10
Native Australians	25	6
Peninsular Arabs	25	6
South Asians	20	5
West Africans	12	3
Northern Europeans	4	1

The global prevalence of type 2 diabetes is projected to increase to >300 million by 2025

Ethnicity

The prevalence of type 2 diabetes varies more than tenfold between the highest- and lowest-risk populations. The lowest prevalence rates (<3%) have been reported in less-developed countries; by contrast, the highest prevalence (30–50% of adults) is observed in populations such as North American Indians, Pacific Islanders and Australian Aborigines that have experienced radical changes from traditional to 'Westernized' lifestyles during the course of the 20th century (Table 1.1). The Pima Indians of Arizona have the highest reported prevalence of type 2 diabetes: >50% in adults aged 35 years or more. In general, the prevalence of type 2 diabetes is about 3–4% in Europe and about 7% in the US.

Social and behavioural changes are regarded as key factors in the recent global explosion of type 2 diabetes. Of these, the most important appear to be:

● decreased levels of physical activity
● over-consumption of energy-dense foods.

Ethnicity is an important determinant of susceptibility to insulin resistance, obesity, type 2 diabetes and other cardiovascular risk factors such as dyslipidaemia. Different patterns of plasma lipids (and apoproteins) that exist independently of obesity and insulin resistance may be seen between some of the ethnic groups listed in Table 1.1. For example:

● South Asians tend to have high triglyceride and low HDL-cholesterol concentrations
● Native Americans generally have high triglycerides and low total cholesterol levels
● Peninsular Arabs generally have high triglycerides and high cholesterol levels.

Thus, while South Asians have high rates of insulin resistance and coronary heart disease, Native Americans (with their low total cholesterol concentrations) are relatively protected, despite having a higher prevalence of type 2 diabetes. Similarly, the fact that West Africans tend to have lower triglyceride levels than South Asians and higher HDL-cholesterol levels than Europeans may help to explain the relatively low incidence of coronary heart disease in West Africa compared with North Europe.

Sex ratios

There are reports that type 2 diabetes is more common in men than women (eg in the United Kingdom Prospective Diabetes Study) but other studies have found the converse. The relative prevalences of the sexes vary from population to population and no clear view has emerged. Methodology can have an important influence on measurement of prevalence rates in epidemiological studies.

Genetic and environmental factors

The thrifty genotype hypothesis

In 1962, Neel proposed that certain populations have a high prevalence of genetic traits which once conferred survival advantages during protracted periods of meagre nutrient supply, but which may now be detrimental due to abundant food supplies and reduced habitual levels of physical activity (Table 1.2). During the early 20th century, for example, rates of obesity and type 2 diabetes among the Pima Indians were both very low, corresponding with a physically active lifestyle and limited food availability, but all this has now changed.

The fetal origins hypothesis

Briefly, this hypothesis, formulated by Barker and Hales (Southampton and Cambridge, UK) provides an alternative to the thrifty genotype hypothesis of type 2 diabetes. It proposes that type 2 diabetes results, at least in part, from relative intrauterine malnutrition and that the latter leads to life-long metabolic 'programming'. This includes a reduced complement of islet β-cells combined with insulin resistance in skeletal muscle. Studies in populations in which birth weight has been carefully recorded have consistently demonstrated a correlation between low birth weight and an increased risk of type 2 diabetes in middle age. The risk appears to be particularly high if obesity (a major environmental factor) develops in adulthood. Other cardiovascular risk factors, including hypertension, have also been linked to low birth weight.

Table 1.2

General comparison of traditional and modern lifestyles of aboriginal peoples (the 'thrifty genotype' hypothesis).

	Traditional	Modern
Lifestyle	Hunter-gatherer	Westernized
Food supply	Erratic	Stable
Energy consumption	Low	Excessive
Physical activity levels	High	Low
Obesity	Rare	Common
Type 2 diabetes	Rare	Common

Other genetic factors

A lifetime concordance of approximately 90% for identical twins is strongly suggestive of a genetic component to type 2 diabetes. Commonly, type 2 patients report a family history of the condition: the lifetime risk associated with having a single parent with type 2 diabetes is approximately 40%; it is 50% or more if both parents are affected. However, due to the multiplicity of factors involved, unravelling the genetics of type 2 diabetes has proved highly problematic.

While studies of an uncommon form of diabetes, Maturity-Onset Diabetes of the Young (MODY, page 32), have yielded important evidence for single gene defects, the genetics of most cases of type 2 diabetes involve a polygenic (multigene) inheritance. Many plausible (candidate) genes, such as that for the insulin receptor, have been excluded and, increasingly, attention is being directed to the regulation of:

- genes encoding signalling intermediates within the intracellular pathways of insulin action
- genes involved in the lifecycle of pancreatic β-cells
- genes involved in the insulin secretory function of pancreatic β-cells.

Difficulties in differentiating the insulin resistance attributable to type 2 diabetes *per se* from that associated with obesity may have hampered the identification of causative or predisposing genes. Although the Barker–Hales hypothesis raises the possibility that genetics are not the sole explanation for familial clustering, recent data suggest that diabetogenic MODY genes may also influence birth weight. Thus, it seems that a complex interaction between specific diabetogenic genes, the background genome (as illustrated by ethnic variations), and the intrauterine environment, contributes to the familial aggregation of type 2 diabetes.

Age-related prevalence

The prevalence of type 2 diabetes increases with age; up to 20% of those over 80 years old develop diabetes (Figure 1.2).

The ageing populations of many societies have contributed substantially to the overall increase in the number of patients with diabetes. Glucose tolerance decreases with age, but the extent of the natural deterioration in insulin sensitivity with age remains uncertain. The weight gain that commonly occurs between the fourth and seventh decades of life creates its own state of insulin resistance, particularly if this adiposity is of central (abdominal) distribution.

Recent years have witnessed the emergence of type 2 diabetes in younger groups, including children, adolescents and young adults. This trend is of particular concern, since the clinical course of type 2 diabetes and the development of long-term tissue complications are largely determined by the duration and the degree of hyperglycaemia.

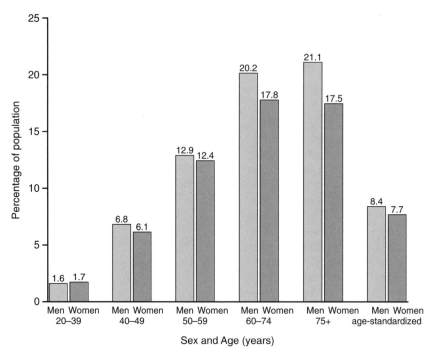

Figure 1.2
Prevalence of diabetes in men and women in the US aged ≥20 years. Included are all diagnosed and previously undiagnosed cases as defined by a fasting plasma glucose ≥7.0 mmol/l (126 mg/dl). Sourced from NHANES III and reproduced with permission from *Diabetes Care* 1998; **21**: 518-24.

> Duration x Degree of hyperglycaemia
> = Severity of complications

Clinical and metabolic characteristics

Since type 2 diabetes is a heterogeneous
disorder, certain features, present in most cases,
are regarded as typical (Table 1.3) – but not all
will necessarily be present in every affected
individual. Factors such as ethnicity, age and
stage in the natural history of the disorder will
also influence its clinical manifestations.

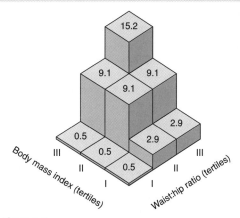

Figure 1.3
Predictive values of tertiles (I is low, III is high) of body
mass index and waist:hip ratio for the development of
type 2 diabetes in a population of middle-aged Swedish
men. The risk of developing type 2 diabetes over a 13-year
period is shown for each pillar. Sourced from Larsson B, in Vague
J, Björntorp P, Guy-Grand P et al (Eds), *Metabolic complications
of the human obesities*. Amsterdam: Elsevier 1985. © 1985.
Massachusetts Medical Society.

Table 1.3
Cardinal clinical and metabolic features of type 2
diabetes.

- Presentation usually in middle-age or later life
- Overweight/obesity common (present in >75%)
- Symptoms often mild, absent or unrecognized
- Relative rather than absolute insulin deficiency
- Insulin resistance commonly present
- Ketosis-resistant (contrast with type 1 diabetes)
- Progressive hyperglycaemia – even with
  antidiabetic therapy
- Insulin treatment frequently required to
  maintain long-term glycaemic control
- Other features of the 'insulin resistance
  syndrome' – eg hypertension, dyslipidaemia –
  often present
- High risk of macrovascular complications –
  which are the main cause of premature mortality
- Hyperglycaemia-related tissue damage may be
  present at diagnosis (microvascular
  complications)

Table 1.4
Age-adjusted relative risk of developing diabetes
among US women aged 30–55 and followed for eight
years. Sourced from Colditz GA, Willett WC, Stampfer MJ *et
al. Am J Epidemiol* 1990; **132:** 501-13.

Relative risk	Body mass index (kg/m²) at baseline
1.0	<22
5.5	25–26.9
20.0	29–30.1
40.2	33–34.9
60.9	≥35

Association with obesity

Associations between obesity and an increased
risk of type 2 diabetes have been documented
both between and within populations (Table
1.4). The anatomical distribution of adiposity
appears to be an important modulator of the
clinical impact of obesity. Thus, type 2 diabetes,
and other cardiovascular risk factors (chapter 7),
are particularly closely associated with visceral
(central abdominal, upper body, truncal)
obesity, rather than lower body adiposity
(Figure 1.3). The waist:hip ratio is a proxy
marker for central obesity that is measured

easily in clinical practice. Visceral adipocytes
display several metabolic differences from their
subcutaneous counterparts that may partly
explain the higher risk of features of the insulin
resistance (or metabolic) syndrome (chapter 2).
According to some recent studies, low hip
circumference may be an independent marker of
insulin resistance.

Dietary composition is also important: several
studies have shown that an increased

proportion of saturated fat in a population's diet is linearly associated with diabetes prevalence. Conversely, the mainly fish diets of the Eskimos and Japanese, rich in omega-3-polyunsaturates, have been reported to improve insulin sensitivity in skeletal muscle.

Other diabetogenic factors

Other factors that may influence the prevalence of abnormal glucose tolerance are presented in Table 1.5. The overall effect of gender is difficult to evaluate and appears to vary between ethnic groups (page 3). The occurrence of diabetes in women increases substantially after the menopause and is positively correlated with parity. Increased circulating concentrations of triglycerides and non-esterified fatty acids are associated with the development of insulin resistance and type 2 diabetes. An accumulation of triglyceride in skeletal muscle, or the increased availability of fatty acids, provides an alternative energy source (to glucose) resulting in decreased cellular glucose use. Chronically raised circulating lipid concentrations also impinge on the intracellular pathways of insulin signalling to reduce insulin sensitivity. A protracted rise in the fatty acid concentration may also impair β-cell function.

Table 1.5
Factors that may influence the prevalence of glucose intolerance and type 2 diabetes.

Age	Diet
Sex	Dyslipidaemia
Ethnicity	History of gestational
Family history of diabetes	diabetes
Obesity	Hyperinsulinaemia
Regional adiposity	Country of residence
Low physical activity	Socio-economic status
Lifestyle	Tobacco smoking

Mortality

Type 2 diabetes has a major impact on health and survival (Figure 1.1). Patients with type 2 diabetes have a reduced life-expectancy – an average five- to 10-year curtailment if they are diagnosed in middle-age (ie between 40 and 60 years). In developed countries, the age-specific mortality rates are approximately twice those of non-diabetic individuals. The principal cause of premature mortality is cardiovascular disease. Myocardial infarction is the most common cause of death, followed by stroke (Table 1.6).

Table 1.6
Age-specific mortality associated with type 2 diabetes (compared with the non-diabetic population). Sourced from Howlett HCS, Bailey CJ, in Krentz AJ (Ed). *Drug treatment of type 2 diabetes*. Auckland: ADIS International, 2000.

Life expectancy*	Reduced by	~ 5–10 years
Mortality rate	Increased	> 2-fold
Fatal coronary heart disease	Increased	~ 2–4-fold
Fatal stroke	Increased	~ 2–3-fold

*Aged 40–60 years at diagnosis

Insulin resistance and cardiovascular risk

Classic risk factors for cardiovascular disease are often already present when type 2 diabetes is diagnosed. The collective impact of these risk factors has been referred to as a 'ticking clock' for atherosclerosis. The presence of diabetes accelerates these adverse effects. Hypertension and dyslipidaemia are more frequently encountered in patients with type 2 diabetes than in age-matched non-diabetic controls. It has been proposed that insulin resistance – defined as a reduced biological effect of insulin – is a fundamental metabolic defect that links these (and other) risk factors.

Although insulin resistance is widely held to be an important, if not primary, defect in type 2 diabetes, the development of significant glucose intolerance implies an additional defect – impaired insulin secretion. While type 2 diabetes is a metabolically heterogeneous condition, insulin resistance and relative insulin deficiency are prominent defects, and both present in most patients.

Insulin resistance + β-cell dysfunction
= Type 2 diabetes

Impaired glucose tolerance

Insulin resistance is also present in subjects with lesser degrees of glucose intolerance. Most patients with type 2 diabetes will have passed from normality through an intermediate stage of impaired glucose tolerance (page 36). The latter state, although not directly associated with a risk of microvascular complications, shares some of the increased risk of atherosclerotic cardiovascular disease that is a feature of type 2 diabetes. In Western societies, more than 5% of younger adults and 20% of those over 65 years of age have impaired glucose tolerance. Since the latter is asymptomatic, most cases remain undiagnosed, but approximately 1–10% of cases will progress to type 2 diabetes each year – the risk is further influenced by factors such as ethnicity, obesity, family history of type 2 diabetes, history of glucose intolerance during pregnancy and the influence of certain drugs with diabetogenic effects (Table 1.5).

The gradual nature of the transition from normal glucose tolerance, through impaired glucose tolerance, to type 2 diabetes, may at least partly explain the absence of marked symptoms in many patients. The absence of the typical osmotic symptoms that accompany the onset of type 1 diabetes, for example, would explain the comparative delay in diagnosis in a high proportion of patients. In turn, the delay in diagnosis helps to explain why evidence of diabetes-related tissue damage can be found in up to 50% of newly diagnosed type 2 patients. Backward extrapolations based on the progression of retinopathy have suggested that the onset of pathological hyperglycaemia frequently occurs several (~5–10) years before the diagnosis is made.

The extent of tissue complications at diagnosis reflects the degree and duration of antecedent hyperglycaemia. Thus, the case for earlier identification of individuals with asymptomatic type 2 diabetes, or glucose intolerance, is strengthened. Population screening is one approach, but its cost-effectiveness remains the subject of debate. Factors such as ethnicity and family history of type 2 diabetes will influence the efficacy of screening.

Morbidity

Macrovascular disease

In addition to the high mortality rate associated with atherosclerotic disease (Table 1.6), there is considerable morbidity associated with macro-vascular disease (Table 1.7). For some associated conditions, such as heart failure, the risk is much higher for diabetic patients than matched non-diabetic control subjects. The prevalence of the following atherosclerotic risk factors is increased in patients with type 2 diabetes:

- hypertension is increased approximately 1.5-fold
- dyslipidaemia is increased approximately two-fold.

Table 1.7
Age-specific morbidity from atherosclerotic disease and related disorders in patients with type 2 diabetes. Sourced from Howlett HCS, Bailey CJ, in Krentz AJ (Ed). *Drug treatment of type 2 diabetes*. Auckland: ADIS International, 2000.

Coronary heart disease	Increased ~2–3-fold
Cerebrovascular disease	Increased >2-fold
Peripheral vascular disease	Increased ~2–3-fold
Cardiac failure	Increased ~2–5-fold

Microvascular complications

Patients with type 2 diabetes are also at risk of developing specific long-term microvascular and neuropathic complications:

- retinopathy
- nephropathy
- peripheral and autonomic neuropathy.

Respectively, these may lead ultimately to visual impairment, end-stage renal failure and foot ulceration. In fact, diabetes is now the largest single cause of adult blindness, end-stage renal failure, and non-traumatic amputation in Western societies.

The high, and increasing, prevalence of type 2 diabetes has ensured that microvascular complications make a major contribution to the overall public health burden now associated with diabetes (Table 1.8). Types 1 and 2 diabetes now contribute approximately equal numbers of patients to renal replacement programmes, for example. The relationship between microvascular disease and atherosclerosis is complex and tight. For example, patients who develop diabetic nephropathy are particularly prone to accelerated cardiovascular disease. This explains why most patients with type 2 diabetes who develop proteinuria due to diabetic nephropathy will actually die from coronary heart disease before they reach end-stage renal failure.

Table 1.8

Approximate prevalence of microvascular complications in type 2 diabetes. Sourced from Howlett HCS, Bailey CJ, in Krentz AJ (Ed). *Drug treatment of type 2 diabetes*. Auckland: ADIS International, 2000.

Clinical nephropathy (ie >300 mg/24 hour albuminuria)	~30%
Retinopathy at diagnosis	~20%
Retinopathy (lifetime risk)	~80%
Retinopathy leading to blindness	~2%
Peripheral neuropathy	~60%
Foot ulceration	~5%

Impact of therapeutic interventions

Hyperglycaemia

Results from the 20-year, randomized United Kingdom Prospective Diabetes Study and other prospective studies have confirmed that therapeutic interventions to reduce the level of hyperglycaemia delay the onset, reduce the progression and so reduce the severity of microvascular complications. The beneficial effects of improved glycaemic control on

atherosclerosis were less impressive. For this reason, other risk factors for cardiovascular disease must be assessed and treated with lifestyle advice and specific drugs, as necessary (chapters 7 and 8).

Non-pharmacological measures, including dietary management, weight reduction where required, and increased levels of physical exercise, are the cornerstones of diabetes treatment, acting primarily to counter insulin resistance. Several classes of antidiabetic drug are also available. These are required by most patients. Sulphonylureas and other insulin secretagogues raise plasma insulin concentrations; metformin and the thiazolidinediones improve insulin action in certain tissues; α-glucosidase inhibitors reduce the rate of carbohydrate digestion, thus slowing carbohydrate absorption from the gastrointestinal tract. Agents from different classes can often be usefully combined to increase glucose-lowering efficacy.

The United Kingdom Prospective Diabetes Study also demonstrated the difficulties of reinstating near-normal long-term glycaemic control in most patients diagnosed in middle-age. Even insulin treatment was ineffective in maintaining normoglycaemia in the long term. The development of novel oral agents and insulin analogues, combined with a greater understanding of how and when to use these agents, offers the prospect of improved results in the future. It is important to remember that the sulphonylureas, metformin, thiazolidinediones and insulin are also associated with unwanted side-effects and that occasionally these can be serious, even fatal. A careful assessment of the potential risks and benefits of pharmacotherapy must be made for each drug, particularly since diabetic complications such as nephropathy can increase the risks associated with some drugs.

Hypertension

Tight control of blood pressure has been identified as another important therapeutic goal in patients with type 2 diabetes, influencing microvascular complications (notably retinopathy) as well as atheroma. Not only is the prevalence of hypertension increased in type 2 diabetes compared with the non-diabetic population, but the magnitude of overall risk reduction when hypertension is controlled is generally greater in diabetic than non-diabetic individuals. This reflects the higher absolute risk of cardiovascular disease in the diabetic population. Several classes of antihypertensive drug have been shown to confer benefit, but the level of blood pressure attained appears to be more important than the class of agent. The results of a recent clinical trial (MICRO-HOPE; page 109) suggest that the angiotensin converting enzyme (ACE) inhibitors may have cardioprotective effects that are independent of their blood-pressure lowering effects, but this is controversial.

Although the results of several large, comparative trials of antihypertensive agents are awaited, it is anticipated that the excess cardiovascular risk attributable to hypertension may not be fully reversible using the current range of drugs. Furthermore, current blood pressure reduction targets present a major therapeutic challenge; combination therapy using several agents from different classes is often required, thus adding to the polypharmaceutical burden faced by patients with type 2 diabetes. The issue of compliance, long-neglected in diabetes, is at last receiving greater attention.

Dyslipidaemia

In the past few years a considerable body of evidence has accumulated from observational studies and randomized intervention trials that have focused attention on the importance of dyslipidaemia and other modifiable risk factors for atherosclerosis. Many middle-aged patients with type 2 diabetes have a 10-year risk of cardiovascular events that equals or exceeds that associated with overt atherosclerotic disease in non-diabetic subjects. In the latter group, the role of drugs such as statins is well-established as

a secondary preventative measure. For patients with type 2 diabetes, the distinction between primary prevention (of cardiovascular disease) and secondary prevention is less clearcut, due to the elevated risk of fatal and non-fatal events. Moreover, those patients with type 2 diabetes who survive a first myocardial infarction have a much poorer prognosis than their non-diabetic counterparts.

For these reasons, patients with type 2 diabetes are regarded as potential candidates for therapeutic interventions such as:

- specific lipid-modifying drugs (statins and fibrates)
- low-dose aspirin (and other antiplatelet drugs, especially following surgical coronary intervention)
- ACE inhibitors or angiotensin receptor blockers (usually as part of antihypertensive therapy or in the treatment of heart failure).

In the UK, the National Service Framework for Coronary Heart Disease (2000) highlighted patients with type 2 diabetes as a group whose absolute 10-year risk will often justify the use of these drugs, in addition to specific antidiabetic and antihypertensive therapy.

Prediction and prevention

It is currently difficult to predict accurately who will develop type 2 diabetes – particularly in populations with a relatively low prevalence of the disorder. Before we improve our predictive skills, major lacunae in our understanding of the aetiology of this heterogeneous disorder need to be filled. However, it is currently possible to define groups at higher-than-average risk. The related factors identified to date include:

- having a first-degree relative (parent or sibling) with type 2 diabetes
- belonging to certain high-risk ethnic groups (page 2)
- being middle-aged or older (earlier rather than later in the high-risk ethnic groups)

- having impaired glucose tolerance (IGT) or impaired fasting glucose (IFG)
- obesity (especially visceral adiposity)
- having certain endocrinopathies (eg Cushing's syndrome or acromegaly)
- receiving treatment with diabetogenic drugs (eg high-dose glucocorticoids)
- a sedentary lifestyle
- having had gestational diabetes
- exhibiting features of the insulin resistance syndrome (page 24)
- small birth weight (Barker–Hales fetal origins hypothesis)
- cigarette smoking.

About 5% of people with IGT progress to type 2 diabetes each year. Several intervention studies have shown that the risk of progression from a high-risk category such as IGT to type 2 diabetes may be averted, or at least deferred, by supervised physical training, dietary advice and weight loss if overweight. These measures can more than halve the number of people who progress from IGT to type 2 diabetes. Large trials evaluating the impact of pharmacological agents (eg the US Diabetes Prevention Program) have shown that metformin can reduce the progression of IGT to type 2 diabetes (Table 1.9). The efficacy and safety of other potential drug interventions for IGT remain to be clarified, and a pharmacological approach is not currently recommended.

For now, sensible 'lifestyle' advice for higher-risk individuals includes:

- a prudent diet
- avoidance of obesity
- regular aerobic exercise
- avoidance of cigarettes
- avoidance of diabetogenic drugs.

Further reading

American Diabetes Association. Standards of medical care in diabetes. Position statement. *Diabetes Care* 2004; **27 (suppl 1):** S15-S35.

Diabetes Atlas, 2nd edn. International Diabetes Federation, Brussels 2003.

Engelgau MM, Geiss LS, Saaddine JB et al. The evolving diabetes burden in the United States. *Ann Intern Med* 2004; **140:** 945-50.

Fagot-Campagna A, Narayan K. Type 2 diabetes in children. *BMJ* 2001; **322:** 377-87.

Grundy SM, Brewer B, Cleeman JI et al. Definition of metabolic syndrome. *Circulation* 2004; **109:** 433-8.

Hales CN, Barker DJ. Type 2 (non-insulin dependent) diabetes mellitus: The thrifty phenotype hypothesis. *Diabetologia* 1992; **35:** 595-601.

Harris MI (Ed). Diabetes in America, 2nd edn. Bethesda, MD: National Institutes of Health, NIH Publication No. 95–1468, 1995, 782pp.

Table 1.9
Controlled studies showing reduced progression of IGT to type 2 diabetes with lifestyle or pharmacological interventions.

Abbreviated name	Duration (years)	Treatment	% decrease (↓) type 2 diabetes
Da Qing	6.0	Diet ± exercise	↓33-47%
Finnish DPS	3.2	Lifestyle	↓58%
DPP	2.8	Lifestyle	↓58%
		Metformin	↓31%
STOP-NIDDM	3.3	Acarbose	↓25%
XENDOS	4.0	Orlistat	↓45%*

Finnish DPS, Finnish Diabetes Prevention study; DPP, Diabetes Prevention Program; Xendos, Xenical in the prevention of diabetes in obese subjects. *Value for obese IGT subjects only.
Tripod study reported a 56% decreased incidence of type 2 diabetes during 31 months follow-up of women with gestational diabetes treated with troglitazone, a thiazolidinedione now discontinued.
DPS. N Engl J Med 2001; 344(18): 1343-50. DPP. N Engl J Med 2002; 346(6): 393-403. STOP-NIDDM. JAMA 2003; 290:486-94. XENDOSs. Diabetes Care 2004; 27: 155-61. TRIPOD. Diabetes 2002; 51: 2796-803.

Harris MI, Flegal KM, Cowie CC *et al.* Prevalence of diabetes, impaired fasting glucose, and impaired glucose tolerance in US adults. The Third National Health and Nutrition Examination Survey, 1988-1994. *Diabetes Care* 1998; **21**: 518-24.

McKeigue PM. Ethnic variation in insulin resistance and risk of type 2 diabetes. In: Reaven G, Laws A (Eds). *Insulin resistance. The metabolic syndrome X*. Totowa, NJ: Humana Press, 1999; 19-33.

Reaven GM. Role of insulin resistance in human disease. *Diabetes* 1988; **37**: 1595-607.

The Expert Committee on the diagnosis and classification of diabetes mellitus. Report of the Expert Committee on the diagnosis and classification of diabetes mellitus. *Diabetes Care* 1997; **20**: 1183-97.

Tuomilehto J, Lindstrom J, Eriksson JG et al. Prevention of type 2 diabetes mellitus by changes in lifestyle among subjects with impaired glucose tolerance. *N Engl J Med* 2001; **344**: 1343–50.

Zimmet P, Alberti KGMM, Shaw J. Global and societal implications of the diabetes epidemic. *Nature* 2001; **414:** 782-7.

2. Pathophysiology

Insulin secretion
Insulin action
Insulin resistance

Defects in insulin secretion and insulin action are evident in subjects with type 2 diabetes. Although the temporal sequence of early pathophysiological events has not yet been resolved, the available evidence suggests that a decrease in insulin sensitivity is likely to precede a significant decrease in insulin secretion in most cases. The debate over whether insulin resistance or subtle abnormalities in insulin secretion comes first continues. However, the issue is confused by the fact that defects in secretion can aggravate reduced action, and vice versa. This conundrum is essentially why investigators have shown so much interest in the precursor stage of diabetes, impaired glucose tolerance (pages 28 and 36).

Impaired insulin action and disturbances of islet β-cell function are already evident during the impaired glucose tolerance stage, and while recent insights from uncommon monogenic forms of diabetes have clarified some points, many aspects of the pathophysiology of type 2 diabetes require further elucidation. This chapter outlines the normal physiology of insulin secretion and insulin action before reviewing the main biochemical defects that characterize type 2 diabetes.

Insulin secretion

Insulin (Figure 2.1) is the principal anabolic hormone of the body. It has a multiplicity of acute (within minutes) actions on the regulation of intermediary metabolism. Effects on the cellular transport of nutrients and ions are also prominent and there are many longer-term effects on gene expression (Table 2.1). Insulin is a 51-amino acid peptide composed of two chains, A and B, joined by disulphide bonds and arranged in a complex tertiary structure. Insulin molecules aggregate in pairs (dimers) which then aggregate with zinc to form the hexamers that comprise the insulin granules in the pancreatic β-cells.

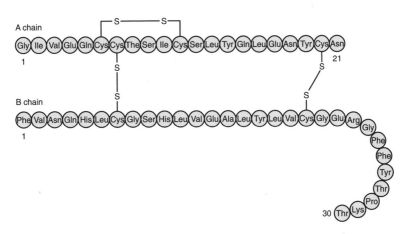

Figure 2.1
Primary structure (amino acid sequence) of human insulin.

Table 2.1
Physiological actions of insulin.

a) Metabolic actions:
   - Suppression of hepatic glucose production
   - Stimulation of glucose uptake by muscle and adipose tissue
   - Promotion of glucose storage as glycogen
   - Suppression of lipolysis and hepatic ketogenesis
   - Regulation of protein turnover
   - Effects on electrolyte balance
b) Other actions (longer-term):
   - Regulation of growth and development (*in utero* and *post-utero*)
   - Regulation of expression of certain genes

Control of insulin secretion

The pre-proinsulin gene is located on the short arm of chromosome 11. Transcription produces pre-proinsulin which is cleaved to proinsulin. Within the Golgi apparatus, proinsulin is then converted via intermediates to the final secretory products, insulin and C(connecting)-peptide (Figure 2.2).

Within the β-cells, insulin molecules associate as hexameric crystals around two zinc ions. When insulin secretory granules fuse with the cell membrane to release their contents, insulin and C-peptide are released in equimolar quantities.

Insulin secretion is tightly matched to circulating glucose concentrations. While insulin is constantly secreted in regular pulses at a low background (basal) level (this accounts for approximately 50% of daily secretion), it is also secreted in close temporal association to the rise in portal plasma glucose after meals. Glucose is transported into the β-cells by the GLUT-2 glucose transporter protein. Within the cell, it is initially phosphorylated to glucose-6-phosphate by the enzyme glucokinase and subsequently metabolized by the glycolytic pathway and tricarboxylic acid cycle to produce adenosine triphosphate (ATP) (Figure 2.3). ATP generation is proportional to the quantity of glucose entering the cell, which, in turn, is proportional to the extracellular glucose concentration.

ATP serves to close ATP-sensitive potassium channels in the β-cell membrane, leading to depolarization of the cell and an influx of extracellular calcium ions through voltage-gated channels (Figure 2.3). The resulting increase in intracellular calcium concentration activates calcium-sensitive proteins which trigger insulin granule translocation towards the membrane. Finally, fusion of these granules with the cell membrane enables insulin secretion.

Insulin is also secreted in response to other secretagogues such as amino acids. Its secretion is inhibited by certain hormones, notably adrenaline (epinephrine) and somatostatin, and enhanced by others, such as glucagon, glucagon-like peptide 1 (7-36 amide) and gastric inhibitory polypeptide. Insulin is also known to exert autocrine effects: excess may inhibit its own secretion but possibly assist the growth and division of local islet cells.

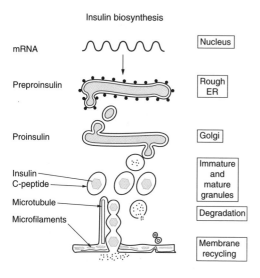

Insulin biosynthesis

mRNA — Nucleus

Preproinsulin — Rough ER

Proinsulin — Golgi

Insulin / C-peptide — Immature and mature granules

Microtubule — Degradation

Microfilaments — Membrane recycling

Figure 2.2
Insulin biosynthesis and processing within a pancreatic β-cell. Insulin and C-peptide are released in equimolar quantities. ER = endoplasmic reticulum.

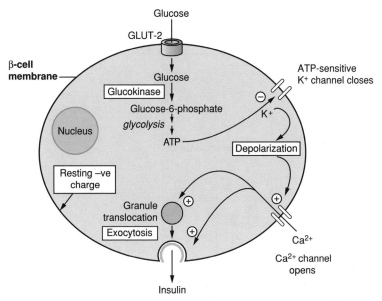

Figure 2.3
Synthesis–secretion coupling model of insulin secretion by a pancreatic β-cell. GLUT-2 = glucose transporter-2.

Defective insulin secretion

Islet β-cells normally adapt to insulin resistance in target tissues with a compensatory increase in insulin secretion. In obese people, for example, insulin secretion may be several times higher than normal. As long as insulin secretion is unimpaired, glucose tolerance can be well-maintained – even in rare genetic syndromes of severe insulin resistance such as Leprechaunism. Marked hyperinsulinaemia is the consequence of such resistance to the actions of insulin.

While cross-sectional and prospective studies in animals and humans have shown that insulin secretion increases in line with plasma glucose concentrations, in many individuals the pancreatic β-cells appear to reach their maximum adaptive capability when plasma glucose exceeds approximately 7–8 mmol/l two hours after a 75 g oral glucose challenge. Protracted hyperglycaemia is associated with no further adaptation of β-cell function and, eventually, insulin secretion starts to decline and the hyperglycaemia escalates. At this stage of impaired glucose tolerance, patients are still generally hyperinsulinaemic, but not sufficiently

so to normalize their metabolism. Subsequent progression to type 2 diabetes is associated with progressive failure of β-cell compensation (Figure 2.4a). Absolute insulinopenia becomes apparent with more marked hyperglycaemia; at this stage, the normal phasic responses of insulin secretion have been lost (Figure 2.4b).

Defective insulin secretion kinetics

Advocates for the primacy of β-cell dysfunction in the development of type 2 diabetes point to subtle defects in insulin secretion in 'pre-diabetic' individuals at high-risk of developing the disorder. Some first-degree relatives of subjects with type 2 diabetes have defects in the dynamics of insulin secretion, including loss of the normal pulsatility (usually about every 13 minutes). Impairment of the first phase (two to five minutes) of insulin secretion (probably the release of pre-formed insulin adjacent to the cell membrane) is also an early abnormality in the development of type 2 diabetes.

Non-diabetic first-degree relatives of people with type 2 diabetes have been shown to have impaired first-phase (and second-phase) insulin

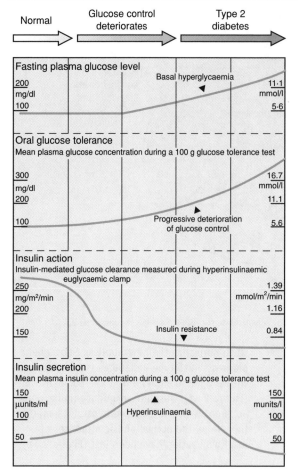

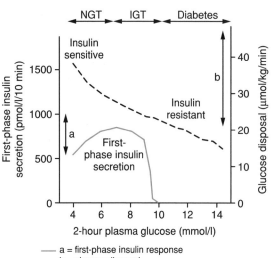

a = first-phase insulin response

b = glucose disposal

Figure 2.4a
Pathogenesis of type 2 diabetes: changes in glucose and insulin concentration and insulin action during the progression from normal through impaired glucose tolerance (IGT) to type 2 diabetes. To convert munits/l to pmol/l, multiply by 6. Sourced from DeFronzo RA. *Diabetes* 1988; **37**: 667-87.

Figure 2.4b
Relationship between insulin resistance (insulin-mediated glucose disposal) and first-phase insulin secretion and two-hour post-challenge glucose levels in subjects with normal glucose tolerance (NGT), impaired glucose tolerance (IGT) and type 2 diabetes. Reproduced with permission from Groop LC, Widén E, Ferrannini E. *Diabetologia* 1993; **36**: 1326-31.

release in response to a glucose challenge compared with matched healthy controls (Figure 2.5). It is noteworthy that these first-degree relatives are also prone to below-average sensitivity to insulin.

Experimental evidence suggests that defects in the dynamics of insulin secretion may lead to impaired metabolic action in target tissues. Thus, insulin lowers blood glucose more effectively when delivered in pulses rather than as a continuous infusion. Loss of the first phase of insulin secretion has been implicated in the pathogenesis of insulin resistance in target tissues; in particular, the suppression of endogenous (mainly hepatic) glucose production is more efficient when the rapid first-phase of

insulin secretion is present (or is compensated for by exogenous infusion). This has therapeutic implications because failure to suppress endogenous glucose production sufficiently can lead to early post-prandial hyperglycaemia (endogenous glucose production is normally inhibited by the insulin surge at the beginning of a meal). Impaired post-prandial suppression of circulating glucagon concentrations may help to sustain inappropriately normal to high rates of hepatic glucose production in patients with type 2 diabetes. If the post-prandial plasma glucose concentrations remain elevated, they then continue to stimulate the β-cells, and an extended, later (second-phase) hyperinsulinaemia is produced. In turn, this can lead to down-regulation of tissue insulin receptors.

Defective β-cell proinsulin processing

In the course of synthesis of insulin from proinsulin, partially processed intermediates (mostly 32-33 split proinsulin) are also produced (Figure 2.6a). Since proinsulin and its intermediates cross-react to variable degrees with many of the anti-insulin antibodies used in conventional insulin radioimmuno- and ELISA assays, this can lead to overestimates of the degree of hyperinsulinaemia. Increased circulating concentrations of proinsulin and partially processed proinsulin molecules – all of which have lower biological activity than insulin – have been reported in people with type 2 diabetes or impaired glucose tolerance. Studies using highly specific antibodies and immunoradiometric assays have demonstrated increased proportions of proinsulin and 32-33 split proinsulin in these groups (Figure 2.6b). These abnormalities are detectable even in the absence of the confounding effects of obesity or fasting hyperglycaemia.

Hyperproinsulinaemia in subjects with type 2 diabetes is not corrected by treatment with sulphonylureas, which suggests that ameliorating the detrimental effect of hyperglycaemia per se on β-cell function (so-called 'glucose toxicity', page 26) does not

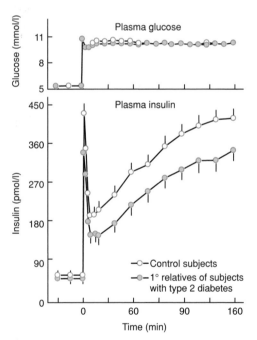

Figure 2.5
Plasma glucose (top) and insulin (bottom) concentrations during hyperglycaemic clamps in 100 non-diabetic first-degree relatives of subjects with type 2 diabetes and a control group of 100 matched healthy volunteers. All were of European ancestry. Note that first- and second-phase insulin secretion in response to hyperglycaemia is impaired in the non-diabetic relatives. Reproduced with permission from Pimenta W et al. JAMA 1995; **273**: 1855-61.

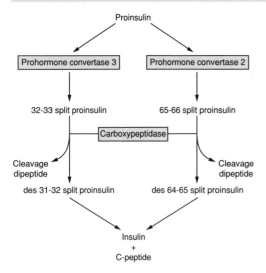

Figure 2.6a

Insulin biosynthesis and intermediates. Proinsulin is
processed via prohormone convertase 2 and prohormone
convertase 3. The latter is predominant; plasma levels of 65-66
split proinsulin and des 64-65 proinsulin are quantitatively
very low.

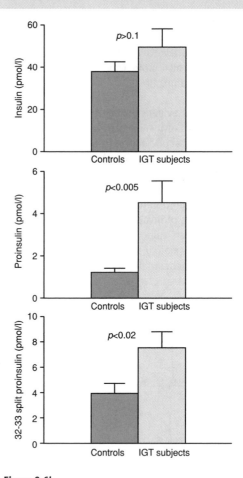

Figure 2.6b

Fasting plasma concentrations of insulin, intact
proinsulin and 32-33 split proinsulin (mean + SEM) in
eight non-obese men with recently diagnosed impaired
glucose tolerance (WHO, 1985; shaded bars) and eight
control subjects (all men; solid bars) matched for age
and body mass index. p values refer to differences between
the groups by unpaired t-test. Reproduced with permission from
Krentz AJ et al. Clin Sci 1993; **85**: 97-100. © The Biochemical
Society and the Medical Research Society.

normalize β-cell proinsulin processing.
Regardless, the reduction of plasma glucose
levels through pharmacological or non-
pharmacological measures will produce useful
secondary improvements in β-cell function.

The molecular mechanisms responsible for
impaired insulin secretion in type 2 diabetes are
still incompletely delineated. The possibility of
defective stimulation of secretion through
defective gut-derived factors ('incretins') is
given credence by the fact that exogenous
glucagon-like peptide 1 (7-36 amide) enhances
the endogenous insulin response to meals. The
inhibitory effect of chronically raised fatty acid
concentrations on β-cell insulin secretion
('lipotoxicity') contrasts with the enhanced
glucose-stimulated insulin secretion seen during
acute elevations of plasma fatty acids. Further,
fatty acids can induce β-cell apoptosis under
experimental conditions. The pathogenic role of
fatty acids in type 2 diabetes may not have been
fully appreciated and it has been suggested that
failure of insulin secretion to suppress lipolysis
may be a crucial step in the natural history of
this disorder. Since fatty acids provide an energy
supply for the process of gluconeogenesis, this
could exacerbate fasting hyperglycaemia by
accelerating endogenous glucose production.

Fatty acids also provide an alternative substrate to glucose for energy production in muscle (page 21). Additionally, insulin resistance may be aggravated by progressive β-cell failure in a spiral of metabolic decompensation.

Islet cell amyloid

Histological changes in the islets have long been recognized in subjects with type 2 diabetes. These often include an initial hypertrophy associated with hyperplasia of the β-cells and glucagon-secreting α-cells but, in cases of established duration, there may be a loss of β-cell mass and a relative increase in glucagon-secreting α-cell numbers. Accelerated accumulation of islet amyloid is a prominent histological feature, but the role of amyloid deposition in the deterioration of β-cell function which occurs over time remains uncertain.

β-cell failure

In the United Kingdom Prospective Diabetes Study, mathematical modelling demonstrated a progressive failure of β-cell function, despite treatment with oral antidiabetic agents or insulin. This finding has obvious therapeutic implications, suggesting that, once the process of β-cell failure has become advanced, it proceeds in an apparently unmodifiable or 'programmed' manner – at least with the treatments used in this study.

Susceptibility to subtle abnormalities in β-cell function during the early pathogenesis of type 2 diabetes is believed to reflect the combined effects of genetics and environment. Genetic factors might, for example, include reduced levels of expression of the genes encoding GLUT-2, glucokinase, or the other enzymes of glucose metabolism and energy production. The genes encoding potassium and calcium channels and other signalling components of the insulin secretion pathway may also be subject to limited expression, as may those encoding enzymes involved in the processing of proinsulin to insulin. While the loss of acute glucose–insulin stimulus-secretion coupling is an early recognized defect of β-cell function, it is not yet clear how this defect occurs. Persistent environmental influences relating to glucotoxicity, lipotoxicity and β-cell overactivity undoubtedly contribute to the early adaptive changes in β-cell function and increased β-cell mass, but the genetic constraints that underlie subsequent failure to maintain either individual β-cell performance or total β-cell population (apoptosis exceeds division and neogenesis) are still unknown.

Summary

Defects in insulin secretion are prominent in subjects with impaired glucose tolerance and type 2 diabetes (Table 2.2); subtle abnormalities in β-cell function can be demonstrated in non-diabetic first-degree relatives of subjects with type 2 diabetes, but the importance of these abnormalities in the aetiology of type 2 diabetes remains unresolved. This may reflect limitations in the techniques available for the assessment of insulin secretion in humans and the failure of some studies to match for important variables such as obesity

Table 2.2
Early defects and potential metabolic consequences of islet β-cell dysfunction in impaired glucose tolerance and type 2 diabetes.

Diminished or absent first-phase insulin release
Impaired suppression of hepatic glucose production with resulting post-prandial hyperglycaemia leads to late (second-phase) hyperinsulinaemia

Abnormal pulsatility of insulin secretion
Present in first-degree relatives of subjects with diabetes; diminished glucose-lowering effect of insulin

Increased secretion of proinsulin-like molecules
Marker of early β-cell dysfunction; pathological significance uncertain, but plasma levels correlate with certain metabolic risk markers for atherosclerosis

Progressive β-cell failure
Failure to compensate for insulin resistance in target tissues; defective regulation of lipolysis and glucose metabolism; progressive fasting and post-prandial hyperglycaemia

and the absolute level of glycaemia. Impaired insulin secretion is a major therapeutic target in type 2 diabetes (chapter 8).

Insulin action

The insulin receptor

The actions of insulin are mediated through the high-affinity binding of insulin to specific receptors located in the membranes of almost all mammalian cells. Certain cells, which show profound acute metabolic responses to insulin, are regarded as classic targets for this hormone. They include:

- hepatocytes
- skeletal muscle cells
- adipocytes.

Other cell types such as erythrocytes do not show matched acute responses to insulin, but this has not deterred investigators from studying insulin–receptor binding in them.

Key post-binding events include conformational alterations and autophosphorylation at tyrosines within the β-subunit of the receptor (Figure 2.7). The phosphorylated β-subunit of the insulin receptor acts as a kinase enzyme, initiating several cascades of post-receptor signalling events, the details of which are only partially elucidated. There are at least six intracellular substrates for the insulin receptor, the best characterized of which is insulin receptor substrate-1 (IRS-1). The various pathways of phosphorylation and dephosphorylation reactions leading from these substrates result in the activation or suppression of insulin-sensitive enzymes – the activation of glycogen synthase, for example, which converts glucose-6-phosphate to glycogen. Other pathways result in the genomic effects of insulin – the deinduction (repression) of phosphoenolpyruvate carboxykinase (PEPCK), for example, a key enzyme in the pathway of

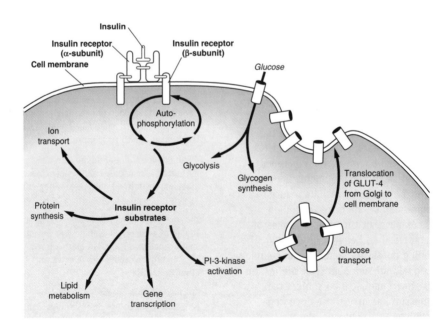

Figure 2.7
Cellular binding of insulin to its receptor and major post-binding events. Sourced from Krentz AJ. *Churchill's Pocketbook of Diabetes*. Edinburgh: Churchill Livingstone, 2000. GLUT-4 = Glucose transporter-4; PI-3-kinase = Phosphatidylinositol-3 kinase.

gluconeogenesis, which converts oxaloacetate to phosphoenolpyruvate.

There are four main mechanisms for impaired insulin action within cells: prereceptor defects, receptor defects, post-receptor defects or effector defects (Figure 2.8). In most cases these reflect a mix of genetic susceptibilities and environmental factors. Inherited susceptibility is conferred by altered expression levels of genes encoding receptors, transporters, signalling intermediates and metabolic enzymes involved in insulin signalling and nutrient metabolism. Environmental factors include nutrient levels, cytokines, hormones, drugs and other agents that impede the biochemical pathways of insulin signalling and action.

Prereceptor defects

Prereceptor defects, such as reduced insulin access to the target cells, may be due to local changes in tissue perfusion, alterations in transcapillary insulin transfer, the presence of

insulin antibodies, or a structurally defective insulin molecule. However, these defects do not make a clinically significant contribution to the common form of type 2 diabetes.

Receptor defects

Receptor defects, such as a reduced number of receptors or a reduced receptor affinity for insulin, may occur in response to chronic hyperinsulinaemia (so-called 'down-regulation'). Although obesity and lesser degrees of glucose intolerance are associated with reduced insulin-receptor binding, mainly by reducing receptor numbers, this is largely reversible on treatment. Inherited severe receptor defects (such as those experienced in Leprechaunism) are very rare and do not necessarily result in diabetes.

Post-receptor defects

Defective intracellular events that occur after insulin has bound to its receptor seem to be mainly responsible for insulin resistance in

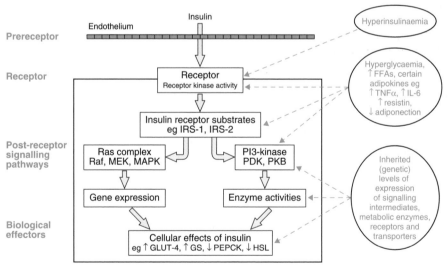

Figure 2.8
Four levels of impaired insulin action: prereceptor, receptor, post-receptor and effector.
IRS, insulin receptor substrate; Ras, rat sarcoma protein; Raf-1, mitogen-activated protein kinase kinase kinase; MEK, mitogen-activated protein kinase kinase; MAPK, mitogen-activated protein kinase; PI3-kinase, phosphatidylinositol-3-kinase; PDK, phosphoinositide-dependent kinase; PKB, protein kinase B; GLUT-4, glucose transporter isoform-4; GS, glycogen synthase; PEPCK, phosphoenolpyruvate carboxykinase; HSL, hormone-sensitive lipase; FFAs, free fatty acids; TNFα, tumour necrosis factor alpha; IL-6, interleukin 6; ↑, increase; ↓, decrease.

type 2 diabetes. Not only is the maximal response to insulin impaired, but this effect is usually only partially reversible with current treatments. The exact nature of these intracellular defects has not yet been resolved, but reductions in the insulin-stimulated tyrosine phosphorylation of IRS-1 and decreased activity of the subsequent signalling intermediates – such as phosphatidylinositol-3 kinase (PI3K) and protein kinase B (PKB) – have both been noted in the muscle of patients with type 2 diabetes. The known signalling intermediates of insulin action seem to be structurally normal in type 2 diabetes, rather it is the cumulative impact of small changes in the levels of expression and activities of some of these intermediates that seems to impact on insulin sensitivity in obesity and type 2 diabetes.

Effector defects

Effector defects are defects in the final products of the insulin signalling pathways, such as glucose transporters and key glucoregulatory enzymes. The insulin-stimulated translocation of the main insulin-sensitive glucose transporter (GLUT-4) to the plasma membrane of muscle cells is impaired in patients with type 2 diabetes, while the transporters themselves remain structurally normal. Likewise, key insulin-sensitive enzymes remain intact. These facts support the view that the insulin-signalling pathways governing the translocation of glucose transporters to the plasma membrane and the activities of key gluco-regulatory enzymes are the main sites of defective function responsible for insulin resistance.

Chronic hyperglycaemia (glucotoxicity) and raised lipid concentrations (lipotoxicity) may also contribute to insulin resistance by damaging mitochondrial function. This in turn increases reactive oxygen species (ROS) within cells and the oxidative stress impairs insulin signalling, glucose metabolism and lipid metabolism.

The metabolic actions of insulin at tissue level may be antagonized by the classic counter-regulatory

hormones: glucagon, the catecholamines, glucocorticoids and growth hormone. These hormones exert their anti-insulin actions through direct effects on insulin signalling, glucose transporters, and glucoregulatory enzymes in target tissues.

Glucoregulatory disturbances of insulin resistance

In normal, healthy individuals, venous plasma glucose concentrations are strictly maintained at approximately 5–7 mmol/l. At any time, this concentration reflects a net balance between the rate of appearance of glucose in the circulation and its rate of disappearance from the circulation. The glucose-lowering effects of insulin (Figure 2.9) are primarily:

- suppression of hepatic glucose production (ie reducing the rate of glucose supply into the circulation)
- stimulation of glucose disposal (ie clearance from the circulation, principally by skeletal muscle, but also by adipose tissue).

Hepatic glucose production

In the post-absorptive state (ie after an 8–12-hour overnight fast) the rate at which glucose enters the circulation from the liver is the main determinant of the plasma glucose concentration. Initially, this glucose is derived mainly from the breakdown of stored glycogen. As hepatic glycogen stores become depleted (usually after about 24 hours), there is increasing synthesis of de novo glucose from 3-carbon precursors such as lactate and various amino acids (gluconeogenesis). Suppression of hepatic glucose production is a major regulatory action of insulin and, in type 2 diabetes, the excessive hepatic glucose production is mainly due to inadequate suppression of gluconeogenesis.

> Hepatic glucose production is the principal determinant of fasting blood glucose concentration

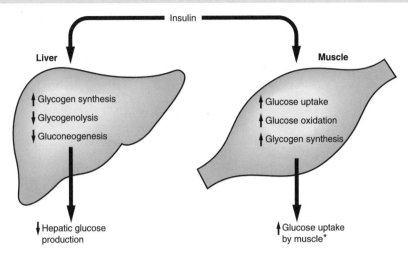

Figure 2.9
Direct actions of insulin on glucose metabolism. Sourced from Krentz AJ. *Churchill's Pocketbook of Diabetes*. Edinburgh: Churchill Livingstone, 2000. *Insulin also stimulates glucose uptake by adipose tissue. However, during a hyperinsulinaemic euglycaemic clamp, ~90% of insulin-mediated glucose disposal occurs in muscle. This is regarded as the 'gold standard' technique for measuring insulin action in humans, but may not accurately reflect normal physiology.

Glucose disposal

Stimulation of glucose uptake (with subsequent entry into the glycolytic pathway or storage as glycogen) requires higher plasma insulin concentrations than are necessary to suppress hepatic glucose production. The stimulation of intracellular translocation of GLUT-4 glucose transporters to the cell membrane for this purpose is a key function of insulin (Figure 2.7). GLUT-4 is strongly expressed in skeletal and heart muscle, and also in adipose tissue. Other isoforms of glucose transporters do not require insulin for translocation to the cell membrane: GLUT-1 is widely distributed and facilitates a continual basal (low) level of glucose uptake; GLUT-2 is found mainly in liver and islet β-cells, where it facilitates a high rate of glucose transport that fluctuates according to changes in extracellular glucose concentration; GLUT-3 provides a steady low rate of glucose transport into tissues that are strongly dependent on glucose, particularly the brain; GLUT-5 is a high-affinity fructose transporter found mainly in the small intestine and testes.

Lipolysis and ketone body metabolism

Another crucial role of insulin is to inhibit the breakdown of adipose tissue stores of triglyceride into non-esterified fatty acids and the gluconeogenic precursor, glycerol. The products of glucose metabolism via glycolysis are lactate (through anaerobic metabolism) and CO_2 (through aerobic metabolism) – the latter is the primary route to energy production. In turn, lactate can be transferred to the liver and there enter the gluconeogenic pathway, leading to glucose formation (the Cori cycle).

Since fatty acids are the principal substrate for ketogenesis within the liver, insulin can suppress ketogenesis by controlling plasma fatty acid levels (Figure 2.10). Both fatty acids and ketones can be used by many tissues as alternative fuels to glucose (eg during starvation and prolonged exercise). The appearance of ketones in the urine of a subject with diabetes indicates severe insulin deficiency. Although ketosis is uncommon in type 2 diabetes, it can develop during severe

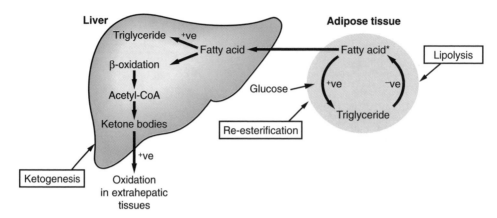

Figure 2.10
Major points of direct regulation of lipolysis and ketone body metabolism by insulin. Sourced from Krentz AJ. *Churchill's Pocketbook of Diabetes*. Edinburgh: Churchill Livingstone, 2000. ⁺ve = Increased by insulin; ⁻ve = Decreased by insulin. *The gluconeogenic precursor glycerol is also liberated by lipolysis.

intercurrent illness and is an indication for prompt insulin treatment.

Insulin resistance

Insulin resistance is a cardinal metabolic feature of type 2 diabetes. It may be defined in generic terms as 'a reduced biological response to a physiological amount of insulin'. The presence of insulin resistance is implied when there is normo- or hyperglycaemia alongside hyperinsulinaemia. For research purposes, insulin action can be quantified using labour-intensive techniques such as the hyperinsulinaemic euglycaemic clamp (also known, more simply, as the glucose clamp), which is widely regarded as the gold standard for quantifying whole-body insulin action. Essentially, it involves simultaneous infusions of insulin and dextrose. The principle is straightforward: the greater the quantity of dextrose that is required to maintain euglycaemia during the sustained hyperinsulinaemia produced by the insulin infusion, the more insulin-sensitive the individual (and *vice versa*).

> Fasting hyperinsulinaemia in the presence of a normal or elevated plasma glucose level implies insulin resistance

In non-diabetic individuals, insulin resistance is usually inferred from the presence of obesity (although there is evidence of heterogeneity within the obese population). It is generally asymptomatic if compensated by hyperinsulinaemia.

> Insulin resistance *per se* is asymptomatic

Clinical features

Severe insulin resistance may be accompanied by physical signs such as:

- Acanthosis nigricans – this dermatological feature is found in the axillae, around the nape of the neck, and elsewhere.
- Acrochordons – multiple skin tags.

Other features, present to variable degrees, include:

- Hyperandrogenism – (ie acne, hirsutism) in women of reproductive age.
- Syndrome-specific features – present in some rare congenital syndromes, such as Leprechaunism, Rabson–Mendenhall syndrome, and the lipodystrophic syndromes.

- Acromegaloid features – have also been reported in the absence of elevated growth hormone concentrations.

> Insulin resistance is a prominent feature of type 2 diabetes

Polycystic ovary syndrome

Polycystic ovary syndrome (PCOS) deserves particular mention because it is probably the most common endocrine disorder in young women. It is often associated with obesity and insulin resistance and typically presents with features of hyperandrogenism such as hirsutism, acne, and a history of menstrual and conception problems (oligomenorrhoea). Other biochemical features of the insulin resistance syndrome (page 27) are common in women with PCOS, implying that the risk of cardiovascular disease may be increased in women with PCOS. Retrospective studies also suggest that the risk of developing type 2 diabetes is higher in affected women.

PCOS overlaps with the much less common type A severe insulin resistance syndrome. Hirsutism and cystic ovarian changes are common accompaniments. The insulin resistance of polycystic ovary syndrome is thought to be independent of obesity (although obesity is an important modifier). It is hypothesized that the resulting hyperinsulinaemia stimulates ovarian androgen production.

> Insulin acts as a gonadotrophin in polycystic ovary syndrome

Plasma levels of sex hormone-binding globulin are reduced in the presence of insulin resistance because hyperinsulinaemia inhibits the hepatic production of this carrier protein. This increases target tissue exposure to free (unbound) androgens, mainly testosterone. Weight loss increases plasma levels of sex hormone-binding globulin, reducing free testosterone levels, and may lead to improved insulin action, lowering of insulin levels and reduced hirsutism. Reduced levels of sex hormone-binding globulin are regarded as a biochemical marker for subclinical insulin resistance. While recent studies have suggested a potential role for metformin and the thiazolidinediones (chapter 10) in the management of PCOS, their efficacy and safety require further evaluation.

Insulin resistance in healthy populations

Some insulin resistance also seems to exist in apparently healthy populations. In fact, up to 25% of otherwise normal individuals are thought to have unrecognized insulin resistance to degrees similar to those seen in patients with glucose intolerance or type 2 diabetes. While the significance of this insulin resistance is presently uncertain, the prevalence of cardiovascular risk factors is known to increase with increasing plasma insulin concentration.

Reduced insulin sensitivity is observed in certain physiological situations, notably puberty and the second and third trimesters of pregnancy. Insulin resistance may also be induced by drug treatment (eg with glucocorticoids). Compensatory insulin secretion from the pancreatic β-cells (page 15) usually ensures that such episodes of insulin resistance remain subclinical. Other factors that may influence insulin sensitivity include:

- *Gender* – although men and women normally have broadly similar insulin sensitivities if differences in body composition (women have more adipose tissue) and aerobic capacity (lower in women) are taken into account.
- *Ageing* – ageing is reportedly associated with reduced insulin sensitivity. However, this has been disputed, and the contribution of age-related insulin resistance to the decline in glucose tolerance commonly observed in the elderly remains uncertain.

Mechanisms of acquired insulin resistance 1: glucose toxicity

There is evidence that chronic hyperglycaemia *per se* adversely affects insulin action – an effect known as 'glucotoxicity'. Persistently high glucose levels reduce insulin-stimulated tyrosine kinase activity of the insulin receptor. The detrimental effect of glucotoxicity on endogenous insulin secretion has been discussed (page 19). The clinical implication is that reducing the level of hyperglycaemia (whether by non-pharmacological measures, oral antidiabetic agents or insulin) may produce secondary improvements in insulin action.

Mechanisms of acquired insulin resistance 2: lipotoxicity

Disturbed fatty acid metabolism is well documented in type 2 diabetes (and lesser degrees of glucose intolerance). Chronically elevated fatty acid concentrations, mainly due to impaired suppression of lipolysis, may be considered to have the following 'toxic' effects:

- impaired insulin-mediated glucose disposal and oxidation (via the glucose–fatty acid or Randle cycle)
- accelerated hepatic glucose production
- suppressed endogenous insulin secretion
- hypertriglyceridaemia (chapter 7).

Increased accumulation and metabolism of fatty acids in muscle and liver impedes post-receptor insulin signalling and reduces mitochondrial function. Excess production of the cytokine tumour necrosis factor-α (TNF-α) by adipocytes also aggravates insulin resistance through inhibitory effects on insulin signalling and GLUT-4 translocation. Elevated circulating fatty acid concentrations have also been implicated in the pathogenesis of hypertension (page 104), but the clinical relevance of the latter observations is uncertain.

Mechanisms of acquired insulin resistance 3: regional adiposity

Insulin action is often reduced in the presence of obesity, but glucose clamp studies have revealed inverse correlations between insulin sensitivity and visceral or intra-abdominal fat deposits, independent of total adiposity (as judged by body mass index). Abdominal obesity is commonly observed in men – although many women also have upper-body obesity with or without lower-body or gynaecoid obesity. Abdominal obesity is strongly associated with an increased risk of type 2 diabetes. The link is believed to result from the increased metabolic activity of visceral adipocytes compared with subcutaneous depots. Visceral adipocytes are not only relatively resistant to the actions of insulin, but exhibit greater sensitivity to the lipolytic effect of the catecholamines. This combination serves to increase the rate of lipolysis resulting in increased portal delivery of non-esterified fatty acids to the liver (page 23). However, some investigators have not confirmed a unique contribution of visceral adiposity to whole-body insulin sensitivity. Adiponectin and resistin, two recently described hormones from adipose tissue, have been proposed as links between obesity and insulin resistance. Adiponectin acts to improve insulin action, but interestingly this hormone is released in smaller amounts in obesity. Resistin impairs insulin action and is increased in obesity.

Hypertension and insulin resistance

Hypertension is very common among patients with type 2 diabetes (page 104). Moreover, many patients with essential hypertension have features of the insulin resistance syndrome. Hypotheses linking insulin resistance with hypertension in patients with type 2 diabetes include:

- Insulin-induced sympathetic activation – which could lead to vasoconstriction and increased peripheral vascular resistance
- Insulin-stimulated renal sodium retention.

Both are speculative and the cause of hypertension in patients with type 2 diabetes – the prevalence of which is also influenced by factors such as age and obesity – remains uncertain. There is evidence that insulin-sensitizing drugs such as thiazolidinediones (chapter 10) can lower blood pressure.

Insulin resistance is associated with reduced vasodilator activity, possibly due to decreased nitric oxide (NO) production by the endothelium. Insulin resistance appears to increase activity of nuclear factor kappa B (NF-κB) in endothelial cells, allowing greater production of adhesion molecules and monocyte attractant proteins. These effects are likely to facilitate local atherogenesis. Additionally, insulin resistance promotes a procoagulant state through impaired fibrinolysis, with increased endothelial production of plasminogen-activator inhibitor-1 (PAI-1) and increased platelet aggregation.

The metabolic (insulin resistance) syndrome

Metabolic syndrome has a number of synonyms: insulin resistance, 'dysmetabolic syndrome', 'syndrome X' and 'Reaven's syndrome'. Insulin resistance has been implicated in a number of pathological states which frequently co-segregate in affected individuals and which are associated with an increased risk of atherosclerotic disease, principally coronary heart disease (Figure 2.11). Key features of the syndrome, originally described by Reaven in 1988 (and refined in 1995) include:

- insulin resistance (defined as decreased insulin-mediated glucose disposal)
- hyperinsulinaemia
- visceral obesity
- glucose intolerance or type 2 diabetes
- dyslipidaemia (hypertriglyceridaemia, low plasma HDL-cholesterol levels and raised small dense LDL-cholesterol levels)
- raised blood pressure
- a pro-coagulant state
- atherosclerosis.

Since there is currently no consensus on the full ramifications of the syndrome, the following may also be included:

- hyperuricaemia
- microalbuminuria
- hyper-homocysteinaemia
- chronic low-grade inflammation
- increased reactive oxygen species.

Environmental factors such as high-fat diets and low levels of physical activity may exacerbate insulin resistance.

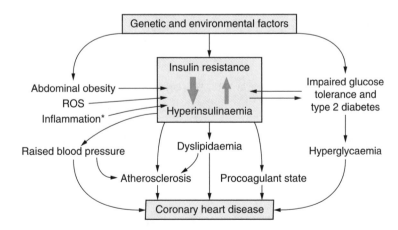

Figure 2.11
Proposed association of key components of the insulin resistance syndrome (metabolic syndrome). Each component is a risk factor for coronary heart disease. Several components are often manifest together in each individual, leading to a substantial increase in the risk of coronary heart disease. ROS, reactive oxygen species; * chronic low-grade inflammation.

Non-alcoholic steatohepatitis (NASH)

Recently, it has been suggested that fatty infiltration of the liver is associated with other features of the insulin resistance syndrome (such as glucose intolerance and dyslipidaemia) in some patients. The contribution of non-alcoholic fatty liver disease (NAFLD) is increasingly being appreciated. A proportion of patients develop inflammatory elements that can lead to fibrosis and cirrhosis in a minority of individuals with non-alcoholic steatohepatitis (NASH).

Working definitions of metabolic syndrome

The following criteria have been proposed by the European Group for the study of Insulin Resistance (1999):

A fasting plasma insulin level in the highest 25% of the population in question, together with two of the following:

- a fasting plasma glucose ≥6.1 mmol/l
- hypertension (blood pressure ≥140/90 mmHg, or treated)
- dyslipidaemia (plasma triglycerides >2.0 mmol/l or HDL-cholesterol <1.0 mmol/l)
- central obesity (waist circumference ≥94 cm in men and ≥80 cm in women).

The National Cholesterol Education Program (NCEP) in the USA proposed three of the risk factors listed in Table 2.2.

There are practical difficulties with such definitions, however, particularly in relation to the lack of population-derived reference ranges. For example waist circumference is normally smaller in people of Asian origin. If the NCEP ATPIII criteria are applied to the American population, 21.8% of adult men and 23.7% of adult women would have 'metabolic syndrome'. Prevalence is age-related, ranging from <7% in those aged 20–29 years and >40% in those aged 60–69 years.

Clinical implications of insulin resistance

Components of the insulin resistance syndrome are frequently present in combination in subjects with impaired glucose tolerance and type 2 diabetes. Whether tissue insulin resistance is the fundamental metabolic defect which links these abnormalities together is not yet known. However, there is considerable epidemiological and experimental evidence to show that insulin resistance is associated with an increased risk of cardiovascular disease. More importantly, the cumulative effects may be synergistic – ie the magnitude of the risk associated with a combination of factors can be greater than would be expected by simple addition. There is also evidence from longitudinal studies that these metabolic risk factors (a) worsen continuously across the spectrum of glucose intolerance and (b) are

Table 2.2
Definition of Metabolic Syndrome by NCEP, ATPIII: three or more of the following risk factors*

Risk factor	Defining level
● Abdominal obesity waist circumference	Men >102 cm (>40 in) Women >88 cm (>35 in)
● Triglycerides	≥150 mg/dl (≥1.7 mmol/l)
● HDL-cholesterol	Men <40 mg/dl (<1.04 mmol/l) Women <50 mg/dl (<1.29 mmol/l)
● Blood pressure	≥130/≥85 mmHg
● Fasting plasma glucose	≥110 mg/dl (≥6.1 mmol/l)

*3rd report of National Cholesterol Education Program (NCEP) expert panel, Adult Treatment Panel III (ATPIII). *Circulation* 2002; **106**: 3143–421.

present even before diagnosis of type 2 diabetes in high-risk individuals.

> Cardiovascular risk factors magnify the risk of atherosclerosis when present in combination

Taking a different perspective, many patients with essential hypertension have one or more additional components of the insulin resistance syndrome which contribute to their risk of cardiovascular events. Accordingly, it is recommended that management of high-risk patients, such as those presenting with hypertension plus other components of the syndrome, takes account of all vascular risk factors detectable in these individuals. Reduction of cardiovascular risk demands attention to all modifiable risk factors (chapter 7).

> Components of the insulin resistance syndrome should be sought and treated in subjects with abdominal obesity, diabetes, hypertension or dyslipidaemia

Further reading

Barker DJ, Hales CN, Fall CHD et al. Type 2 (non-insulin-dependent) diabetes mellitus, hypertension, and hyperlipidaemia (syndrome X): relation to reduced fetal growth. Diabetologia 1993; 36: 62-7.

Beltowski J. Adiponectin and resistin – new hormones of white adipose tissue. Med Sci Monit 2003; 9: RA55-61.

Carn DB, Utzschneiden KM, Hull RL et al. Intra-abdominal fat is a major determinant of the National Cholesterol Education Program Adult Treatment Panel III criteria for metabolic syndrome. Diabetes 2004; 53: 2087-94.

Clark A, Nilsson MR. Islet amyloid: a complication of islet dysfunction or an aetiological factor in type 2 diabetes? Diabetologia 2004; 47: 157-69.

Ford ES, Giles WH, Dietz WH. Prevalence of the metabolic syndrome among US adults. JAMA 2002; 287: 356-9.

Gerich JE. Insulin resistance is not necessarily an essential component of type 2 diabetes. J Clin Endocrinol Metab 2000; 85: 2113-5.

Grundy SM, Cleeman JI, Merz CNB et al. Implications of recent clinical trials for the National Cholesterol Education Program Adult Treatment Panel III Guidelines. Circulation 2004; 110: 227-39.

Iourno MJ, Nestler JE. The polycystic ovary syndrome: treatment with insulin sensitizing agents. Diabetes Obesity Metab 1999; 1: 127-36.

James O, Day C. Non-alcoholic steatohepatitis: another disease of affluence. Lancet 1999; 353: 1634-6.

Khan SE. The relative contributions of insulin resistance and beta-cell dysfunction to the pathophysiology of type 2 diabetes. Diabetologia 2003; 46: 3-19.

Krentz AJ. Insulin resistance. Br Med J 1996; 313: 1385-9.

Pratley RE, Weyer C. The role of impaired early insulin secretion in the pathogenesis of type II diabetes mellitus. Diabetologia 2001; 44: 929-45.

Reaven GM. Pathophysiology of insulin resistance in human disease. Physiol Revs 1995; 75: 473-86.

Saltiel AR, Khan CR. Insulin signalling and the regulation of glucose and lipid metabolism. Nature 2001; 414: 799-806.

Shepherd PR, Kahn BB. Glucose transporters and insulin action. N Engl J Med 1999; 341: 248-57.

Shulman GI. Cellular mechanisms of insulin resistance. J Clin Invest 2000; 106: 171-6.

3. Classification

American Diabetes Association and World Health Organization classification systems
Secondary forms of diabetes
  Drug induced diabetes
  Endocrinopathies
  Genetic syndromes

In 1980, the World Health Organization (WHO) proposed a classification of diabetes mellitus based on the recommendations of the US National Diabetes Data Group. This classification (revised in 1985), reflected advances in understanding of the aetiology and pathogenesis of diabetes. Notably, the descriptive terms 'juvenile-onset' and 'maturity-onset' diabetes were replaced with the terms 'insulin-dependent' and 'non-insulin dependent' diabetes respectively. A new category – impaired glucose tolerance (IGT) – was also introduced to describe the intermediate zone of diagnostic uncertainty between normal glucose tolerance and diabetes.

In 1997, the American Diabetes Association (ADA) again reclassified diabetes, revised the diagnostic criteria and introduced another new category – impaired fasting glucose (IFG). This most recent classification attempts to categorize according to disease aetiology rather than treatment. The WHO revised its 1980/1985 classification similarly at about the same time.

The 1997 American Diabetes Association classification system is based on aetiology, rather than therapy

ADA and WHO classification systems

The 1997 ADA classification of diabetes, subsequently endorsed by the WHO, recognizes four main categories.

Type 1 diabetes

Previously known as 'insulin-dependent' or 'juvenile onset' diabetes – characterized by selective islet β-cell destruction, absolute

Table 3.1
Aetiological classification of diabetes mellitus (American Diabetes Association, 1997).

I.   Type 1 diabetes
     Islet β-cell destruction usually leading to absolute insulin deficiency:
     A. Immune-mediated
     B. Idiopathic.
II. Type 2 diabetes
     Heterogeneous – ranging from predominantly insulin resistance with relative insulin deficiency to predominantly insulin deficiency with insulin resistance.
III. Other specific forms
     A. Genetic defects of β-cell function, eg MODY syndromes*
     B. Genetic defects in insulin action, eg Leprechaunism
     C. Diseases of the exocrine pancreas, eg pancreatitis
     D. Secondary to endocrinopathies, eg acromegaly
     E. Drug- or chemical-induced, eg by glucocorticoids
     F. Infections, eg congenital rubella.
     G. Uncommon forms of immune-mediated diabetes, eg anti-insulin receptor antibodies
     H. Other genetic syndromes associated with diabetes, eg Down's syndrome.
IV. Gestational diabetes
     Diabetes or impaired glucose tolerance diagnosed in pregnancy – includes pre-existing diabetes.

NB. All patients with type 1 diabetes require life-long insulin treatment. Patients in categories II, III and IV may also require insulin treatment. Thus, use of insulin *per se* can no longer be used to subcategorize diabetes.
*MODY = maturity-onset diabetes of the young due to specific genetic defects of glucokinase, or hepatic nuclear factors.

insulin deficiency and reliance on exogenous insulin to preserve life.

Type 2 diabetes

Previously known as 'non-insulin dependent' or 'maturity-onset' diabetes – occurs mostly in later life, but recent reports of occurrence in children highlight the importance of classifying according to aetiology.

Other specific types

Diabetes may be secondary to a variety of diverse conditions, including specific genetic or acquired syndromes and the use of certain drugs. All are now clearly defined and classified under this subheading.

Gestational diabetes

When diabetes mellitus or IGT is diagnosed during pregnancy, it is referred to as gestational diabetes. Gestational diabetes is pathophysiologically most similar to type 2 diabetes, but insulin is often required for adequate glycaemic control. Gestational diabetes usually resolves post-partum.

Impaired glucose tolerance

The 1980 WHO reclassification introduced the intermediate category of IGT in recognition of the area of diagnostic uncertainty between normality and diabetes. Patients with impaired, but stable, glucose tolerance are not at risk of developing the microvascular complications of diabetes (chapter 6). However, they are at increased risk of developing type 2 diabetes and macrovascular disease (chapter 7). Both IGT and the more recently defined category of IFG are usually asymptomatic, and both are discussed in more detail in chapter 4.

> Impaired glucose tolerance represents an intermediate stage between normality and diabetes

Secondary forms of diabetes

Diabetes mellitus is a feature of various hereditary and acquired diseases and may arise during treatment with certain drugs. Patients with secondary forms of diabetes are just as susceptible to chronic complications as those with primary forms of this disorder.

> Patients with secondary diabetes are also at risk of long-term complications

Pancreatic disease

Acute pancreatitis

Transient hyperglycaemia may require insulin therapy, but permanent diabetes is unlikely to follow a single episode of pancreatitis unless massive pancreatic destruction occurs.

Chronic pancreatitis

Chronic pancreatitis is frequently complicated by glucose intolerance or diabetes and, at least in Western countries, is often attributable to alcoholism. Pancreatic calcification may be evident on radiographs or computerized tomographs. While sulphonylurea treatment may suffice in some patients with an adequate number of functioning β-cells, insulin therapy is often required. Associated intestinal malabsorption and variable degrees of glucagon deficiency (due to α-cell destruction) may predispose to troublesome hypoglycaemia.

Carcinoma of the pancreas

The diagnosis should be suspected in elderly patients presenting with a short history of diabetes including the following features:

- marked and rapid weight loss (especially if disproportionate to the hyperglycaemia)
- upper abdominal pain (especially radiating to the back)
- jaundice with features of biliary obstruction.

Diabetes developing *de novo* alongside pancreatic carcinoma is not, as may be thought, a consequence of insulin deficiency due to islet destruction. Insulin resistance is implicated and glucose tolerance may improve with resection of the tumour. Pancreatic carcinoma may occur more commonly in patients with pre-existing type 2 diabetes.

Pancreatectomy

Pancreatectomy is sometimes required to relieve chronic pancreatitis-associated pain. If more than 80–90% of the pancreas is excised, life-long insulin therapy will be needed – large doses (>30–40 units/day) are rarely necessary in the absence of obesity, because insulin resistance is not usually a feature. Sulphonylureas (chapter 9) are ineffective. Partial distal resection (including that performed on the related donors of segmental pancreatic graft recipients) causes variable degrees of glucose intolerance, including diabetes.

Cystic fibrosis

Diabetes mellitus may complicate cystic fibrosis. Since patients with cystic fibrosis are now living longer, diabetes is emerging as an important complication. Diabetes usually appears in the late teens or early 20s. The recurrent chest infections and intestinal malabsorption associated with cystic fibrosis may complicate diabetes management. Insulin is eventually required in most patients, but sulphonylureas may be useful as an interim measure.

Haemochromatosis

This autosomal dominant inborn error of metabolism is characterized by excessive iron deposition in various organs. Diabetes, for which insulin therapy is often required, also develops in approximately 50% of cases. However, haemochromatosis is an uncommon cause of diabetes. Its alternative name 'bronzed diabetes' describes the associated cutaneous pigmentation (partly due to melanin). Diagnosis should be suspected in patients with hepatomegaly, suspicious pigmentation, pituitary or testicular failure, cardiomyopathy or chondrocalcinosis – a search for the most common mutations causing this disorder is now possible. Hepatocellular carcinoma develops in

approximately 15% of cases. Investigations include measurement of serum iron and ferritin, hepatic imaging and liver biopsy. Family members of a proband should be screened. Treatment is by regular venesection and the prognosis good if adequate treatment is begun before cirrhosis develops.

Malnutrition-related diabetes

Malnutrition-related diabetes encompasses the rare ketosis-resistant subtypes of 'fibrocalculous' or 'protein-deficient pancreatic' diabetes that are encountered in the tropics. Cyanide (derived from the cassava plant) toxicity has been hypothesized, but this has been challenged. Some subjects require high doses of insulin (>200 units/day).

Drug-induced diabetes

Many drugs are associated with the development of glucose intolerance or type 2 diabetes in predisposed individuals. A deterioration in glycaemic control in patients with pre-existing diabetes is also a common clinical problem. Anti-inflammatory doses of corticosteroids, for example, may necessitate the use of insulin in type 2 diabetes previously controlled by oral agents. In fact, major metabolic decompensation, such as hyperosmolar pre-coma or coma can ensue. Post-receptor insulin resistance and activation of the glucose–fatty acid cycle (chapter 2) are implicated.

Individuals with a personal history of glucose intolerance, eg gestational diabetes, are at particular risk from corticosteroid therapy, but the latter may also precipitate diabetes in middle-aged or elderly individuals who have no personal history of glucose intolerance. The typical scenario involves the development of insulin resistance which can progress to diabetes in individuals with a subclinical partial defect in insulin secretory capacity. This is difficult to predict, but a family history of type 2 diabetes should alert the clinician. Whenever high-dose corticosteroids are begun, plasma glucose monitoring is a sensible precaution.

High-dose corticosteroids may precipitate diabetes mellitus in predisposed individuals

For some other drugs, degrees of insulin resistance and/or impairment of endogenous insulin secretion are implicated in the development of glucose intolerance or type 2 diabetes:

Diuretics

Diuretics, particularly high-dose thiazides, have been associated with insulin resistance and hypokalaemia-induced impairment of insulin secretion. Modern prescribing of lower doses of thiazide ($\leq$2.5 mg bendrofluazide, or equivalent) minimizes the adverse metabolic effects. Loop diuretics, such as furosemide, are held to be less diabetogenic.

β-blockers

Beta-blockers can reduce insulin secretion and increase the risk of type 2 diabetes. Moreover, patients with hypertension often have several features of the insulin resistance syndrome (chapter 2). Both β-blockers (non-selective agents, particularly) and thiazide diuretics have been implicated in the development of type 2 diabetes in people with essential hypertension, particularly when used in combination. However, the clinical benefits of lowering elevated blood pressure are likely to outweigh the metabolic disadvantages (chapter 7). Note that β-blockers can interfere with the recognition of hypoglycaemia and the counter-regulatory response in diabetes (chapter 11).

ACE inhibitors

Angiotensin converting enzyme (ACE) inhibitors may actually reduce the risk of type 2 diabetes development in hypertensive subjects. Certain angiotensin II receptor blockers also protect against diabetes.

β-adrenergic agonists

β_2-adrenergic agonists increase hepatic glucose production. Thus ritodrine (used in premature labour), carry a risk of metabolic decompensation in women who have diabetes, or who had gestational diabetes, particularly when given parenterally.

β-blockers and thiazide diuretics can promote the development of type 2 diabetes

Oral contraceptives

Minor metabolic effects have been noted with the use of modern, low-dose oestrogen preparations. Progesterone-only preparations also have very little effect.

Cyclophilin immunosuppressants

Immunosuppression is required for organ transplantation (eg renal transplantation for diabetic nephropathy, chapter 6). Cyclosporin is associated with insulin resistance and β-cell toxicity; similar but greater metabolic derangements have been observed with tacrolimus. Concomitant corticosteroid therapy exacerbates these effects.

Diazoxide

Diazoxide is an infrequently used antihypertensive vasodilator with an inhibitory effect on insulin secretion. It has been exploited in the medical management of insulinoma and severe sulphonylurea-induced hypoglycaemia (chapter 9), but can have potent diabetogenic effects in non-diabetic individuals.

Protease inhibitor-associated lipodystrophy

Recently, a syndrome has been described in patients with human immunodeficiency virus-1 (HIV-1), also receiving treatment with protease inhibitors or nucleoside-analogue reverse transcriptase inhibitors. The cardinal features of this syndrome are:

- peripheral acquired lipoatrophy (face, limbs)
- central adiposity (abdomen and dorsocervical spine)

- hyperlipidaemia
- glucose intolerance
- insulin resistance.

Some suggest that this syndrome represents a programmed adipocyte death (apoptosis) induced by antiretroviral drugs; others suggest mitochondrial toxicity. Type 2 diabetes has been reported in <10% of cases, some in the absence of antiretroviral therapy.

Other drugs

Excess amounts of calcium channel blockers and phenytoin may reduce insulin secretion and impair glucose tolerance, but do not appear to precipitate diabetes at normal doses. Some atypical antipsychotics (such as clozapine and olanzapine) can induce insulin resistance and may increase the risk of diabetes.

Endocrinopathies

Pathological and chronic hypersecretion of hormones that antagonize insulin action (ie the counter-regulatory hormones, page 22) are frequently associated with glucose intolerance and/or type 2 diabetes mellitus. Deteriorating glycaemic control in a subject with pre-existing diabetes may be the presenting feature of such endocrinopathies.

- *Thyrotoxicosis*: is the most common endocrinopathy encountered in patients with type 2 diabetes. Excess thyroid hormones antagonize the effects of insulin. Increased lipolysis is implicated in the impairment of glycaemic control.
- *Acromegaly*: approximately 30% of patients with acromegaly have IGT and another 30% have diabetes mellitus.
- *Cushing's syndrome*: post-receptor insulin resistance is seen, especially when there are very high cortisol levels secondary to ectopic corticotrophin (ACTH) secretion.
- *Conn's syndrome*: glucose intolerance is reported in about 50% of cases of primary hyperaldosteronism – the effects of hypokalaemia on insulin secretion are implicated.

- *Phaeochromocytoma*: insulin resistance and α-adrenergic inhibition of insulin secretion by adrenaline (epinephrine) are associated with this uncommon endocrinopathy.
- *Glucagonoma*: this very rare metabolic syndrome includes a necrolytic migratory erythema rash associated with insulin resistance.
- *Somatostatinoma*: this also very rare syndrome includes cholelithiasis and is associated with inhibition of endogenous insulin secretion.
- *Hyperparathyroidism*: is associated with subclinical insulin resistance.
- *Prolactinomas*: are the most common functioning pituitary tumours. Hyperprolactinaemia can be associated with hyperinsulinaemia, but glucose tolerance is rarely affected.

In contrast to these endocrinopathies, certain autoimmune disorders are associated with enhanced insulin sensitivity. (These, incidentally, are more frequently encountered in patients with type 1 diabetes as part of a pluriglandular syndrome). There is a tendency to fasting hypoglycaemia in non-diabetic patients with untreated hypoadrenalism.

- *Primary hypothyroidism*: this common autoimmune disorder is associated with a reduced metabolic rate and impaired insulin clearance.
- *Addison's disease*: is rare but requires life-long corticosteroid replacement therapy.
- *Hypopituitarism*: will lead to increased insulin sensitivity (in a sulphonylurea- or insulin-treated patient), thus increasing the risk of hypoglycaemia.

Genetic syndromes

The incidence of diabetes – mainly diabetes with ketosis-resistant, non-insulin dependent phenotypes – is also increased in a number of inherited syndromes. These include:

Chromosomal defects

- *Down's syndrome*: trisomy/translocation of chromosome 21
- *Turner's syndrome*: karyotype 45 XO, mosaics
- *Klinefelter's syndrome*: 47, XXY, mosaics
- *Prader-Willi syndrome*: deletion/translocation of chromosome 15

- *Bardet-Biedl syndrome*: autosomal recessive disorder – main features are retinitis pigmentosa, polydactyly, central obesity, mental retardation, diabetes and hypogonadism; genetic loci on chromosome 11 have been described
- *Alström syndrome*: pigmentary retinal degeneration associated with sensorineural deafness, obesity, diabetes, hyperlipidaemia and nephropathy; disease-causing defect mapped to chromosome 2p.

Neurodegenerative disorders

- *Myotonic dystrophy*: this autosomal dominant, multisystem disorder arises as a result of expansion of a trinucleotide repeat on chromosome 19. It is associated with insulin resistance, but overt diabetes is relatively uncommon. The mutation codes for a putative serine–threonine protein kinase.
- *Friedreich's ataxia*: this autosomal recessive disorder is associated with diabetes; insulin resistance and impaired insulin secretion are reported.

Mitochondrial syndromes

Mitochondria are intracellular organelles responsible for the generation of energy by oxidative phosphorylation. Defects in the mitochondrial genome associated with diabetes were first recognized in the 1990s. Mitochondrial DNA is exclusively maternally inherited.

Wolfram syndrome

This is a rare autosomal recessive neurodegenerative syndrome comprising diabetes insipidus, diabetes mellitus (with a tendency to ketosis), optic atrophy and (sensorineural) deafness (hence, also known as DIDMOAD). The deafness may not be clinically evident and many patients also develop hydronephrosis, ataxia and psychiatric disturbances. Death occurs in the third to fifth decades. Although autosomal recessive inheritance has been proposed, mitochondrial defects have been described.

Maternally inherited diabetes

Syndromes associated with mitochondrial DNA mutations account for just a small proportion (<1%) of diabetes in the UK. However, families in which the maternal transmission of non-insulin dependent forms of diabetes (category III diabetes according to the 1997 reclassification) is associated with sensorineural deafness have also been described. A point mutation in mitochondrial DNA at position 3243 in the tRNA[LEU(UUR)] gene has been identified. While the same mutation is responsible for another rare syndrome – 'myopathy, encephalopathy, lactic acidosis and stroke-like episodes (MELAS)' – diabetes mellitus is not usually a feature of the latter syndrome.

Maturity-Onset Diabetes of the Young (MODY)

This uncommon form of diabetes is a heterogeneous autosomal dominant disorder characterized by hyperglycaemia and relative insulinopenia that presents before the age of 25 years. Offspring with both parents affected by type 2 diabetes have generally been excluded from the molecular genetic studies that have elucidated the aetiology of this heterogeneous syndrome. MODY and the common form of type 2 diabetes differ in several important respects and the main features which distinguish them are presented in Table 3.2.

> There is a 50% risk of diabetes in the offspring of a patient with MODY

Several distinct genetic subtypes have been identified to date, the first having been discovered in 1992:

Table 3.2
A comparison of type 2 diabetes and MODY syndromes.

	Type 2 diabetes	MODY
Age of onset	Predominantly in middle- to old-age, but increasingly recognized in children too*	Childhood to young adulthood
Pathophysiology	Insulin resistance and β-cell dysfunction	β-cell dysfunction
Role of environment	Considerable	Minimal
Associated obesity	Common	Uncommon
Inheritance	Polygenic/heterogeneous	Monogenic/autosomal dominant

*Usually associated with obesity in children, and in those belonging to high-risk ethnic groups. Sourced from Hattersley AT. *Diabetic Med* 1998; **15**: 15-24.

- *MODY 1* – mutations in the gene encoding hepatic nuclear factor 4α (~5% of cases)
- *MODY 2* – mutations in the gene encoding the 'glucose-sensing' β-cell enzyme glucokinase (~10% of cases)
- *MODY 3* – mutations in the gene encoding hepatic nuclear factor 1α (~65% of cases)

Mutations in other transcription factors, some with phenotypic associations, have been found.

In MODY-2, it seems that mutations in the gene encoding for β-cell (and liver) glucokinase lead to a reduction in insulin secretion involving a shift in the dose–response curve for glucose-stimulated insulin secretion. Thus, at any specified plasma glucose concentration, less insulin is secreted. Fasting plasma glucose concentrations are typically around 7 mmol/l, with post-prandial levels <10 mmol/l; this is a stable defect which is probably present from birth and which shows little progression with time. Patients who are started on insulin at diagnosis appear to be in a chronic 'honeymoon' state, and require less than 0.5 units/kg/day of insulin.

Glycaemic control is good in many individuals without drug therapy; the major exception to this rule is pregnancy where insulin may be required temporarily to ensure optimal control (many cases are, in fact, diagnosed during pregnancy). Use of sulphonylureas in the

treatment of MODY has to be undertaken cautiously because of the marked responsiveness of individuals with mutations of the hepatic nuclear factor 1α gene. Short-acting sulphonylureas or meglitinides (chapter 9) may be more suitable. The minor biochemical disturbance associated with MODY 2 is not usually associated with a significant risk of chronic microvascular complications. This relatively stable subtype contrasts with the hepatic nuclear factor mutations which cause progressive hyperglycaemia. Accordingly, oral agents and even insulin may be necessary and there is a significant risk of long-term complications. The precise molecular mechanisms responsible for diabetes in MODY 1 and MODY 3 remain uncertain. Interference with insulin secretion through altered expression of other genes has been postulated. Since approximately 20% of affected families do not have any of the MODY mutations identified to date, it seems that additional mutations are still to be discovered.

Molecular genetic testing

If genetic testing is negative, no screening will be necessary during childhood. Women with MODY 2 are often diagnosed when screened for diabetes during pregnancy; earlier diagnosis of females of reproductive age with MODY would allow steps to be taken to attain excellent glycaemic control prior to conception. Family members of patients with MODY should be aware of the symptoms of diabetes. If unaffected offspring of a proband are found to have a MODY 1 or MODY 3 genotype, testing through childhood, adolescence and into adulthood may be required. Around 80% of patients with MODY 3 are diagnosed by the age of 35 years. Lifestyle measures may be helpful in controlling diabetes. More information is available at www.ex.ac.uk/diabetesgenes/mody/info.htm.

Further reading

Alberti KGMM, Zimmet P, for the WHO. Definition, diagnosis and classification of diabetes mellitus and its complications. Part 1. Diagnosis and classification of diabetes mellitus. Provisional report of a WHO consultation. *Diabetic Med* 1998; **15**: 539-53.

American Diabetes Association. Position statement. Diagnosis and classification of diabetes mellitus. *Diabetes Care* 2004; **27 (suppl 1)**: S5-10.

The Expert Committee on the Diagnosis and Classification of Diabetes Mellitus. Follow-up Report on the Diagnosis of Diabetes Mellitus. *Diabetes Care* 2003; **26**: 3160-7.

The Expert Committee on the Diagnosis and Classification of Diabetes Mellitus. Report of the Expert Committee on the Diagnosis and Classification of Diabetes Mellitus. *Diabetes Care* 1997; **20**: 1183-97.

Hattersley AT. Maturity-onset diabetes of the young: clinical heterogeneity explained by genetic heterogeneity. *Diabetic Med* 1998; **15**: 15-24.

Krentz AJ. *Churchill's Pocketbook of diabetes.* Edinburgh: Churchill Livingstone, 2000.

Stride A, Hattersley AT. Different genes, different diabetes: lessons from maturity-onset diabetes of the young. *Ann Med* 2002; **34**: 202–16.

4. Diagnosis and assessment

Clinical presentation
Establishing the diagnosis
Diagnostic criteria
Initial assessment
Initial management
Hyperosmolar, non-ketotic coma
Influence of co-morbidity
Gestational diabetes

Clinical presentation

Most patients with type 2 diabetes are diagnosed in the relatively late stages of a long and complex pathological process. They have often had pathological degrees of hyperglycaemia for several years before the diagnosis is made. The pathogenic process of diabetes has its origins in the patient's genotype, and may be influenced by intrauterine experience, before being moulded throughout life by environmental factors. The condition itself is typically only recognized once symptoms are established or secondary organ damage becomes apparent (Table 4.1).

> Type 2 diabetes is usually diagnosed in the late stages of a complex and progressive pathological process

The presenting clinical features of type 2 diabetes range from surprisingly few symptoms in some patients to the dramatic and life-threatening hyperglycaemic emergency of hyperosmolar non-ketotic coma (page 46). Patients with lesser degrees of hyperglycaemia, whose symptoms may pass unnoticed for many years, may well carry a greater risk of insidious, unnoticed tissue damage.

> Approximately 50% of patients in developed countries with type 2 diabetes are undiagnosed

So, although classic osmotic symptoms are the rule in type 2 diabetes (with the notable exception of significant weight loss compared with type 1 diabetes), a high index of clinical suspicion must be maintained if asymptomatic cases are to be identified (Table 4.1).

Table 4.1
Presenting features of type 2 diabetes.

Minimal	Asymptomatic patients are identified by screening*
Osmotic symptoms	Thirst
	Polyuria
	Nocturia
	Blurred vision
	Fatigue/lassitude
Infection	Recurrent fungal infection (eg genital candidiasis)
	Recurrent bacterial infections (eg urinary tract infection)
Macrovascular complications	Coronary artery disease (angina pectoris, acute myocardial infarction)
	Cerebrovascular disease (transient ischaemic episodes, stroke)
	Peripheral vascular disease (intermittent claudication, rest pain, ischaemic ulceration)
Microvascular and neurological complications	Retinopathy (acute or progressive visual impairment)
	Nephropathy (microalbuminuria/proteinuria, hypertension, nephrotic syndrome)
	Neuropathy (symptomatic sensory polyneuropathy, foot ulceration, amyotrophy, cranial nerve palsies, peripheral mononeuropathies, entrapment neuropathies)
Associated conditions	Glaucoma (disputed association)
	Cataract (occurs earlier in diabetes)

*Usually opportunistic in the UK.

Although its validity has not been confirmed through clinical trials, type 2 diabetes satisfies the accepted criteria for a disorder suitable for screening on a population-wide basis. Screening of individuals with recognized risk factors for type 2 diabetes or the insulin resistance syndrome (page 27) certainly makes sense. The American Diabetes Association (ADA) (1997) recommends that testing (fasting plasma glucose measurements) be performed every three years in all individuals over the age of 45 and in selected high-risk groups of younger people (Table 4.2), but the cost-effectiveness of universal testing is uncertain. Costs would vary according to the demographics of the population screened (chapter 1) and the screening methods used.

The principal determinant of the clinical presentation of diabetes is the degree to which insulin, or insulin action, is deficient (chapter 2). A high renal threshold for glucose, which is particularly common in elderly subjects, may attenuate diabetic symptoms. Glycosuria, and hence osmotic symptoms, are minimal or even absent in the presence of hyperglycaemia in such cases.

> A high renal threshold for glucose may prevent the manifestation of osmotic symptoms, particularly in elderly subjects

The metabolic actions of insulin may be impaired at the cellular level by the direct or indirect actions of counter-regulatory hormones, ie glucagon, the catecholamines, cortisol and growth hormone (chapter 2) – all of which are secreted in response to physical and psychological stresses. The catecholamines are also able to inhibit endogenous insulin secretion and the combination of effects imparted may lead to marked metabolic decompensation in patients with limited insulin reserves. Conditions such as myocardial infarction, acute left ventricular failure or severe sepsis rapidly expose undiagnosed diabetes. Note that patients with type 2 diabetes are predisposed to such complications.

Table 4.2
Criteria for periodic testing for diabetes in asymptomatic individuals aged <45 years. Sourced from the American Diabetes Association, 1997.

- A first-degree relative with diabetes
- Overweight or obesity (especially abdominal obesity)
- Impaired glucose tolerance (on previous testing)
- Impaired fasting glucose
- Previous gestational diabetes or large baby (>4.5 kg)
- Polycystic ovary syndrome
- Essential hypertension
- Hypertriglyceridaemia
- Low HDL-cholesterol levels
- High-risk ethnic origin
- Premature cardiovascular disease
- Corticosteroid, β-blocker, high-dose thiazide therapy
- Primary hyperuricaemia or gout
- Specific endocrinopathies (eg Cushing's syndrome, acromegaly, phaeochromocytoma)
- Certain inherited disorders (eg Turner's syndrome, Down's syndrome)

Impaired glucose tolerance

Since, by definition, plasma glucose levels are not raised to diabetic levels in people with IGT, osmotic symptoms are usually absent. Asymptomatic glycosuria can result (as with type 2 diabetes), but other causes of glycosuria must be excluded (Table 4.3).

> Impaired glucose tolerance is generally asymptomatic

The diagnosis of IGT essentially relies on the performance of a 75 g oral glucose tolerance

Table 4.3
Causes of glycosuria.

- Diabetes mellitus
- Impaired glucose tolerance (IGT)
- Lowered renal threshold for glucose (eg during pregnancy, in children)

NB: fluid intake, urine concentration and certain drugs may all influence results.

test (page 43). The reproducibility of the test has been questioned since a small proportion of individuals seem to revert to 'normal glucose tolerance' on retesting, but it is still the most expedient, in fact only, means of detecting IGT.

Although individuals with stable IGT are not at direct risk of developing chronic microvascular disease, they do seem to suffer an increased incidence of atheromatous disease (chapter 7). Co-segregation of IGT with the classic risk factors for atheroma (eg dyslipidaemia and higher blood pressure) probably accounts for much of this increase. IGT (and even asymptomatic type 2 diabetes) should be considered a potentially co-existent condition in patients presenting with macrovascular disease – ie ischaemic heart disease, cerebrovascular disease and peripheral vascular disease.

Comparative cross-sectional studies currently suggest that IGT and the more recently introduced category of impaired fasting glucose (IFG) (page 43) are not entirely synonymous in terms of their pathophysiology or long-term implications. The contribution of impaired β-cell function, relative to insulin resistance, appears to be greater in subjects with IFG, while insulin resistance seems to be more prominent in individuals with IGT.

Establishing the diagnosis

While a urine test revealing glycosuria is suggestive of diabetes, a positive urine test alone is insufficient evidence on which to base a diagnosis. Glycosuria may occur in the absence of diabetes and *vice versa* (Table 4.3).

> Diabetes cannot be diagnosed from glycosuria alone; reliable blood glucose measurement is also necessary

Neither the confirmation nor exclusion of diabetes should rest solely on the measurement of glycated haemoglobin or fructosamine. Although these assays provide highly specific, longer-term indications of blood glucose levels,

they are not yet adequately standardized or sufficiently sensitive. False negative results are particularly likely with less marked degrees of hyperglycaemia and neither IGT nor IFG can be inferred. However, more recently commercially available HbA_{1c} assays – which have been more rigorously standardized – can be useful in confirming suspected cases of diabetes.

Venous plasma glucose

A blood or plasma glucose measurement is the essential investigation in the diagnosis of diabetes. This should be performed by a clinical chemistry laboratory using a specific glucose assay to ensure accuracy. An appropriate sample of venous plasma is collected in fluoride oxalate to inhibit glycolysis.

Reagent test strips for monitoring capillary glucose (most of which give an adjusted reading equivalent to plasma glucose) are convenient and readily available, but the results should be independently confirmed – especially if the result is borderline and the patient asymptomatic. A laboratory-based test *must* be performed to confirm a diagnosis based on a test-strip result. A random or fasting plasma glucose measurement is not only appropriate in such cases, but usually sufficient to establish diagnosis if diabetic symptoms are also present. If the result is borderline, the diagnosis should be confirmed by repeat measurement on a separate day. Repeat testing is particularly important in individuals with no or minimal symptoms of diabetes.

> The diagnosis of diabetes should always be confirmed by a repeat plasma glucose measurement in asymptomatic individuals

An oral glucose tolerance test is infrequently required to confirm a diagnosis and should not be regarded as a first-line investigation. Glucose tolerance tests are time-consuming, relatively labour-intensive and less reproducible than fasting plasma glucose measurements.

A diagnosis of diabetes can usually be established using random or fasting glucose measurements; glucose tolerance testing is not often required

Diagnostic criteria

The revised diagnostic criteria for diabetes (according to the ADA, 1997) are as follows:

- random plasma glucose $\geq$11.1 mmol/l (200 mg/dl)
- fasting plasma glucose $\geq$ 7.0 mmol/l (126 mg/dl).

The diagnostic fasting plasma glucose level is lower than that previously specified by the National Diabetes Data Group (1979) and World Health Organization (WHO) (1980, 1985): $\geq$7.8 mmol/l (140 mg/dl). The new, lower threshold reflects the results of cross-sectional and prospective studies that focused on the association with microvascular complications, mainly retinopathy. The ADA has proposed that fasting glucose measurement is the principal means of diagnosis, and now places emphasis on the equivalence of fasting glucose concentrations and at two hours after a 75 g oral glucose challenge. In contrast, the WHO has argued for retention of the oral glucose tolerance test in its reclassification, so the issue is by no means universally agreed. Studies to date suggest that the ADA criteria are more likely to identify patients who are: middle-aged, more obese and relatively more insulin-deficient. Moreover, the overall prevalence of diagnosed diabetes within populations seems to increase when reliance is placed on fasting plasma glucose levels alone.

Impaired fasting glucose

The 1997 ADA criteria introduced a new intermediate category of impaired fasting glucose (IFG), originally defining it as a fasting venous plasma glucose 6.1–6.9 mmol/l (110–125 mg/dl). IFG has recently been redefined as a fasting venuous plasma glucose $\geq$5.6 mmol/l (100 mg/dl) but <7.0 mmol/l (126 mg/dl) since this equates

more closely with the population of people showing IGT.

IFG denotes an abnormally high fasting glucose concentration, falling just short of the diagnosis of diabetes. False positive diagnoses of diabetes or IFG may arise if the subject has prepared inadequately (Table 4.4). This is even more relevant now, following the reduction in the diagnostic threshold for diabetes based on fasting plasma glucose to $\geq$7.0 mmol/l (126 mg/dl). Cross-sectional studies in the US and Europe indicate that there is only ~20–40% concordance between IFG and IGT [diagnosis of the latter is based on 120-minute glucose concentrations $\geq$7.8 mmol/l (140 mg/dl) but <11.1 mmol/l (200 mg/dl) – following a 75 g oral glucose challenge]. The situation is complicated further by overlap between these two diagnostic categories – some individuals with IGT will have fasting glucose concentrations that lie within the normal range [<5.6 mmol/l (100 mg/dl)], others will have values that lie within the IFG range. Several US and European studies suggest that post-prandial hyperglycaemia identified using the glucose tolerance test may predict cardiovascular mortality more accurately through identification of patients with IGT. In a large, multinational European study, the Diabetes Epidemiology Collaborative analysis Of Diagnostic criteria in Europe (DECODE) study, IGT (but not IFG) predicted mortality from cardiovascular and non-cardiovascular causes.

Table 4.4
Preparation for a fasting blood test.

- The subject should refrain from consuming any food or drink from midnight before the morning of the test
- Water alone is permitted for thirst
- Regular medication can generally be deferred until the sample has been taken
- The venous blood sample is taken between 0800 hours and 0900 hours the following morning

NB: This preparation is also required for a 75 g oral glucose tolerance test or for measurement of fasting blood lipids. The patient should refrain from smoking before and during the latter test.

Impaired glucose tolerance

A diagnosis of IGT can only be made on the basis of a 75 g oral glucose tolerance test giving a 120-minute plasma glucose $\geq$7.8 mmol/l (140 mg/dl) but <11.1 mmol/l (200 mg/dl). An equivocal random plasma glucose level (ie less than but close to 11.1 mmol/l) simply points to the need for a glucose tolerance test.

> Diagnosis of impaired glucose tolerance requires a 75 g oral glucose tolerance test

The oral glucose tolerance test

The oral glucose tolerance test is regarded as the most robust means of establishing a diagnosis of diabetes. Note, however, that the test is contraindicated if there is severe (and, by definition, diagnostic) hyperglycaemia. In individuals (as opposed to epidemiological surveys) the WHO (1998) emphasized that the oral glucose tolerance test was the gold standard, taking both fasting and 120-minute values into consideration.

> The World Health Organization (1998) consultation on the revised diagnostic criteria reaffirmed the importance of the oral glucose tolerance test

Glucose tolerance tests should be carried out under controlled conditions after an overnight fast (page 176). Patient preparation is detailed in Table 4.4. The process is otherwise summarized as follows:

- Subject should be consuming a diet containing adequate amounts of complex carbohydrate (>150g daily)
- Subject can generally defer regular medication on the morning of the test until after the test
- Subject should be encouraged to travel to the clinic by transport (minimal exercise) and to arrive at least 30 minutes before the test to allow time to relax and receive information about the test

- Subject should sit quietly throughout the test
- 75 g anhydrous glucose is dissolved in 250 ml water; flavouring with sugar-free fruit essence and chilling increase palatability and may help reduce associated nausea
- A venous line may be inserted if preferred, and kept patent by flushing with 1.5–2.0 ml sterile isotonic saline. The line should be withdrawn and discarded immediately before subsequent sampling
- Venous blood is sampled before (time 0) and 120 minutes after ingestion of the drink (which should be completed within five minutes)
- Plasma (preferred) or whole-blood glucose samples are taken
- Urinalysis may also be performed every 30 minutes (but is only undertaken if a significant alteration in renal threshold for glucose is suspected).

Interpretation of the results of a 75 g oral glucose tolerance test are presented in Table 4.5. Note that these results apply to venous plasma and that whole blood values are about 15% lower, provided the haematocrit is normal. For capillary whole blood, the diagnostic boundaries for diabetes are $\geq$6.1 mmol/l (fasting) and $\geq$11.1 mmol/l (120 minute – ie the same as for venous plasma) (Table 4.5).

Table 4.5
Interpretation of 75 g oral glucose tolerance test.

	Venous plasma glucose, mmol/l (mg/dl)	
	Fasting	120 minutes after glucose load
Normal	<5.6 (<100)	<7.8 (<140)
Impaired fasting glucose	5.6–<7.0 (100–<126)	–
Impaired glucose tolerance	–	7.8–<11.1 (140–<200)
Diabetes mellitus	$\geq$7.0 ($\geq$126)	$\geq$11.1 ($\geq$200)

NB: In the absence of symptoms, a diagnosis of diabetes must be confirmed by a second diagnostic test, ie a fasting, random, or repeat glucose tolerance test, on a separate day.

Note that marked carbohydrate depletion can impair glucose tolerance; the subject should have received adequate nutrition in the days up to the test.

> The type of glucose sample must be known; diagnostic levels vary according to specimen

Impact of acute intercurrent illness

Patients under physical stress (eg surgical trauma, acute myocardial infarction) may experience transient elevations in their plasma glucose, but these often settle rapidly without specific antidiabetic therapy. Such clinical situations are also likely to unmask asymptomatic pre-existing diabetes or to precipitate diabetes in predisposed individuals.

This acute, transient hyperglycaemia should not be dismissed, particularly where it occurs in association with ketonuria in acutely ill patients in whom rigorous treatment is indicated; oral antidiabetic agents (especially metformin) should be avoided. If reassessment six to eight weeks after recovery from the acute illness indicates that glucose tolerance has normalized, it may be that the temporary insulin treatment can be withdrawn (chapter 11). However, patients do appear to benefit from continued treatment after a myocardial infarction and, if appropriate (and in the absence of troublesome hypoglycaemia), insulin should be continued. The management of diabetes during myocardial infarction is described in detail in chapter 7.

Initial assessment

A thorough history and physical examination should be performed:

- Record the mode of diagnosis and presence of symptoms, if any.
- Review the family history of diabetes carefully. Enquire into the obstetric (still births, large babies, gestational diabetes) and menstrual history (oligomenorrhea, especially with features of hyperandrogenism) of women.
- Enquire in detail about drug history, smoking habits and alcohol consumption, and about habitual physical activity and sports interests.
- Measure height and weight and calculate body mass index. Measure waist circumference and/or waist:hip ratio. A waist circumference >102 cm (40 in) for men or >88 cm (35 in) for women, and/or waist:hip ratio >0.95 for men and >0.85 for women are considered undesirable (pages 5, 28 and 191). Note any major weight changes in recent months.
- Identify associated conditions, predisposing and aggravating factors.
- Always investigate occupational, home and family-related factors, and concomitant medical conditions that might influence the prognosis and treatment of type 2 diabetes.
- Remember that features of other endo-crinopathies (page 35) may occasionally be evident, that signs of marked insulin resistance are relatively uncommon and that specific diabetic syndromes, such as the lipodystrophies, are rare.
- Measure blood pressure carefully; lying and standing pressures should be recorded if there is any suggestion of postural hypotension arising from autonomic neuropathy.
- Seek evidence of established diabetic complications at diagnosis – examine for retinal, renal, neuropathic, cardiac and peripheral vascular disorders (chapters 6 and 7).
- Investigate symptoms and signs of neuropathy, including autonomic dysfunction where appropriate, and foot disease (chapter 6).
- Examine the fundi (through pharmacologically dilated pupils, unless there are contraindications).
- Consider biochemical testing. A case can be made for routine haematology, blood lipids and hepatic, renal and thyroid function assessment. Abnormal liver and kidney function tests are relatively common and may influence choice of therapy.

Ocular complications

Diabetic retinopathy is discussed in chapter 6. Cataract and possibly glaucoma are more common in patients with diabetes.

Nephropathy

Microalbuminuria (<300 mg/day) or overt (Albustix-positive) proteinuria are hallmarks of diabetic nephropathy. As with the other microvascular complications of diabetes, the development of nephropathy is closely related to the duration and severity of hyperglycaemia. As well as indicating early nephropathy, the presence of microalbuminuria reflects a higher risk of macrovascular disease (chapter 7). Since nephropathy can develop during the asymptomatic phase preceding diagnosis, plasma creatinine should be checked on diagnosis, especially if the new patient is Albustix-positive (has urinary protein loss $\geq$500 mg/day).

Neuropathy and foot disease

Evidence of these complications should be carefully evaluated at diagnosis (chapter 6).

Macrovascular disease

The close relationship between the components of the metabolic (insulin resistance) syndrome (page 27) should prompt the identification of associated risk factors for atherosclerosis such as:

- hypertension
- dyslipidaemia
- microalbuminuria.

Clinical stigmata of hyperlipidaemia should be sought, pedal pulses palpated and signs of vascular insufficiency noted. Further investigations may be warranted (chapter 7).

Initial management

The pressing clinical consideration is whether or not insulin treatment is required at once. In patients under 35 years with acute symptoms,

weight loss and ketonuria, the need to start insulin is clearcut – such cases are likely to have type 1 diabetes. Serious intercurrent illness at diagnosis may also point to insulin being the initial treatment of choice. On the other hand, the overweight or obese middle-aged or elderly patients with typical type 2 diabetes are more likely to be candidates for initial aggressive dietary management. Sulphonylureas or metformin might also be given to the latter group at diagnosis, where the patient is severely hyperglycaemic or symptomatic.

> In newly diagnosed diabetic patients, the first consideration is whether or not insulin treatment is immediately required

Because it is not always possible to assign diagnosed diabetes to a particular subcategory, the choice of initial therapy does not necessarily reflect the aetiology (chapter 3). The problem arises because of unpredictable endogenous insulin deficiency at diagnosis and the rate at which the latter progresses. As already mentioned, patients with type 2 diabetes may need insulin temporarily following diagnosis.

> Initial treatment with insulin does not necessarily confirm a diagnosis of type 1 diabetes

It is sometimes particularly difficult to decide whether a newly presenting, middle-aged, non-obese patient with moderately severe hyperglycaemia has type 1 or type 2 diabetes. Although relatively uncommon in the elderly, type 1 diabetes can present in any age group.

> Type 1 diabetes may present at any age – even in the very old

Even the presence of marked obesity does not guarantee a diagnosis of type 2 diabetes; occasionally obese patients present with marked osmotic symptoms and/or ketonuria indicative of insulin dependence. An insulin trial is probably the most sensible option under these circumstances, with insulin use reviewed after two to three months.

> Features of type 1 diabetes sometimes develop in patients with marked obesity; insulin is indicated

The situation is complicated as our knowledge of the subtypes of diabetes increases. In many cases, insulin deficiency is the predominant feature but presents less dramatically than in the classic type 1 condition. This has been termed latent autoimmune diabetes in adults (LADA). The diagnosis usually becomes clear retrospectively following the primary failure of treatment with oral antidiabetic agents. However, useful clinical pointers include:

- unintentional weight loss immediately preceding diagnosis
- normal or low body weight for height at diagnosis
- presentation with osmotic symptoms of short duration
- marked fasting hyperglycaemia (eg >15 mmol/l).

Of these, unintentional weight loss is perhaps the most important. Dietary manipulation with or without drug treatment can produce dramatic improvements in this respect. The issue of insulin dependence is particularly vexed in patients of African ancestry, who may present with ketosis, even frank ketoacidosis, yet ultimately prove to have diabetes which is controllable – possibly even with diet alone. Ketonuria (together with hyperglycaemia) is usually indicative of a marked degree of insulin deficiency and requires insulin treatment. However, in patients with otherwise typical features of type 1 diabetes, especially weight loss, the

absence of ketonuria at diagnosis should not be taken as unequivocal evidence that insulin therapy is not required. When deciding whether to withdraw insulin, considerable caution is always required (page 186).

> Ketonuria in concert with hyperglycaemia suggests marked insulin deficiency

> Significant ketosis in Caucasian subjects with diabetes means that insulin is required

A few young European patients with hyperglycaemia but no ketonuria prove to have relatively uncommon inherited forms of diabetes, such as MODY (page 36). In the past, such patients often received insulin therapy from diagnosis, under the assumption that they had type 1 diabetes.

Hyperosmolar, non-ketotic coma

Hyperosmolar, non-ketotic coma is a life-threatening metabolic complication of type 2 diabetes. Patients presenting with marked hyperglycaemia (>25–30 mmol/l – the upper detection limit of glucose oxidase test strips) should therefore be assessed carefully for a history or evidence of:

- marked osmotic symptoms (such as thirst and polyuria) during preceding days
- dehydration (reduced skin turgor, hypotension)
- impaired consciousness
- acute intercurrent illness (especially sepsis).

This constellation of clinical features should alert the clinician to the possibility of hyperosmolar non-ketosis, a medical emergency requiring prompt hospital admission for iv rehydration and insulin administration (Table 4.6). Patients may be moribund, even comatose, by the time of admission, to the extent that a misdiagnosis of stroke or shock is not uncommon. Hyperosmolar non-ketosis can also

Table 4.6

Guidelines for the management of diabetic hyperosmolar, non-ketotic coma in adults. Sourced from Krentz AJ. Diabetic ketoacidosis, hyperosmolar coma and lactic acidosis. In: Föex P, Garrard C, Westaby S (Eds). *Principles and practice of critical care.* Oxford: Blackwell Science, 1997; 637-48.

a) Fluids and electrolytes

Volumes:	1 l/hour for 2–3 hours, thereafter adjusted according to requirements.
Fluids:	Isotonic ('normal') saline (150 mmol/l) is routine.
	Hypotonic ('half-normal') saline (75 mmol/l) if serum sodium exceeds 150 mmol/l (no more than 1–2 l – consider 5% dextrose with increased insulin if marked hypernatraemia).
	5% dextrose 1l 4–6-hourly when blood glucose has fallen to 10–15 mmol/l (severely dehydrated patients may require simultaneous saline infusion).
Potassium replacement:	No potassium in first 1l, unless initial plasma potassium <3.5 mmol/l.
	Thereafter, add following dosages to each 1l of fluid:
	If plasma potassium is <4.0 mmol/l, add 40 mmol KCl (severe hypokalaemia may require more aggressive KCl replacement)
	If plasma potassium is 3.5–5.5 mmol/l, add 20 mmol KCl
	If plasma potassium is >5.5 mmol/l, add no KCl but repeat measurement of plasma potassium within 1–2 hours.
	Particular care is required in pre-renal uraemia.
	NB: Rhabdomyolysis may cause acute renal failure (rare).

b) Insulin

Using continuous iv infusion:	Give 6 units/hour soluble insulin until blood glucose has fallen to 15 mmol/l.
	Thereafter, adjust rate (usually down to 1–4 units/hour) during dextrose infusion to maintain blood glucose at 5-10 mmol/l until patient is eating again.
	Transfer to subcutaneous insulin.
	Review as outpatient after 1–2 months – withdrawal of insulin may be possible.
	A sulphonylurea or even diet alone may suffice.

c) Other points

Search for and treat precipitating cause (eg sepsis, myocardial infarction).
Hypotension usually responds to adequate fluid replacement.
Monitor for central venous pressure in elderly patients or if cardiac disease present.
If level of consciousness is impaired, pass nasogastric tube to avoid aspiration of gastric contents.
If level of consciousness is impaired, or no urine passed within ~4 hours of start of therapy, insert urinary catheter.
Thromboembolic complications are relatively common. Some clinicians recommend routine anticoagulation; others treat clinically evident thromboses as they arise. Low-dose heparin is a reasonable option, but there are no data from randomized trials.

develop in patients already receiving treatment for type 2 diabetes. Typical biochemical features include:

- severe hyperglycaemia (plasma glucose often >50 mmol/l)
- hyperosmolarity (see below)
- severe volume depletion with pre-renal uraemia
- electrolyte depletion
- minimal or absent ketosis.

Consciousness is usually depressed when plasma osmolality has exceeded ~340 mosmol/l. Plasma osmolality may be determined by freezing-point depression or estimated using a formula based on plasma concentrations:

2 x (sodium + potassium) + urea + glucose
(where sodium, potassium, urea and glucose are in mmol/l).

Hyperosmolar non-ketosis is associated with a relatively high case–fatality rate. As many as two-thirds of cases are previously undiagnosed patients and the syndrome tends to be confined to middle-aged and elderly patients – black patients are over-represented in some reports. Precipitating factors are thought to include diabetogenic drugs such as high-dose corticosteroids and infection, both of which antagonize insulin action. The quenching of thirst through carbonated drinks with a high sugar content may also contribute in some cases.

In cases that recover, diabetes can often be controlled by antidiabetic tablets or even dietary measures, which is taken to indicate that patients still have relative rather than absolute insulin deficiency. If insulin is administered for one to two months after recovery, the possibility of successful withdrawal can then be assessed (page 173). Drugs with diabetogenic potential (including high-dose thiazides and non-selective β-blockers) should be used with caution.

While ketonuria is not usually a feature of type 2 diabetes, ketosis, and sometimes ketoacidosis, can be precipitated by acute severe intercurrent illness.

> Patients with type 2 diabetes of African ancestry may present with hyperosmolar non-ketosis or even diabetic ketoacidosis

Influence of co-morbidity

Significant concurrent physical or psychological disease modifies the presentation and management of diabetes. To use an extreme example, alongside a condition such as advanced malignancy (limited life-expectancy), the primary goals of diabetes management would be relief of the osmotic symptoms and prevention of major metabolic decompensation – long-term microvascular complications would not be considered. Insulin may still be the most appropriate therapy in such a case – not only is it likely to provide the quickest relief of osmotic symptoms, but other drugs may be contraindicated, eg because of concomitant

renal or hepatic impairment. Use of high doses of potent corticosteroids such as dexamethasone is a relatively common reason for using insulin preferentially in such patients.

> Diabetic patients are frequently affected by significant co-morbidity

Psychological considerations

A diagnosis of diabetes often has a major emotional impact on the patient (and his or her immediate family). Fears about complications such as blindness and amputation are accompanied by significant immediate restrictions on daily life. Factors that may influence the psychological response to diagnosis include: age, the treatment required, the degree and type of self-monitoring required, the presence of complications, co-morbidity, the implications for employment, the impact on recreational activities, and the degree of family and social support.

Furthermore, certain psychosocial characteristics have a bearing both on the initial reaction and on the patient's subsequent success in managing their disease: personality, temperament, health beliefs, cultural or religious conditioning, acute and chronic co-existent psychological states, intelligence, educational achievement, occupation, philosophical leaning. These factors also influence the success of diabetes education. A sympathetic approach, tailored to the individual, is required.

Depression

The overall prevalence of depression in type 2 diabetes is similar to that observed in other chronic diseases. Psychosocial pressures are often cited by patients as reasons for failure to attain or sustain their glycaemic targets, and issues such as compliance are certainly influenced by anxiety and depression. Serious psychiatric disturbance obviously demands expert psychiatric assessment, and chronic psychoses, habitual drug abuse and alcoholism can all place considerable obstacles in the path of successful self-management.

> Depression is more common in patients with diabetes

Recall that some atypical antipsychotic agents can aggravate glycaemic control (page 35).

Gestational diabetes

The 1997 reclassification of diabetes (page 27) recognized gestational diabetes – diabetes first diagnosed in a woman during pregnancy – as a specific sub-category. Diabetes or IGT which is actually precipitated by the pregnancy, and pre-existing diabetes or IGT are now all included in this category. In most women with gestational IGT or diabetes precipitated by their pregnancy, glucose tolerance returns to normal post-partum. The long-term risk of permanent type 2 diabetes is substantially increased, usually in line with the frequency of type 2 diabetes in the relevant population and ethnic group. In the UK, the incidence of gestational diabetes is low (1–2%) in white Europeans and highest (4–5%) in South Asians. Women with MODY are often diagnosed during pregnancy.

> Impaired glucose tolerance in pregnancy is classified as gestational diabetes mellitus

Diagnosis

There is no consensus on the diagnostic criteria for gestational diabetes. In the absence of an unequivocal elevation of blood glucose, diagnosis will rest on the results of an oral glucose tolerance test. A higher risk of gestational diabetes is conferred by the clinical factors presented in Table 4.7.

Glycosuria is common during pregnancy, but one or more random blood glucose tests may

Table 4.7
Groups of women associated with a higher risk of gestational diabetes.

- Older women
- Women with a history of glucose intolerance
- Women with a history of large-for-gestational-age babies (birthweight >4.5 kg or >90th centile for gestational age)
- Women from certain high-risk ethnic groups
- Women who have had glycosuria during pregnancy in the past
- Women who are overweight or obese
- Women with a pregnancy complicated by polyhydramnios
- Women with a family history of diabetes in a first-degree relative

be sufficient to allay concerns about diabetes in the absence of other risk factors. In high-risk populations a case can be made for screening for pre-existing diabetes early in pregnancy. A fasting plasma glucose >7 mmol/l (126 mg/dl) or a random plasma glucose >11.1 mmol/l (200 mg/dl) confirms a diagnosis of diabetes.

Fasting plasma glucose concentrations tend to decline during the first trimester, which may render these tests unsuitable for detection of all cases. In fact, a complex literature has built up around the issue of gestational diabetes. Expert opinions about the importance of its detection and clinical implications have become polarized. Concerns have been voiced that diagnosis may lead to a higher rate of Caesarian section in the absence of clear clinical indications, but there is an opposing view that some form of screening for glucose intolerance is appropriate. Screening usually takes the form of a blood test between 24 and 28 weeks' gestation. Glycated proteins are not sufficiently sensitive for this purpose. The test described by O'Sullivan is the most widely used in the US.

The O'Sullivan screening test

This test has a cutoff value of ≥7.8 mmol/l 60 minutes after an oral 50 g glucose challenge and a high sensitivity and specificity (>80% for each) for glucose intolerance at 20–28 weeks. It may also be applied to high-risk populations in the first trimester, but it is worth bearing in mind that it was designed to determine the risk of subsequent diabetes in the mother, rather than predict the outcome of the index pregnancy.

Management

The detection of gestational diabetes raises important questions about the aims of treatment. It has been argued that there are insufficient data to justify universal screening for gestational diabetes because there is no reliable evidence that subsequent intervention is effective – except perhaps in reducing the proportion of babies with macrosomia (but macrosomia is confounded by maternal obesity). Dietary measures may suffice.

Calorie restriction

A 30% reduction in the daily calorie consumption of obese women will reduce hyperglycaemia. The US National Academy of Science recommends that the total weight gain during pregnancy for obese women should be limited to <6 kg:

Body mass index (kg/m²)	Recommended weight gain (kg)
20–26	11.5–16.0
26–29	7.0–11.5
>29	<6.0

Oral antidiabetic agents

Oral drug treatment is usually avoided, although fears about teratogenicity have not been clearly substantiated. Metformin, for example, has not shown any evidence of teratogenicity *in vitro*. Early experience with the first-generation sulphonylureas, eg chlorpropamide, was marred by reports of profound hypoglycaemia in the neonates of diabetic mothers. However, the role of second-generation sulphonylureas has recently been re-examined. In a US study, glibenclamide

(glyburide) was used, apparently safely. This drug does not cross the placenta, but caution must still be exercised and more research is needed before the sulphonylureas can be recommended for gestational diabetes. Thiazolidinediones should be substituted with other antidiabetic therapy (usually insulin) after pregnancy is established, as animal studies have suggested that thiazolidinediones impair fetal growth in late gestation.

Insulin

Insulin is required in approximately 30% of women with gestational diabetes. The merits of attempting to judge control by comparing pre-prandial with post-prandial blood glucose levels have been debated, however no clear answer has emerged with respect to preventing fetal macrosomia. Rapid-acting insulin analogues have been used successfully in gestational diabetes, but in a relatively small number of women. There is a suggestion that the incidence of associated hypoglycaemia may be lower than with conventional short-acting insulin. Lispro is not detectable in cord blood, but further studies are required to establish the safety of insulin analogues during embryogenesis. Ironically, the risk of producing underweight babies as a result of strict maternal glycaemic control has raised theoretical concerns about programming a higher risk of diabetes in the offspring (page 3).

Post-pregnancy follow-up

Follow-up and counselling of mothers with gestational diabetes should include advice about avoiding obesity and the protective effect of regular exercise. Follow-up studies suggest that if body weight is successfully managed during pregnancy, the risk of conversion to type 2 diabetes might be reduced by approximately 50%.

> Maintenance of ideal body weight reduces the risk of future development of type 2 diabetes

In the weeks following delivery, a 75 g oral glucose tolerance test should be performed. Most patients (>90%) will revert to normal glucose tolerance post-partum.

An annual fasting plasma glucose test and instructions to present for additional testing if symptoms of diabetes are experienced are the minimal follow-up requirements. In high-risk populations, such as Hispanic American women, as many as 40% of cases that resolve immediately after the index pregnancy will become re-established as permanent diabetes within six years. In European populations, the rate of progression is much lower, which makes systematic follow-up that much harder. A 31-month follow-up of women with GDM reverting to normal after parturition (TRIPOD study), found that treatment with the thiazolidinedione troglitazone (now withdrawn) decreased the incidence of type 2 diabetes by 56%. Trials with current thiazolidinediones are in progress.

A small proportion of women with gestational diabetes subsequently develop type 1 diabetes. It is suggested that these patients have slow-onset autoimmune β-cell destruction which is unmasked by the insulin resistance of pregnancy.

Planning pregnancy

Since there is a strong relationship between glycaemic control at conception and the risk of congenital malformations, the importance of planned pregnancy in women with diabetes should be stressed and reminders given whenever the opportunity arises. For the reasons outlined in Table 4.8, diabetic pregnancy is regarded as high risk and should be managed with appropriate specialist diabetic and obstetric supervision. A combined clinic, in which the mother is reviewed at frequent intervals, is favoured by many units.

> Pregnancy should be planned wherever possible in women with diabetes

> Pregnancy in women with diabetes carries additional risks for both mother and child

Table 4.8
Risks associated with diabetic pregnancy.

a) Maternal risks
- Metabolic control deteriorates in the 2nd and 3rd trimesters (insulin may be required)
- Pre-existing complications such as retinopathy and nephropathy may progress
- Risk of pre-eclamptic toxaemia is increased two-fold
- Subclinical coronary heart disease may be unmasked
- Increased risk of urinary tract infection
- Increased rates of Caesarian section

b) Fetal risks
- Risk of congenital malformations is increased
- Rates of stillbirth are increased
- Perinatal mortality is increased
- Incidence of neonatal complications (eg hypoglycaemia, birth trauma) is increased
- Lifetime risk of diabetes in offspring is increased

Certain drugs, eg ACE inhibitors and angiotensin II receptor blockers, should be avoided in women at risk of pregnancy and during pregnancy. Such drugs are used more frequently in diabetic women. Pre-pregnancy counselling and attainment of excellent glycaemic control (which may necessitate insulin treatment) are aims for all women contemplating conception.

Contraception

Contraception is an important component of planned pregnancy. Selecting appropriate contraception should not present a problem to most pre-menopausal women with type 2 diabetes. Marked obesity, uncontrolled hypertension and the presence of cardiovascular disease may, however, contraindicate the use of combined oestrogen–progestogen oral contraceptives.

The main contraceptive options are as follows; standard contraindications should be observed:

- *Oral combined contraceptive* – metabolic side-effects are usually minimal with the modern, low-dose oestrogen preparations, but there is a reluctance to use the oral combined pill in women with vascular complications of diabetes because of adverse changes in plasma lipid profiles. Hypertriglyceridaemia, in particular, may be aggravated. The progesterone-only pill or other methods are preferred. An associated prothrombotic state is well recognized, and certain progestogens (desogestrel, gestodene) are associated with somewhat higher risks.
- *Progesterone-only pill* – there are no appreciable metabolic side-effects and reports of reduced efficacy may simply reflect non-compliance. These preparations may be used during breast-feeding.
- *Long-acting depot progestogens* – these may be particularly useful if compliance is a problem. There is potential for menstrual irregularity, however, as well as adverse effects on plasma lipids (page 111).
- *Intrauterine contraceptive devices* – effective, without metabolic side-effects, and no specific contraindications in diabetic women.
- *Mechanical barrier methods* – as effective as in non-diabetic patients.

- *Surgical sterilization or vasectomy* – may be preferred by some couples. In the few situations in which pregnancy is contraindicated, eg severe maternal coronary heart disease, sterilization offers definitive long-term protection.

Further reading

American Diabetes Association. Position statement. Diagnosis and classification of diabetes. *Diabetes Care* 2004; **27 (suppl 1)**: S5-10.

Davies M. New diagnostic criteria for diabetes: are they doing what they should? *Lancet* 1999; **354**: 610-1.

The DECODE study group on behalf of the European Diabetes Epidemiology Group. Glucose tolerance and mortality: Comparison of WHO and American Diabetes Association diagnostic criteria. *Lancet* 1999; **354**: 617-21.

The Expert Committee on the Diagnosis and Classification of Diabetes Mellitus. Follow-up report on the diagnosis of diabetes mellitus. *Diabetes Care* 2003; **26**: 3160-7.

Greene MF. Oral hypoglycaemic drugs for gestational diabetes. *N Engl J Med* 2000; **343**: 1178-9.

Jarrett RJ. Should we screen for gestational diabetes? *Br Med J* 1997; **315**: 736-7.

Metzger BE, Coustan DR (Eds). Proceedings of the fourth international workshop-conference on gestational diabetes. *Diabetes Care* 1998; **21**(2): B1-B167.

O'Sullivan JB, Mahon CM, Charles D, Dandrow RV. Screening criteria for high-risk gestational diabetes patients. *Am J Obstet Gynecol* 1973; **116**: 894-5.

5. Principles of management

Aims and objectives
Organization of care
Diabetes in primary care
Education
Review schedule
Importance of glycaemic control
Maintaining standards of care
The economics of diabetes care

Aims and objectives

The aims of treatment for type 2 diabetes are focused on optimizing quality of life. They are approached through symptom management, together with measures to both prevent and limit complications and associated disorders. A key aim is to return metabolic control to as near-normal as possible in each individual.

The objectives and priorities of individual care plans will vary with the circumstances of the patient, but a typical list of objectives is given in Table 5.1. It is pertinent to recall that type 2 diabetes is part of the metabolic or insulin

resistance syndrome of cardiovascular risk factors detailed in chapter 2 and that the main cause of premature mortality is macrovascular disease. Much of the morbidity is due to microvascular complications and the treatment objectives therefore emphasize the importance of detecting and containing those vascular risk factors that can be modified with proven benefit. Glycaemic control, as a means of improving general metabolic status, must not be compromised, and assiduous attention should be given to atherothrombotic risks including abdominal obesity, hypertension and dyslipidaemia. Helping the patient to understand and contribute fully to the management of their condition ('empowerment') through education and support measures is a valuable means of realizing diabetes control and other objectives. The concept of 'expert patients' has been endorsed by the World Health Organization (WHO) in relation to diabetes.

> Patients should be empowered to self-manage their diabetes wherever possible

Organization of care

Since the treatment of type 2 diabetes can encompass a broad spectrum of disciplines, not just within medicine, but allied professions, it is generally acknowledged that a multidisciplinary team approach offers considerable advantages. A 'diabetes team' will ideally include all the skills and specialisms listed in Table 5.2, but some members may well contribute more than one requirement. The diabetes team will extend links with social workers, community nurses and psychological counselling expertise, and involve substantial administrative commitment.

Table 5.1
Aims and objectives in the management of type 2 diabetes.

General aim	Enhance quality of life through relief and prevention of symptoms
Key objectives	Manage existing symptoms and complications
	Optimize glycaemic control
	Detect and control other risk factors for micro- and macrovascular diseases
	Provide education for healthy living and self-management

Table 5.2
Core members of a type 2 diabetes care team.

Diabetologist	Ophthalmologist
Primary care physician*	Podiatrist
Diabetes nurse specialist/educator	Pharmacist
Dietician	

*Preferably with a special interest in diabetes.

> Diabetes care requires a multidisciplinary team approach

In the UK, for example, the concept of 'shared care' is promoted through close liaison between primary (family general practitioner) and secondary (hospital-based specialist) care. Care teams within a hospital setting are customarily built around specialist physicians, but as the organization of diabetes care moves towards the greater involvement of primary care, geographically adjacent community-based practices are being encouraged to combine resources and build community diabetes teams. Initiatives to bring together appropriate expertise within the primary care setting are usually facilitated by primary care physicians with a particular interest in diabetes. The hospital-based diabetes specialist can serve as a link between a number of teams in primary care, so that overlap is minimal and the best healthcare is delivered. Treatment strategies are usually agreed under the direction of the hospital-based specialist, who also handles all aspects of local diabetes care that cannot be undertaken within the primary care team.

The practicalities of organizing and integrating the breadth of disciplines participating in diabetes care presents a major challenge. Many different structures have been shown to work effectively and there is no single ideal system. Detailed help with setting up a diabetes care team is available from the sources given in Table 5.3. The constraints of healthcare provision (budgets, personnel, other resources and services) and the special needs of different communities (eg the elderly and ethnic groups) means that customization of generalized schemes will best reflect the requirements of the local patients.

Open access (walk-in without appointment) clinics, available on a daily basis and staffed by a diabetes nurse specialist have proved highly successful. These are practicable where large communities are served, provide a valuable opportunity to troubleshoot problems, a forum for patients to help each other and share

Table 5.3
Organization of diabetes care: sources of guidance.

European Diabetes Policy Group 1998-1999. Guidelines for diabetes care. A desktop guide to type 2 diabetes mellitus. *Diabetic Med* 1999; **16**: 716-30.

American Diabetes Association. 2004 Clinical Practice Recommendations. *Medical Management of Type 2 Diabetes, 5th edn*. Web address is www.diabetes.org

Delivery and organization of diabetes care. In: Pickup J and Williams G (Eds). *Textbook of Diabetes*, volume 2, 3rd edn. Oxford: Blackwell Science, 2003 (section 19, pages 70.1–71.9).

Diabetes UK (formerly the British Diabetic Association) – has several helpful documents, including *Recommendations for the management of diabetes in primary care* (2nd edn) and *Recommendations for the structure of specialist diabetes care services*. Address: 10 Parkway, London NW1 7AA. Web address is: www.diabetes.org.uk

Clinical Governance Support Team. NHS Modernisation Agency, 2004. Web address is: www.cgsupport.nhs.uk

National Service Framework. Web address is: www.doh.gov.uk/nsf/diabetes

difficulties and solutions, and reinforcement of the ethos of diabetes care. A local diabetes telephone helpline can also be very useful for patients, particularly early on in treatment when questions and uncertainties are most common.

Deficiencies and inequalities in the provision of care for people with diabetes in England and Wales were highlighted in an Audit Commission report (*Testing Times*, Audit Commission Publications, 2000). This report informed the first National Service Framework (NSF) for Diabetes (see page 66). The NSF is a national programme conceived to improve diabetes healthcare. It comprises three phases: first, a mission statement of 12 fundamental 'standards' for the prevention and management of diabetes (published in 2001); second, a delivery strategy to optimize the organization of care on a local and regional basis (published in 2002); third, a 10-year implementation phase in which the former two phases are brought into effect – see www.doh.gov.uk/nsf/diabetes.

Diabetes in primary care

The long-term management of diabetic patients in the UK is increasingly supervised in part or entirely in primary care – which is particularly appropriate for patients with type 2 diabetes who have satisfactory glycaemic control and no significant diabetic complications. Problems with metabolic control and/or the detection of complications should prompt consideration of specialist advice.

Various models of care have been described:

- *miniclinics* – run in general practice but based on hospital clinics
- *integrated care systems* – patient management is shared between the primary and secondary sectors – but local circumstances will influence the arrangements within a particular health district. Most require close co-operation between hospital-based and primary care, since ready access to the hospital service and diabetes specialist nurses are prerequisites. An effective patient register and recall system are also essential components. Regular audit of process and outcome is required.

> A dynamic and regular process of audit is required to identify deficiencies and ensure improvements in practice

Some studies have shown that specialist-directed management of diabetes in primary care can result in good rates of patient attendance, satisfactory collection of data (blood pressure, retinal examination), and suitable record-keeping. In contrast, unstructured care can lead to losses to follow-up, inferior glycaemic control, inadequate attention to complications and, potentially, increased mortality.

> A specialist-directed recall system is regarded as a prerequisite for successful primary care

In parts of the UK, Local Diabetes Service Advisory Groups have been established with the aim of coordinating general practice, hospital services and other professionals and – crucially – patients involved in diabetes care. Consensus guidelines may help to ensure consistency and minimum standards of care, allowing, for example, a district-wide policy for retinal screening or foot care to be established. The 'annual review' is central to patient care in the UK: this encompasses an assessment of current management, metabolic control and the status of chronic complications, and allows treatment amendments and arrangements for future review to be made.

Information technology

Information technology is increasingly important in data management; paper records may well become obsolete and a district diabetes database should now be regarded as essential. Electronic transfer of clinical and laboratory information between general practice and diabetes centres is becoming more established, but the standardization and complicity of software need further development. Information technology has the potential to:

- review record systems annually using built-in data prompts and risk-assessment programs
- capture digital images thus enabling photographs of retinal and foot lesions to be incorporated into the electronic record
- assist appropriate management by practice nurses and general practitioners (GPs) through decision support
- assist education through interactive computer programs.

> Information technology is an essential component of structured diabetes management

The care plan

Preparing a care plan involves the application of principles and protocols for diabetes management to the local strategy for the provision of care. A checklist of items that need to be covered during the first consultation with a newly diagnosed patient is given in chapter 4, page 44. Based on the first consultation, a care plan can be devised. The care plan should

Table 5.4

Example of key components of a care plan for type 2 diabetes.

- Actions required following initial assessment:
  - initial management of existing symptoms and complications
  - immediate referrals, as required
  - further tests, as required
- Antidiabetic treatment
- Monitoring
- Other treatments (new and ongoing)
- Initial advice on living with diabetes
- Initiation of education programme
- Communication with other care team members
- Review schedule

Table 5.5

Agenda for a diabetes education programme.

Initial
- What is diabetes?
- How will diabetes affect my life?
- My diabetes care plan
- Meet the diabetes care team

Ongoing
- Understanding diabetes
- Coping strategies (special counselling if necessary)
- Healthy living (including exercise and stress reduction)
- Dietary management and weight control
- Taking medication (including hypoglycaemia)
- Self-monitoring of blood glucose
- Starting insulin
- Foot care
- Special issues (eg driving, sport, holidays, intercurrent illness)

Occasionally thereafter
- Care update (revision, reinforcement and motivation)
- Dealing with complications

identify the general and specific needs of the individual patient, and set out the treatment programme in a format which is familiar to all members of the diabetes care team. A sample list of headings for a care plan is given in Table 5.4.

All care plans should be 'negotiated' and agreed with the patient concerned so that the patient is suitably empowered within the limitations of the plan. It is essential that the patient views the plan as a conjoint effort and loose contract, and it is the responsibility of the nurse specialist and/or educator to emphasize this point. Patient involvement will encourage commitment and compliance, and assist self-management.

Education

Education is a key component of every treatment programme for type 2 diabetes, and may be arbitrarily divided into two stages. First, the patient will require an immediate and straightforward explanation of their diagnosis – ie what it is, how it will affect their life, and what will be involved in their care plan. Second, an ongoing programme should be established to provide more details as and when the patient needs them, and to establish a forum for discussion and the trouble-shooting of problems encountered.

A typical agenda of education programme topics is listed in Table 5.5. An initial barrage of

information might be overwhelming, and care must be taken that facts are meted out in digestible quantities, at an appropriate pace. Although the ideal is that all members of the diabetes care team (Table 5.2) are involved in patient education, one figure, usually the specialist nurse, will provide continuity throughout.

Diabetes is inevitably a family affair, affecting all those in close contact with the patient and requiring their understanding, support and encouragement. Including family or friends within a diabetes education programme can enhance a patient's ability to implement the knowledge and experience gained. Meeting with and sharing experiences with other patients is valuable, and patients are often generous and enthusiastic with their time and commitment to helping their peers.

The manner in which an education programme is best delivered is the subject of debate. However, provided it is patient-centred, adaptable and fulfils its objectives, it seems logical to accept that it can take on whatever format best reflects local needs, resources and opportunities. Education must be complemented by motivation and personalization to ensure success and lasting impact. Ideas for the structure, content and delivery of diabetes education can be obtained from the Diabetes Education Study Group in Switzerland, the American Association of Diabetes Educators, the American Diabetes Association and Diabetes UK (details of these groups are given in Table 5.3 and at the end of the chapter).

Continuing education, possibly linked in with clinic appointments, can be used to maintain rapport between patient and care team, and help to sustain patient motivation, compliance and commitment to the care plan. The availability of psychological expertise is increasingly regarded as a bonus. There is evidence that interventions, such as counselling, cognitive behavioural therapy and psycho-dynamic therapy, may improve glycaemic control.

Review schedule

The future schedule of appointments will be incorporated into the care plan. Obviously this schedule must be flexible to take account of unforeseen developments.

Table 5.6
Check-list for each consultation with a patient with type 2 diabetes.

I. *Contact frequency*
  ● Daily for initiation of insulin or change in regimen
  ● Weekly for initiation of oral glucose-lowering agents or change in regimen
  ● Routine diabetic visits:
    Quarterly for patients who are not meeting goals
    Biannually for other patients
	IV. *Laboratory evaluation*
	  ● Glycated haemoglobin or fructosamine assessed every three to six months
	  ● Fasting plasma glucose (optional)
	  ● Fasting lipid profile annually for lipid treatment – follow up profiles as needed and monitor progress towards target
	  ● Urinalysis for protein annually
	  ● Microalbuminuria measurement annually (if urinalysis negative for protein)

II. *Medical history*
  ● Assess treatment regimen
    Frequency/severity of hypo-/hyperglycemia
    SMBG results
    Patient regimen adjustments
    Adherence problems
    Lifestyle changes
    Symptoms of complications
    Other medical illnesses
    Medications
    Psychosocial issues
	V. *Review of management plan*
	  ● Evaluate at each visit:
	    Short- and long-term goals
	    Glycaemia
	    Frequency/severity of hypoglycaemia
	    SMBG results
	    Complications
	    Control of dyslipidaemia
	    Blood pressure
	    Weight
	    Medical nutrition therapy
	    Exercise regimen
	    Adherence with self-management training
	    Follow-up of referrals
	    Psychosocial adjustment
	  ● Evaluate annually:
	    Knowledge of diabetes
	    Self-management skills

III. *Physical examination*
  ● Physical examination annually
  ● Dilated eye examination annually*
  ● Evaluate at each visit:
    Weight
    Blood pressure
    Previous abnormalities on physical examination
    Feet	

*In patients with well-controlled diabetes and blood pressure and little or no background retinopathy, slightly longer intervals may be safe. Extending the intervals between retinal examinations may ease the burden on district-wide screening programmes.
SMBG = self-monitoring of blood glucose.

A checklist for ongoing consultations with the clinician is given in Table 5.6. Since co-morbidity may impact both on choice of therapy and therapeutic targets, a careful general medical assessment should always be made, including a thorough check for vascular risk factors and diabetic complications (chapters 6 and 7). New diagnoses in existing patients should prompt screening of first-degree relatives, where appropriate, especially if they are already known to have one or more of the risk factors.

> Since comorbidity may impact both on choice of therapy and therapeutic targets, a careful general medical assessment should always be made

The annual review

The following checklist is recommended for annual review in primary care; aspects of the review are often shared between a practice nurse and doctor and the date of the review is prompted by the computerized practice register. The checklist should form the basis of practice audit and be supplemented periodically by questionnaire surveys of patient perceptions and satisfaction with care.

> A comprehensive annual review is the cornerstone of structured diabetes management

Interview

- Review general state of health (physical and psychological).
- Review results of self-monitoring.
- Enquire about episodes of hypoglycaemia (where appropriate).
- Reinforce patient commitment to self-management – especially diet, exercise, foot care, and drug compliance.
- Enquire about tobacco and alcohol use.
- Discuss other diabetes-related problems, eg complications, status of co-existing conditions and intercurrent illness.

Physical examination

- Body weight; calculation of body mass index (kg/m^2).
- Waist circumference.
- Blood pressure measurement (sitting).
- Assessment of visual acuity.
- Detailed fundal examination.
- Inspection of feet and footwear.
- Insulin injection sites (where appropriate).

Laboratory investigations

- Glycated haemoglobin (HbA_{1c}) concentration (or alternative).
- Urinalysis for protein (or albumin/creatinine ratio) and glucose.
- Serum creatinine and electrolyte concentrations.
- Lipid profile.

Management

- Glycaemic control – review of diet, exercise, weight, lifestyle, and antidiabetic medication.
- Assessment of co-existing conditions.
- Review of ancillary medication.
- Attention to modifiable cardiovascular risk factors – antihypertensive therapy, lipid-lowering therapy, aspirin.
- Management of long-term complications – consider specialist referral where appropriate.
- Agree targets and care plan.
- Arrange review date – patients with complications, suboptimal glycaemic control, uncontrolled hypertension, or other unresolved problems will require earlier review.

Importance of glycaemic control

Glycaemic control is the accepted yardstick for assessing metabolic control in diabetic patients. The justification for optimizing glycaemic control to delay the onset and reduce the severity of microvascular and macrovascular complications is discussed below.

Microvascular complications

All forms of diabetes, be they primary or secondary (chapter 3), are characterized by a risk of the development of long-term microvascular complications (chapter 6). While some patients seem more susceptible than others – perhaps reflecting genetic or other influences – the most important factors determining the risk of development and progression of chronic complications are:

- the duration of the diabetes
- the degree of the hyperglycaemia.

Subclinical (or functional) abnormalities, such as increased retinal blood flow or delayed peripheral nerve conduction velocity, may be present at diagnosis. These usually remain asymptomatic (ie detectable only with specialized techniques) and tend to improve as the hyperglycaemia is controlled. In the longer term, sustained hyperglycaemia will cause tissue damage through a number of postulated mechanisms (chapter 6).

> The risk of chronic microvascular complications is closely related to the degree and duration of the hyperglycaemia

The glucose hypothesis

According to the glucose hypothesis of diabetic complications, permanent – and effectively irreversible – tissue damage is attributable to chronic exposure to pathological degrees of hyperglycaemia. This process usually takes years to become clinically apparent and may be influenced by additional genetic or environmental factors.

> Prognosis of the diabetic patient will be improved not just by treating the hyperglycaemia, but by treating all associated conditions and complications as effectively as possible

Justification for aiming towards the best possible long-term metabolic control derives not just from clinical observation, but builds logically on the results of randomized, controlled clinical trials. The observational Wisconsin Epidemiologic Study of Diabetic Retinopathy supports the view that the basic relationship between degree and duration of hyperglycaemia and the specific microvascular complications of diabetes is similar in both the type 1 and type 2 disease.

Appropriately controlled clinical trials were required to evaluate the risks and benefits of intensified therapy specifically in patients with type 2 diabetes and the results first appeared in the early 1990s. The randomized Kumamoto trial, conducted in 110 lean, insulin-treated Japanese patients with type 2 diabetes, showed that better glycaemic control reduced microvascular complications. The United Kingdom Prospective Diabetes Study was of longer duration and much larger. A summary of the main points of this trial, the largest of its kind, are presented in Table 5.7. The design and results of the Hypertension in Diabetes study – which was embedded within the main trial – are outlined in more detail on page 107.

The key messages to emerge from the United Kingdom Prospective Diabetes Study were:

1. Improved glycaemic control with either sulphonylureas or insulin is associated with beneficial long-term effects, principally in retarding the appearance and progression of microvascular complications. The benefits are continuous until normal glycaemic control is achieved.

2. Very few patients with type 2 diabetes achieve and maintain good metabolic control with dietary modification alone, and most will require drug treatment within three years of diagnosis.

3. Glycaemic control deteriorates with duration of diabetes, even when treated intensively with an oral antidiabetic agent or insulin. Most patients will eventually require a combination of oral antidiabetic agents and/or insulin to maintain glycaemic control (Figure 5.1).

Table 5.7
United Kingdom Prospective Diabetes Study details.

Set up to establish:
a) whether intensive therapy using oral antidiabetic agents or insulin reduced the risk of macrovascular or microvascular complications relative to conventional measures (ie diet)
b) whether any particular therapy is advantageous (or disadvantageous).

Study design:
Between 1977 and 1991, 5102 patients (58% male) with newly diagnosed type 2 diabetes were recruited in 26 centres. Patients were stratified according to ideal body weight (<120% or >120%).
- Non-overweight patients. If, after three months' dietary run-in, patients had a fasting plasma glucose 6.1–15 mmol/l and no symptoms of hyperglycaemia, they were randomly assigned to either:
  – conventional policy: dietary therapy aiming for fasting glucose <15 mmol/l
  – intensive policy: aiming for fasting glucose <6 mmol/l using either sulphonylureas (initially chlorpropamide or glibenclamide, and subsequently glipizide) or insulin (commencing with once-daily ultralente or isophane, with short-acting insulin added if pre-meal glucose >7 mmol/l).
- Overweight patients. 753 of 1704 overweight patients with fasting plasma glucose 6.1–15 mmol/l were randomly assigned to receive either metformin as monotherapy (*n*=342), or continued treatment with diet alone (*n*=411). The residual 951 overweight patients were allocated to intensive glycaemic control with chlorpropamide (*n*=265), glibenclamide (*n*=277) or insulin (*n*=409).
- Protocol amendments. During the study, progressive hyperglycaemia was observed in all groups (Figure 5.1). This led to an amendment allowing the early addition of metformin in asymptomatic patients in the intensive group if their fasting glucose remained >6 mmol/l on maximal doses of a sulphonylurea. In this supplementary randomised controlled trial, 537 non-overweight and overweight patients receiving the maximum dose of sulphonylurea were allocated to either continuing sulphonylurea therapy alone (*n*=269), or the addition of metformin (*n*=268). If marked hyperglycaemia recurred, patients were transferred to insulin.

Results:
UKPDS 33: Effects of intensive control with sulphonylureas or insulin.
- Over 10 years the median HbA_{1c} was 7.0% in the intensive policy group vs 7.9% for the conventional (diet) group. There was no difference in HbA_{1c} levels between the different intensive policy subgroups.
- Compared with the conventional (diet) policy group, the intensive policy group showed:
  – 12% risk reduction for any diabetes-related endpoint (*p*=0.029)
  – 25% reduction in microvascular endpoints (*p*=0.0099; Figure 5.2)
  – reduced need for photocoagulation (*p*=0.0031)
  – better preservation of vibration sense at 15 years (*p*=0.0052)
  – 30% reduction in occurrence of microalbuminuria at 15 years (*p*=0.033)
  – 16% reduction in fatal and non-fatal myocardial infarction (*p*=0.052)
  – no significant reductions in either diabetes-related deaths or all-cause mortality
  – no significant difference between the three main intensive agents (chlorpropamide, glibenclamide or insulin) for any of the three aggregate endpoints (any diabetes-related endpoint, diabetes-related death, or all-cause mortality)
  – hypoglycaemia was more common (*p*<0.0001) in the intensive policy groups whether analysed by intention to treat or actual therapy. The highest rate of hypoglycaemia was observed with insulin treatment
  – weight gain was significantly higher in the intensive policy group (mean increase 2.9 kg) than in the conventional group (*p*<0.001). Weight gain was highest for insulin-treated patients.

UKPDS 34: Effects of metformin in non-overweight and overweight patients.
Diet vs metformin in overweight patients:
- Over 10 years, median HbA_{1c} was lower in the metformin-treated group compared with conventional treatment (7.4% vs 8.0%).
- Compared with conventional treatment, patients initially allocated to metformin showed a:
  – 32% risk reduction for any diabetes-related endpoint (*p*=0.002)
  – 42% risk reduction for any diabetes-related death (*p*=0.017)

- 36% risk reduction for all-cause mortality (*p*=0.011)
- 30% risk reduction for all macrovascular diseases (*p*=0.02)
- 39% risk reduction for myocardial infarction (*p*=0.01).

The reduction in diabetes-related endpoints, mortality and stroke was greater for patients initially allocated to metformin (UKPDS 34) than not (UKPDS 33), alongside intensive therapy with sulphonylureas or insulin.

Protocol amendment supplementary study – addition of metformin to maximal dose sulphonylurea:
- In the substudy, continued therapy with a sulphonylurea alone was associated with a much lower mortality (about one-third) than in the main study, whereas addition of metformin lowered mortality to a lesser extent (about two-thirds of the mortality rate of the main study).

Combined analysis of the metformin studies:
- Combined analysis of these two metformin studies showed that addition of metformin had an effect comparable to that observed with intensive therapy (sulphonylurea or insulin) in UKPDS 33 with a 19% net reduction in any diabetes-related endpoint (*p*=0.033). However, the beneficial effect on cardiovascular outcomes observed after initial randomization to metformin was not substantiated after secondary addition of metformin to sulphonylurea in the supplementary study.
- Metformin improved glycaemic control without inducing weight gain and was associated with fewer reported episodes of hypoglycaemia than the other intensive therapies.

An additional substudy showed minor benefits of acarbose when added to other therapies.

Post-study monitoring:
When the UKPDS ended, all surviving patients returned to routine care according to clinical need, with follow-up for 5 years (1997–2002).
- Mean HbA$_{1c}$ in patients originally randomized to intensive policy rose after 3 years to converge with those originally randomized to conventional policy.
- Mortality in the metformin-sulphonylurea substudy was no longer significantly different between the combination and sulphonylurea alone.

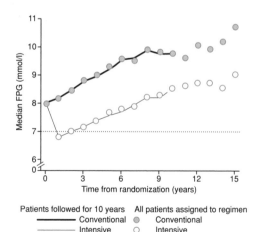

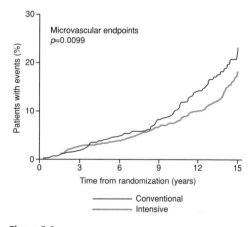

Figure 5.1
Cross-sectional and 10-year cohort data for fasting plasma glucose (FPG) for patients on intensive (sulphonylureas or insulin) or conventional (dietary) therapy in the United Kingdom Prospective Diabetes Study. Reproduced with permission from the *Lancet* 1998; **352:** 837-53.

Figure 5.2
Kaplan-Meier plots of aggregate microvascular endpoints for intensive and conventional treatment groups. Reproduced with permission from the *Lancet* 1998; **352:** 837-53.

4. Intensive therapy with sulphonylureas or insulin carries a risk of hypoglycaemia and weight gain. The risks and benefits of therapy must be carefully considered for each patient. Initial therapy with metformin may reduce the long-term complications independently of glycaemic control.

The results of this complex and lengthy study point to the potential for major health benefits from improved glycaemic control in patients with type 2 diabetes (alongside vigorous treatment of hypertension; chapter 7); and suggest that a combined approach targeting hyperglycaemia, hypertension and other risk factors is particularly advantageous (see Steno 2 study, page 89). During the UKPDS study all antidiabetic therapies had to be titrated up, or additional therapy introduced, to keep up with the progressive nature of the disorder – on average, a major adjustment such as an additional therapeutic agent, was required every four to five years. The small but sustained difference in glycaemic control between the conventional (diet) and intensive policy groups was associated with clinically relevant reductions in microvascular endpoints. Both sulphonylureas and insulin treatment were associated with increases in plasma insulin concentrations and weight gain, but insulin was eventually required in a substantial proportion of patients. The risks and benefits of insulin, including the risk of a higher rate of hypoglycaemia (~2% of patients suffered a major episode each year), require that the circumstances of the individual patient are considered thoroughly before insulin treatment is started. Insulin treatment is customarily reserved for type 2 patients who fail to respond adequately to diet and oral antidiabetic agents alone (in contrast to its use in this study).

Macrovascular disease

Although evidence from observational studies also suggests a link between the magnitude of the hyperglycaemia and the risk of atherosclerotic vascular disease, the United Kingdom Prospective Diabetes Study did not

demonstrate a statistically significant reduction in macrovascular events through improved glycaemic control alone by lowering HbA_{1c} 0.9% over 10 years. To some extent, this may reflect the design, size and patient selection of the trial. A reduction in the incidence of myocardial infarction was noted, but this fell just short of conventional statistical significance ($p=0.052$). However, an epidemiological analysis of the data (UKPDS 35) showed that a 1% reduction in HbA_{1c} would result in an average 14% reduction in myocardial infarction ($p<0.0001$). Thus, the data support the notion that glycaemia is a modifiable risk factor for myocardial infarction, and it is possible that the benefits of glycaemic control on coronary heart disease were underestimated in the United Kingdom Prospective Diabetes Study.

There is additional evidence suggesting that good metabolic control is also important immediately after a myocardial infarction, but it is generally accepted that reducing macrovascular disease – the principal cause of mortality in type 2 diabetes – will also require attention to other major modifiable cardiovascular risk factors such as dyslipidaemia, hypertension and smoking (UKPDS 23). Contrary to theoretical concerns, no adverse cardiovascular effects were observed with either sulphonylurea or insulin use in the United Kingdom Prospective Diabetes Study.

Metformin

The results of this study provided evidence for a beneficial effect on macrovascular complications where metformin was used as initial therapy in overweight patients. However, improved glycaemic control did not explain the more favourable outcome with metformin, and this led to speculation that other actions, such as improved fibrinolysis, might be involved. Metformin's benefits were not sustained when the drug was added-in to the treatment of a more heterogeneous (and relatively small) subgroup of patients already receiving the maximal dose of a sulphonylurea.

The reason for this remains uncertain but it is now widely regarded as a statistical aberration rather than a real effect, particularly since the sulphonylurea subgroup exhibited much lower mortality than the main randomization. Sulphonylureas are considered in more detail in chapter 9 and metformin in chapter 10.

Assessment of glycaemic control: urinalysis (glycosuria)

Semi-quantitative testing for the presence of glucose using reagent-impregnated test strips is of limited value. Urinalysis provides retrospective information about glucose levels over a limited period of time. Other limitations include the effects of renal threshold, urinary concentration, neuropathic bladder and inability to detect hypoglycaemia.

Renal threshold

The renal threshold for the reabsorption of glucose in the proximal convoluted tubule – 10 mmol/l (180 mg/dl) on average – varies between individuals. Thus, patients with a low renal threshold will tend to show glycosuria more readily than patients with a high threshold. In fact, some individuals with a low renal threshold may have glycosuria but normal glucose tolerance ('renal glycosuria') – children are particularly likely to test positive for urinary glucose. Conversely, a high threshold, which is common among the elderly, may give the misleading impression of apparently satisfactory control. The renal threshold of a particular individual will also change with time according to circumstances – it is usually lowered in pregnancy, for example.

Urinary concentration

Recent fluid intake and urine concentration also affect glycosuria. Renal impairment may elevate the threshold for glucose reabsorption.

Neuropathic bladder

Delayed bladder emptying, due to diabetic autonomic neuropathy (page 80), will reduce accuracy of measurements through dilution.

Hypoglycaemia

Hypoglycaemia cannot be detected by urinalysis.

Good, long-term metabolic control requires more accurate information about blood glucose in the range generally below that reflected in urinary glucose measurements. In elderly patients with type 2 diabetes, urinalysis may mislead completely (see above) and pathological degrees of hyperglycaemia go undetected. Urinalysis must be supplemented by tests for glycaemia in all patients in whom the therapeutic objectives extend beyond simply the avoidance of osmotic symptoms.

> Urinalysis alone is an inadequate means of assessing metabolic control in most diabetic patients

Assessment of glycaemic control: glycated haemoglobin

Glycated haemoglobin (HbA_{1c}) is formed by the post-translational non-enzymatic glycation of the N-terminal valine residue of the β-chain of red cell haemoglobin. The process of non-enzymatic glycation (which in other tissues is implicated in the pathogenesis of the long-term complications of diabetes) is considered in more detail in chapter 6, but the proportion of HbA_{1c} to total haemoglobin (normal non-diabetic reference range approximately 4–6%) provides a clinically useful index of average glycaemia over the preceding six to eight weeks. Average HbA_{1c} levels collected over a longer period (ie years) provide an estimate of the risk of microvascular complications. Sustained high concentrations identify patients in whom efforts should be made to improve long-term glycaemic control.

Glycaemic targets

Clearly, targets must be adjusted to suit the circumstances of the individual (chapter 8). As discussed above, a patient with advanced complications might not be expected to gain tangible benefits from tight glycaemic control;

indeed, such an approach might carry unacceptable risks of severe hypoglycaemia.

Frequency of measurement

It is generally recommended that HbA$_{1c}$ should be measured every six months. Monitoring should be more frequent if indicated. Pregnancy, for example, requires monthly monitoring.

Previous sample collection

Blood can be collected by venesection before the clinic visit, in primary care, by the hospital phlebotomy service or even by the district nurse. Alternatives include rapid assays for clinic use, and self-collection of a fingerprick sample (into a capillary tube or onto filter paper) which is then mailed to the laboratory.

Limitations of HbA$_{1c}$ measurement

Although HbA$_{1c}$ levels are a reliable indicator of recent average glycaemic control, they do not provide information about the daily pattern of blood glucose fluctuation, which is required for logical fine-tuning of insulin dosing. Fortunately, this complementary information can be obtained from the patient's self-test results. More recent changes in glycaemia (within the preceding four weeks or so) will influence current HbA$_{1c}$ level more than current glucose level. Spurious HbA$_{1c}$ levels may arise in states of:

- blood loss/haemolysis/reduced red cell survival (low HbA$_{1c}$)
- haemoglobinopathy – elevated levels of HbS (low HbA$_{1c}$) or elevated levels of HbF (high HbA$_{1c}$)
- uraemia due to advanced diabetic nephropathy (page 86) is associated with anaemia and reduced erythrocyte survival , and this may also falsely lower HbA$_{1c}$ level.

Approximate correlations between HbA$_{1c}$ values and either mean daily plasma glucose or fasting plasma glucose values are shown in Figure 5.3.

Fructosamine assay

The generic term 'fructosamine' refers to the protein-ketoamine products that result from the

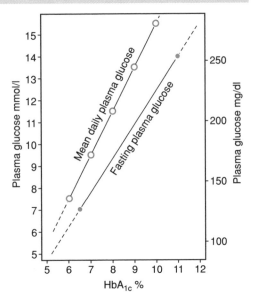

Figure 5.3
Approximate relationship between HbA$_{1c}$ and either mean daily plasma glucose or fasting plasma glucose. Data from Diabetes Control and Complications Trial, and populations screened for trials with Glucovance.

glycation of plasma proteins. The fructosamine assay measures these glycated plasma proteins (mainly albumin) to reflect average glycaemia over the preceding two to three weeks. This shorter period may be particularly useful when rapid changes in control need to be assessed, eg during pregnancy, and fructosamine assessment is also less expensive than an HbA$_{1c}$ assay (an important consideration in some laboratories). The methodology is suitable for automation and rapid results can be obtained for use in the clinic or office, which obviates the need for a prior blood test. Albumin levels can be misleading in certain hypoalbuminaemic states such as nephrotic syndrome, however, and some fructosamine assays are subject to interference by hyperuricaemia or hyperlipidaemia.

Patient self-testing

Patient self-monitoring of capillary blood glucose obtained by fingerprick has become an established method for monitoring glycaemic control. Enzyme-impregnated dry strip methods are available, which give an approximate visual indication of blood glucose. Ideally, these should be used in conjunction with a portable meter for a more accurate measurement. Most colorimetric strips are based on the glucose oxidase reaction:

$$\text{Glucose} + O_2 \xrightarrow[\text{oxidase}]{\text{Glucose}} \text{Gluconic acid} + H_2O_2$$

The hydrogen peroxide generated by this reaction then reacts with a reduced dye in the test strip and produces an oxidized colour proportional to the amount of H_2O_2. This, in turn, reflects the amount of glucose oxidized. In most test strips, there is a separating layer which excludes cells and allows penetration by plasma. Thus, the reading obtained from the blood sample is actually a *plasma* glucose value.

Alternatively, glucose oxidation by glucose oxidase can be linked to the conversion of ferricinium to ferrocene. Ionization of ferrocene back to ferricinium liberates electrons which alter the current passed along a platinum wire, to give an accurate glucose measurement on a portable meter.

Novel devices to continuously or periodically measure interstitial glucose concentrations automatically are advanced in development.

Practical considerations

Many different strips and dedicated meters are available. More expensive options include the storage and retrieval of multiple test results within a memory facility and the ability to download these results into a personal computer. Meters with large digital displays or audio output are available to aid the visually impaired and guidance from trained personnel with up-to-date knowledge of testing systems ensures that patients acquire the most appropriate device for their particular requirements. Supervised instruction of patients (or their carers) in the use of the chosen system should be provided and the manufacturers' instructions must be followed meticulously if reliable measurements are to be obtained.

> Guidance from the diabetes care team is helpful in the selection of an appropriate test system for self-blood glucose monitoring

Some systems use light reflectance to provide readings accurate to 0.1 mmol/l. Factors such as the adequacy of the capillary sample and calibration of the meter require attention. Test strip containers may carry a barcode strip or number which needs to be programmed into the meter. Control solutions of specified concentration are available from manufacturers – their telephone helplines are also useful sources of customer support. Sub-optimal storage of test strips is a potential source of error. It should be emphasized that quality control is essential.

Elderly patients often cope remarkably well with self-testing and many gain reassurance from it, but practical, patient-related limitations to self-testing include:

- inadequate manual dexterity, eg through deforming rheumatoid arthritis or advanced neuropathy or post-stroke
- intellectual inability or incapacity
- visual handicap.

Initiation of self-testing is an important preliminary step in patients who will eventually require insulin, but frequent self-testing has not been clearly demonstrated to improve control in others; testing every few days before breakfast and occasionally at other times (including 1–2 hours post-prandially) will usually suffice.

Efficacy

Self-testing remains a controversial issue. While, intuitively, it would seem that any additional information about glycaemic control would be advantageous, there is little firm evidence to support the assumption that routine self-monitoring improves glycaemic control. The evidence-base for this activity is small though, all the more surprising in view of the data suggesting that glycaemic control is suboptimal in a large proportion of patients

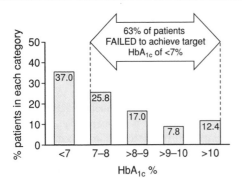

Figure 5.4
Glucose control (to ADA criteria) in diabetic patients in the US NHANES 1999–2000 Survey. Sourced from *JAMA* 2004; **291**: 335-42. Only 37% of patients achieved the target of HbA$_{1c}$ <7%.

(Figure 5.4). There is a need for good randomized trials of self-testing in type 2 diabetes patients.

Maintaining standards of care

Initiatives at local, national and international level are necessary to improve standards of care for patients with diabetes. At national level the interests of patients with diabetes are served by organizations such as Diabetes UK and the American Diabetes Association. These bodies act as advocates for people with diabetes. Generation of funds for research is another important aspect of their activities; both the UK and US national diabetes organizations publish peer-reviewed clinical and scientific papers in their respective journals. Annual scientific meetings under the auspices of these bodies bring together doctors, nurses, other healthcare professionals and scientists to share and evaluate progress in areas ranging from basic science to clinical care. These national meetings are amplified by international gatherings such as that of the European Association for the Study of Diabetes. The International Diabetes Federation, founded in 1950, holds triennial international meetings.

The Saint Vincent Declaration

Inevitably, there is a political dimension to the provision of diabetes care. International collaborations such as the Saint Vincent Declaration in Europe in 1989 represent another facet to the quest for improved patient outcome. This declaration resulted from a meeting of representatives from European government health departments and patient organizations under the aegis of the regional offices of the World Health Organization and the International Diabetes Federation. The meeting produced a unanimous agreement on a series of recommendations of general goals and five-year targets. A demand for formal recognition by policy-makers of the public health problems presented by diabetes was accompanied by recommendations for research and the setting of laudable, if ambitious, targets for improvements in care:

- to reduce new blindness due to diabetes by one-third or more
- to reduce the numbers of diabetic patients entering end-stage renal failure by at least one-third
- to reduce diabetic morbidity and mortality from coronary heart disease
- to improve pregnancy outcome in women with diabetes so that it approximates to that in non-diabetic women.

The 1997 Lisbon Statement acknowledged the initiation of diabetes action programmes in most of the countries that were signatories to the Saint Vincent Declaration. The latter was coupled with a resolution to continue collaborative efforts to improve the healthcare of diabetic patients in Europe.

National Service Framework

In England a rolling programme of National Service Frameworks (NSFs) was launched in 1998 to set national standards for healthcare provision, determine strategies for delivery of that care, and establish performance markers to monitor progress. Diabetes was the fourth NSF (page 54): a mission statement was published in 2001 and implementation started in 2002 (Department of Health website is www.doh.gov.uk/nsf/diabetes/index.html). Separate versions of the diabetes NSF have been prepared in Wales and Northern Ireland.

Scotland has lead the way in developing clear practical national guidance through the Scottish Intercollegiate Guidelines Network (SIGN). This includes several excellent documents on the management of diabetes. Diabetes guidelines were last revised in 2001 (www.sign.ac.uk).

In England and Wales, the National Institute for Clinical Excellence (NICE) publishes opinions on the manner in which health professionals might use antidiabetic medications, based substantially on considerations of cost-effectiveness (www.nice.org.uk).

The economics of diabetes care

Since diabetes is a common and chronic disorder, it consumes a considerable proportion of the healthcare budgets of developed countries. In 2000, data suggested that diabetes was responsible for an estimated 9% of the total direct healthcare costs of the UK and 14% of the total direct healthcare costs of the US. The estimated annual costs of foot ulceration alone have been put at £13m in the UK and $500m in the US. Indirect costs are very difficult to estimate because they include those costs attributable to acute and chronic morbidity and premature mortality leading to loss of occupational productivity.

> Diabetes consumes a disproportionately large part of national healthcare budgets and also incurs an extensive burden in terms of indirect and intangible costs such as social factors and reduced quality of life

The cost-effectiveness of new treatments using relatively expensive therapies is an increasingly important dimension of care. Vigorous treatment of hyperglycaemia, hypertension and the many associated complications of type 2 diabetes

(chapters 6 and 7), demands investment in drugs and effective healthcare delivery systems. This outlay can reasonably be expected to be recouped through a reduced requirement for later interventions against complications such as retinal photocoagulation or renal replacement therapy. However, analyses of the cost-effectiveness of treatment pose considerable difficulties for health economists and this is still a relatively imprecise and speculative discipline. The projected massive global increase in the number of patients with diabetes (page 2) points to a need for even greater expenditure in the future and this will undoubtedly present major challenges, particularly for less economically developed countries.

Further reading

American Diabetes Association. Economic costs of diabetes in the US in 2002. *Diabetes Care* 2003; **26**: 917-32.

American Diabetes Association. Clinical practice guidelines 2003. *Diabetes Care* 2003; **26 (suppl 1)**: S1-S156.

Coster S, Gulliford MC, Seed PT *et al*. Self-monitoring in type 2 diabetes mellitus: a meta-analysis. *Diabetic Med* 2000; **17**: 755-61.

Coutinho M, Wang Y, Gerstein HC, Yusuf S. The relationship between glucose and incident cardiovascular events. *Diabetes Care* 1999; **22**: 233-40.

European Diabetes Policy Group. A desktop guide to type 2 diabetes mellitus. *Diabetic Med* 1999; **16**: 716-30.

Gaede P, Vedel P, Larsen N *et al*. Multifactorial intervention and cardiovascular disease in patients with type 2 diabetes. *N Engl J Med* 2003; **348**: 383-93.

Goldstein DE, Little RR, Lorenz RA *et al*. Tests of glycaemia in diabetes (technical review). *Diabetes Care* 1995; **18**: 896-909.

Ismail K, Winkley K, Rabe-Hesketh S. Systematic review and meta-analysis of randomised controlled trials of psychological interventions to improve glycaemic control in patients with type 2 diabetes. *Lancet* 2004; **363**: 1589-97.

Klein R. Hyperglycemia and microvascular and macrovascular disease in diabetes. *Diabetes Care* 1995; **18**: 258-68.

Sacks DB, Bruns DE, Goldstein DE *et al*. Guidelines and recommendations for laboratory analysis in the diagnosis and management of diabetes mellitus. *Clin Chem* 2003; **48**: 436-72.

Saydah SH, Fradkin J, Cowie C. Poor control of risk factors for vascular disease among adults with previously diagnosed diabetes. *JAMA* 2004; **291**: 335-42.

Selvin E, Marinopoulos S, Berkenbilt G *et al*. Meta-analysis: glycosylated hemoglobin and cardiovascular disease in diabetes mellitus. *Ann Intern Med* 2004; **141**: 421-31.

Stratton IM, Adler AI, Neil AW *et al*. Association of glycaemia with macrovascular and microvascular complications of type 2 diabetes (UKPDS 35): prospective observational study. *Br Med J* 2000; **321**: 405-12.

St Vincent Declaration. Diabetes care and research in Europe. *Diabetic Med* 1990; **7**: 370.

Testing times: a review of diabetes services in England and Wales. London: Audit Commission Publications, 2000. (www.diabetes.audit-commission.gov.uk)

Tuomilehto J. Controlling glucose and blood pressure in type 2 diabetes. *Br Med J* 2000; **321**: 394-5.

UK Prospective Diabetes Study Group. Effect of intensive blood-glucose control with metformin on complications in overweight patients with type 2 diabetes (UKPDS 34). *Lancet* 1998; **352**: 854-65.

UK Prospective Diabetes Study Group. Intensive blood-glucose control with sulphonylureas or insulin compared with conventional treatment and risk of complications in patients with type 2 diabetes (UKPDS 33). *Lancet* 1998; **352**: 837-53.

UK Prospective Diabetes Study Group. Risk factors for coronary heart disease in non-insulin dependent diabetes (UKPDS 23). *Br Med J* 1998; **316**: 823-8.

Contact information

Diabetes Education Study Group. Division of Therapeutic Education for Chronic Diseases, 3HL, University Hospital, 1211 Geneva 14, Switzerland.

American Association of Diabetes Educators, 444 North Michigan Avenue, Suite 1240, Chicago, IL80611, USA

American Diabetes Association at www.diabetes.org/ and www.news@diabetes.org/.

Diabetes UK at www.diabetes.org.uk.

European Association for the Study of Diabetes at www.easd.org.

Medscape at www.medscape.com (endocrinology).

6. Microvascular complications

Biochemistry of diabetic complications
Ocular complications
Diabetic neuropathy
Diabetic foot disease
Diabetic nephropathy

Although the acute symptoms of diabetes can usually be controlled with appropriate therapy, all major forms of diabetes are also associated with the insidious development of specific damage to the small vessels of certain organs. The small vessel (microvascular) complications of diabetes primarily affect the retina, the renal glomerulus and the peripheral nervous system. All of these tissues are freely permeable to glucose and complications are closely linked to glycaemic control. The ultimate clinical consequences of diabetic microvascular disease are failure of the related major systems and visual impairment, chronic renal failure and neuropathic foot ulceration, respectively. Type 2 diabetes is also associated with an increased mortality from atherosclerotic (macrovascular) complications, particularly coronary heart disease, but these will be discussed in the next chapter. Together, the micro- and macrovascular complications of diabetes are major (and growing) causes of diabetic morbidity and mortality on a global scale.

Biochemistry of diabetic complications

Studies in animal models have provided insight into the biochemical mechanisms responsible for the chronic microvascular complications of diabetes. The principal hypotheses which link tissue damage to long-term exposure to high glucose concentrations include the polyol pathway, protein kinase C activity, and non-enzymatic glycation. Oxidative stress may also contribute to the development and progression of diabetic complications.

The polyol pathway

Increased activity of this ubiquitous biochemical pathway leads to intracellular accumulation of osmotically active sorbitol and fructose through the action of the enzyme aldose reductase. Depletion of myo-inositol and impairment of Na^+-K^+-ATPase activity are associated disturbances that have been implicated, particularly in the pathogenesis of diabetic neuropathy. Alterations in cellular redox state, leading to a state of 'pseudo-hypoxia' through the following reactions, may also be relevant:

$$Glucose + NADPH + H^+ \longrightarrow Sorbitol + NADP^+$$
$$Aldose\ reductase$$

$$Sorbitol + NAD^+ \longrightarrow Fructose + H^+$$
$$Sorbitol\ dehydrogenase$$

Protein kinase C activity

Accumulation of diacylglycerol as a result of high intracellular glucose concentrations activates protein kinase C-β in endothelial cells. This alters vascular permeability and increases basement membrane synthesis – an important early histological feature of the microvascular complications of diabetes. Pathological changes result:

$$\uparrow Glucose \rightarrow \uparrow Diacylglycerol \rightarrow \uparrow Protein\ kinase\ C\text{-}\beta$$

Secondary increases in the expression of growth factors with effects on vascular permeability may contribute to neovascularization in the retina.

Non-enzymatic glycation

The long-term modification of proteins such as collagen and nucleic acids by non-enzymatic glycation (ie attachment of glucose to the amino groups of proteins at a rate proportional to the mean glucose concentration) also contributes to tissue damage. Physical cross-linking of biochemically altered proteins modifies their structure and function – in the vascular wall, for example. While the earliest biochemical changes are reversible with restoration of good glycaemic control, the reversibility falters with time, and advanced glycation endproducts (AGEs) are eventually formed.

Glucose + Protein ➤ Schiff base ➤ Amadori product ➤ AGEs

This process is the basis of glycated haemoglobin assays for the determination of medium-term glycaemic control. AGEs are cleared by cellular receptors (RAGEs).

Drug treatment

Drugs such as aldose reductase inhibitors, protein kinase C inhibitors and aminoguanidine block these metabolic pathways independently of glycaemia, and may prevent the development of certain complications in animal models of diabetes. A clinical trial of aminoguanidine in Europe was halted by the manufacturer while the results of a US trial of the drug in nephropathy have not been published to date. Since clinical trials of promising drugs such as the aldose reductase inhibitors have proved disappointing to date, excellent metabolic control remains fundamental to the prevention of microvascular complications. The results of the United Kingdom Prospective Diabetes Study (page 60) reinforced the relationship between glycaemic control and microvascular complications of type 2 diabetes, demonstrating that each 1% reduction in HbA_{1c} for 10 years was associated with a 37% reduction in microvascular complications and a 21% reduction in diabetes-related endpoints and deaths (Figure 6.1). Four important observations were made during analysis of the results (UKPDS 35):

- The lower the glycaemia, the lower the risk of complications
- Any rise in HbA_{1c} above the normal range

carries an increased risk of glycaemic complications (no threshold was identified)

- Any improvement in glycaemia is likely to be beneficial
- Near-normoglycaemia should be the aim for as many patients as possible.

> The microvascular complications of type 2 diabetes increase in line with the extent and duration of the accompanying hyperglycaemia

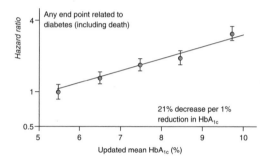

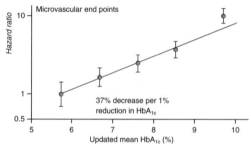

Figure 6.1
United Kingdom Prospective Diabetes Study (UKPDS 35). For each 1% decrease in HbA_{1c} there is a 21% decrease in any diabetes-related endpoint and a 37% decrease in microvascular complications.
Reproduced with permission from *BMJ* 2000; **321**: 405-12.

Ocular complications

Clinical ocular complications associated with type 2 diabetes include:

- transient visual disturbances secondary to osmotic changes
- retinopathy – responsible for >80% of blindness in diabetic patients
- cataracts – these develop earlier in diabetic patients

- glaucoma – which may be primary or secondary to diabetic retinopathy.

Key points about diabetic retinopathy

- Diabetes is the principal cause of partial sight and blind registration in adults in western countries.
- Diabetic retinopathy is asymptomatic until well advanced.
- Effective treatment is available.
- Laser photocoagulation must be applied before the retinopathy becomes too advanced.
- Patients must be screened thoroughly and regularly using sensitive techniques.

> Retinal screening must be undertaken regularly in patients with type 2 diabetes

Population-based studies show that the prevalence of any degree of retinopathy is highest in younger, insulin-treated patients than in non-insulin treated older patients with type 2 diabetes. Severe retinopathy may develop in both major types of diabetes, but with some important differences. Factors other than hyperglycaemia, notably hypertension, have an important influence, particularly in patients with type 2 diabetes, as demonstrated in the Hypertension in Diabetes study (page 106).

> Hypertension has a major influence on the progression of retinopathy in type 2 diabetes

Moreover, studies in the US have shown that the risk of retinopathy is higher among certain ethnic groups, namely Native Americans, Mexican Americans and African Americans. The higher risk in these groups does not appear to be attributable to differences in glycaemic control or other recognized risk factors.

Approximately 20% of patients may have some evidence of retinopathy at diagnosis of their diabetes, but the prevalence increases with age and duration of diabetes. Careful fundoscopy is therefore mandatory in newly presenting patients. Maculopathy is the major cause of visual loss in those with retinopathy at diagnosis, but cataract (page 76) is also relatively common. Control of blood pressure is important in the prevention of visual impairment due to maculopathy. The benefits of long-term tight glycaemic control are well established and this should be carefully explained to the patient. However, several studies (mainly in patients with type 1 diabetes) have shown that pre-existing retinopathy can deteriorate transiently shortly after rapid improvements in glycaemic control and careful expert surveillance – with timely laser photocoagulation if necessary – is therefore required when glycaemic control is improved acutely. Acute reduction in retinal blood flow leading to retinal hypoxia is a postulated mechanism.

> Pre-existing retinopathy may deteriorate transiently when glycaemic control is improved

Ocular symptoms

Until it is very advanced, diabetic eye disease is largely asymptomatic. However, ocular symptoms attributable to diabetes include:

- Transient disturbance of refraction, usually myopia. This may be a presenting symptom of diabetes or may occur with the institution of antidiabetic therapy. Patients are advised to defer eye tests until diabetic control has been stabilized. Osmotic changes within the ocular lens are thought to be responsible.

Other less commonly encountered symptoms include:

- Gradual loss of vision, suggestive of the development of maculopathy or cataract.
- Sudden, painless, loss of vision due to vitreous haemorrhage. Retinal arterial and venous thrombosis may also occur in patients with diabetes.
- Appearance of 'floaters', possibly due to small or recurrent vitreous haemorrhages.

- Chronic pain and redness, due to rubeosis and secondary glaucoma.
- Field defects and impaired night vision, which are sequelae of extensive laser photocoagulation.

In addition, extraocular cranial nerve palsies may cause diplopia.

> Diabetic retinopathy and its sequelae are usually asymptomatic until well-advanced

Screening for diabetic retinopathy

Early recognition of diabetic retinopathy is essential if laser therapy is to be administered early enough for useful vision to be preserved. Annual checks of corrected visual acuity combined with expert evaluation of the fundus are required. In the UK, diabetologists, trained general practitioners or optometrists have generally performed direct fundoscopy in the clinic or surgery. Elsewhere, an ophthalmologist or optometrist might provide this service.

Visual acuity

Corrected best visual acuity is measured at 6 m using a well illuminated Snellen chart. Patients should wear their distance glasses, if required. A pinhole will correct refractive errors to approximately 6/9. Each eye should be tested separately. Visual acuity should be tested before mydriatic eye drops are applied. Impaired visual acuity that does not improve with pinhole testing is suggestive of maculopathy or cataract.

Retinal examination

If direct ophthalmoscopy is employed, the pupils must first be pharmacologically dilated by applying 1% tropicamide 10–15 minutes before the examination. Transient local discomfort is common and the effect of tropicamide may take several hours to wear off. Additionally, the pupils of elderly patients, and particularly patients with overt diabetic neuropathy, may not dilate well; autonomic imbalance is postulated. Cautions and

contraindications to mydriasis (pupil dilation) are few:

- *Driving* – this should be avoided, if possible. Dazzle from headlights and impaired visual acuity (which may fall transiently below legal requirements) carry obvious risks after tropicamide; alternative transport should preferably be arranged in advance. Although pilocarpine is sometimes used to reverse the effect of tropicamide the effect may only be partial, with the pupil becoming fixed in mid-dilatation. Reading may also be temporarily impaired.
- *A history of intraocular surgery* – although this is rarely a problem, the advice of the ophthalmologist should be sought. Some types of intraocular lens implant may dislocate with pupillary dilatation.
- *Precipitation of acute glaucoma* – has long been feared in susceptible patients, but a recent re-evaluation suggests that the risk may have been overstated.

Non-mydriatic retinal photography

Non-mydriatic retinal cameras can provide colour photographs of the optic disc and macula and these have been extensively used in screening programmes in the UK. The photographs obtained require expert evaluation but studies suggest that cameras may improve the detection rate for maculopathy. High-resolution video cameras with digital data capture are a more recent development; digital data have the additional advantage of being suitable for electronic transfer and incorporation into computer-based record systems. Retinal photography is emerging as the screening method of choice in the UK. The National Institute for Clinical Excellence for England and Wales has recommended that tests should have a sensitivity of 80% or higher, a specificity of 95% or higher and a technical failure rate of less than 5%.

Frequency of screening

The possibility that retinopathy may have developed before diagnosis of diabetes and the tendency for maculopathy to develop within a few years of diagnosis means that all patients need to be examined both at diagnosis and annually thereafter. More frequent examination should be considered if retinopathy is detected and patients who default from follow-up should always have their eyes examined when the opportunity presents.

> Patients who have defaulted should always have a detailed eye examination on reattendance

Classification of diabetic retinopathy

For clinical purposes, diabetic retinopathy is classified into several well defined stages (Table 6.1). It is not inevitable that the retinopathy will pass from one stage to the next. The clinical importance of the classification derives from the likelihood of treatment success in the earlier stages. The benefits of photocoagulation have been proven in randomized, controlled studies initially using the xenon arc and later the argon laser.

Maculopathy denotes retinopathy concentrated at the macula, ie within the temporal vessels, approaching the fovea. Maculopathy may threaten central vision, particularly in patients with type 2 diabetes. Advanced diabetic eye disease includes the sequelae of vitreous haemorrhage and secondary rubeotic glaucoma – visual impairment is always present to some degree, and often blindness.

Table 6.1
Classification of diabetic retinopathy.

- Background retinopathy
- Pre-proliferative retinopathy
- Proliferative retinopathy
- Advanced diabetic eye disease
- Maculopathy

Note that these categories are not necessarily mutually exclusive, nor are they as distinct as the classification suggests.

> Proliferative retinopathy and maculopathy are potentially sight-threatening forms of diabetic retinopathy

a) Background retinopathy

Background retinopathy (Figure 6.2) is characterized ophthalmoscopically by microaneurysms, intraretinal blot or (less frequently) flame haemorrhages, and hard exudates (waxy-looking lipid deposits from damaged vessels). In isolation, venous dilatation is not regarded as evidence of retinopathy. All of these features are asymptomatic, and each may fluctuate, with microaneurysms and haemorrhages, for example, sometimes disappearing on re-examination.

- *Surveillance* – careful periodic review is essential and usually recommended about every six months for all but the most minimal or slowly progressive cases. Good control of glycaemia and blood pressure are associated with a lower risk of progression.
- *Explanation* – it is usually appropriate to inform the patient of the discovery of retinopathy, at which stage the importance of regular review can be stressed. Accurate prognosis may be difficult (although risk of serious visual impairment is likely to be greatly reduced by therapy) but a reassuring approach is best.
- *Search for other complications* – carefully, and notably for hypertension and nephropathy. The latter may, in turn, influence progression of retinopathy.
- *Review glycaemic control* – the importance of glycaemic control should be discussed in terms appropriate to the patient, but the setting of unrealistic glycaemic targets is likely to generate anxiety and frustration.

b) Pre-proliferative retinopathy

Pre-proliferative retinopathy (Figure 6.3) is characterized by venous loops, beading or reduplication, arterial sheathing, intraretinal microvascular abnormalities (arteriovenous shunts), cotton wool spots (retinal infarcts), and multiple, extensive haemorrhages. These features denote increasing retinal ischaemia, the extent and degree of which tend to be underestimated by the ophthalmological appearance. Specialist investigations such as fluorescein angiography may be indicated. Pre-proliferative retinopathy, by definition, carries a relatively high risk of progression to new vessel formation within 12 months.

- Ophthalmic referral – a specialist opinion is indicated within four weeks.

c) Proliferative retinopathy

Proliferative retinopathy (Figure 6.4) is characterized by new vessel growth on the optic disc or in the periphery of the retina in response to growth factors released by areas of ischaemic retina. These new vessels are friable and likely to cause pre-retinal or vitreous haemorrhage. Those on the optic disc are the most-feared in this respect. The vessels are asymptomatic in the absence of haemorrhage. When a large haemorrhage occurs, the patient will present with sudden, painless, monocular vision loss. Following a large haemorrhage, there is loss of the normal red reflex on ophthalmoscopic examination. Smaller bleeds may cause the patient to notice 'floaters' in the visual field. On examination, the new vessels appear frond-like, and extend into the subhyaloid space from their origin at the retinal surface. Widespread retinopathy elsewhere is usual, but it may be impossible to discern any retinal features on fundoscopy because of blood in the vitreous humour.

- Urgent ophthalmic referral – immediate expert assessment is indicated for suspected acute vitreous haemorrhage or sudden vision loss.
- Laser photocoagulation – timely argon laser therapy can reduce the risk of severe visual loss by >50% over five years in patients with proliferative retinopathy. Laser therapy must be given before visual loss is too advanced. Panretinal photocoagulation, which may involve thousands of retinal burns, is associated

with potential complications including: impaired night vision, visual field constriction, impaired colour vision and progression of macular oedema. New vessels regress in response to photocoagulation and the stimulus to further new vessel formation is removed by destruction of the ischaemic retina. Successful photocoagulation may induce permanent quiescence of proliferative retinopathy, but this treatment is more appropriately regarded as a palliative procedure. Intraocular haemorrhages must be absorbed before laser treatment can be applied, which may take several weeks.

> Sudden loss of vision necessitates immediate referral to an ophthalmologist

d) Advanced diabetic eye disease

Advanced diabetic eye disease includes retinal detachment due to fibrous traction and rubeosis iridis (new vessels on the iris). Severe panretinal ischaemia may lead to new vessel formation on the iris. Obstruction of the drainage angle by new vessels may then cause painful secondary rubeotic glaucoma. Retinal detachment – a grey elevation of the retina – may be obscured by vitreous haemorrhage. Painless sudden loss of vision is the presenting symptom in both cases. Action:

- Urgent ophthalmic referral – immediate expert assessment is indicated for retinal detachment.
- Panretinal photocoagulation.
- Surgical vitrectomy – this highly specialized procedure may restore useful vision in selected patients with advanced diabetic eye disease. Intraocular microsurgical techniques permit removal of fibrous plaques and re-attachment of areas of retina; direct intraocular laser procedures are also feasible.
- Enucleation – this is the last resort for a painful, blind, rubeotic eye.

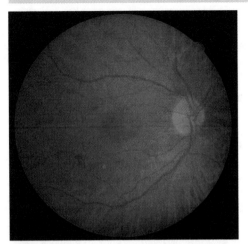

Figure 6.2
Background retinopathy

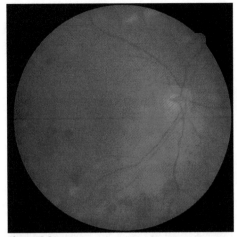

Figure 6.3
Pre-proliferative retinopathy

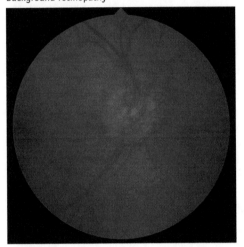

Figure 6.4
Proliferative retinopathy

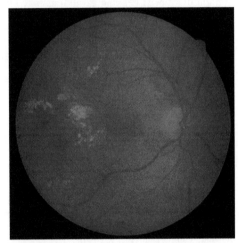

Figure 6.5
Maculopathy

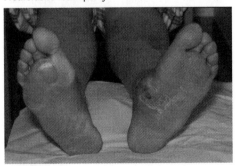

Figure 6.6
Charcot neuroarthropathy: bilateral changes with ulcerating deformity on medial aspect of left foot.

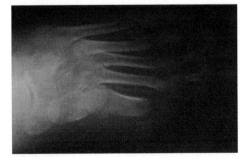

Figure 6.7
Charcot neuroarthropathy: extensive degenerative changes in mid-foot. Note partial surgical removal of first metatarsal and arterial calcification.

Figures 6.2–6.5 reproduced with permission from Krentz AJ. *Churchill's Pocketbook of Diabetes*. Edinburgh: Churchill Livingstone, 2000.

e) Maculopathy

Maculopathy (Figure 6.5) mainly affects patients with type 2 diabetes. Three types are recognized:

- exudative (may develop into circinate plaques)
- oedematous (cystic or diffuse; may be difficult to visualize with direct ophthalmoscopy or photography)
- ischaemic (the least amenable to laser treatment).

Maculopathy should be suspected if a significant reduction in visual acuity (ie by two lines on the Snellen chart) occurs in the absence of an obvious cause, such as cataract. Expert slit-lamp examination may be needed to confirm diagnosis. Leaking capillaries may be more easily identified by fluorescein angiography.

- *Ophthalmic referral* – this is recommended for hard exudates (well defined waxy lesions) within two disc diameters of visual fixation. Unexplained deterioration in visual acuity also merits referral, whether or not retinopathy is apparent – it may be due to treatable macular oedema. If in doubt, always obtain an expert opinion.
- *Photocoagulation* – the focal type is recommended for microaneurysms and the grid type for diffuse macular oedema.
- *Control of hypertension* – hypertension should be sought and treated vigorously.

Visual handicap

Patients with severe visual impairment should be registered as partially sighted (best corrected acuity 6/60) or blind (3/60 or worse), as appropriate. This will trigger financial benefits and social service support. Low vision aids and adapted household appliances are available. Pen injectors and other devices may be useful for patients requiring insulin. Self-monitoring of capillary glucose is possible, with glucose meters modified to give an audible result. Other support might include: braille instruction, large print and audio books, and guide-dog provision. Depression is understandably common, but peer-support, generally arranged through patient organizations, can be helpful.

Cataract

Opacities of the crystalline lens are usually asymptomatic in the early stages of development, but a common cause of treatable visual impairment. Cataracts are features of conditions such as myotonic dystrophy and chronic corticosteroid therapy, which can be associated with diabetes. Type 2 diabetes is a risk factor for cataract formation and the lesions may also progress more rapidly in diabetic patients.

> Cataracts are more common in diabetic patients and appear earlier than in non-diabetic individuals

Treatment is indicated if the cataract is interfering significantly with daily activities or the assessment of retinopathy. Surgical extraction with implantation of an intraocular lens is a routine procedure once the cataract has matured.

Glaucoma

In diabetic patients, glaucoma may be:

- *Primary* – chronic, open-angle glaucoma may be more common in diabetic patients; there is a suggestion that its presence may protect to a degree against retinopathy
- *Secondary* – due to advanced diabetic eye disease (such as rubeosis iridis).

Diabetic neuropathy

Neuropathy is the most common chronic complication of diabetes. It is a cause of considerable morbidity and its contribution to premature mortality may be underestimated. Diagnosis is essentially clinical; specialized techniques are usually unnecessary.

Electrophysiological measurements are often abnormal at diagnosis of diabetes but tend to improve with control of glycaemia; overactivity of the intraneural polyol pathway (page 65) has been implicated. In chronic diabetic neuropathy, however, there appears to be a major contribution from microangiopathy of the vasa nervorum. Only a minority of diabetic patients will go on to develop clinically troublesome neuropathy. Several stages are recognized, the earliest of which are usually asymptomatic:

- Intraneural biochemical abnormalities – sorbitol accumulation and associated myoinositol depletion.

- Impairment of electrophysiological measurements – decreased nerve conduction velocity.

- Clinical neuropathy – may be symptomatic or asymptomatic. Histological changes evident (research tool only).

- End-stage complications – foot ulceration and Charcot neuroarthropathy (page 85) are major and effectively irreversible derangements of neural structure and function.

Classification of established diabetic neuropathy is also essentially clinical, reflecting the differing manifestations and natural histories of the various forms (Table 6.2).

Table 6.2
Classification of diabetic neuropathies.

- Focal neuropathies – eg cranial nerve palsies, carpal tunnel syndrome
- Distal symmetrical polyneuropathy – glove and stocking; may be asymptomatic
- Acute painful sensory neuropathy – uncommon; may follow initiation of insulin treatment
- Motor neuropathies – uncommon; usually resolve
- Autonomic neuropathy – erectile dysfunction is probably the most common manifestation; other forms are rare

Clinical syndromes

a) Focal neuropathies

Focal neuropathy can affect the cranial nerves, eg the third, fourth or sixth. While oculomotor nerve palsies are usually incomplete, diplopia is prominent. However, the pupil is often spared and ptosis is uncommon. It can also affect the peripheral nerves, eg median, ulnar, common peroneal. Localized vascular lesions are thought to be responsible. Mononeuritis multiplex denotes the involvement of several peripheral nerves; distinguishing it from generalized peripheral neuropathy may be difficult. Transient focal neuropathies may also occur occasionally in hyperosmolar non-ketotic coma (page 46).

Spontaneous recovery of cranial nerve lesions within three months is the rule; in the absence of features such as ptosis, the patient can usually be reassured about the likely cause of a third cranial nerve palsy without resort to computed tomographic imaging. Recurrence is recognized. Persistent carpal tunnel syndrome merits investigation with nerve conduction studies; local injection therapy or decompression may help. Foot drop may benefit from an orthopaedic support. Ulnar nerve lesions may cause wasting of the dorsal interossei and hypothenar eminence.

b) Chronic symmetrical distal polyneuropathy

Chronic symmetrical distal polyneuropathy is common but often remarkably asymptomatic. Symptoms, if present, are usually confined to the legs and feet and start distally. Advanced neuropathy may also affect the hands and limit daily activities, such as insulin administration. Symptoms may include:

- *Paraesthesiae* – unpleasant sensations, akin to walking on pebbles, are characteristic.

- *Numbness* – loss of sensation may not be noticed by the patient. Instead, the patient may complain of subjectively cold feet, particularly in bed. The presence of pedal pulses on palpation together with signs of neuropathy will confirm the correct diagnosis.

- *Pain* – unremitting, burning, or lancinating pain.
- *Allodynia* – unpleasant sensations resulting from contact with bedclothes, trousers, etc, are reported.
- *Muscular leg cramps* – again especially in bed.
- *Impaired sense of position* – this may result in unsteadiness of gait and a tendency to trip. This can be a prominent but sometimes underrecognized symptom.

Classic signs of diabetic peripheral neuropathy are, however, easily detected on clinical examination:

- *Absent ankle jerks* – an early feature, but age-related loss is also common in the elderly.
- *Diminished vibration sense* – a 128 Hz tuning fork is applied to a distal prominence, such as the dorsum of the terminal phalanx of the hallux (big toe). If sensation is absent, the fork should be moved progressively proximal to the medial malleolus, then along the upper tibia (avoiding soft or oedematous tissue). Vibration sense may also diminish with age. More quantitative devices, eg the biothesiometer, are available, but are expensive and so usually confined to research studies. Age-related reference ranges are available.
- *Reduction in other sensory modalities* – position, light touch, pain and temperature – may accompany or follow loss of vibration sensation. Insensitivity to the application of a 10 g (5.07) Semmes-Weinstein monofilament will identify patients at high risk of neuropathic ulceration (page 83). This simple and reproducible test involves the perpendicular application of a nylon filament to a callus-free surface of the sole until it buckles under the gentle pressure.
- *Warm, dry skin* – with fissuring due to local sympathetic denervation.

- *Dilated superficial veins* – and sometimes bounding pedal pulses due to vascular shunting.
- *Clawed toes* – denervation of intrinsic foot muscles produces 'clawing' of the toes, exposing the metatarsal heads; this predisposes to ulceration.

Management should involve the following:

- *Education* – insensitive feet may be scalded by hot bathwater or in front of a heater or open fire. Injuries by unperceived foreign bodies in footwear may occur; prevention is paramount. Non-diabetic anatomical abnormalities such as hallux valgus predispose to ulceration. Basic elements of foot care are presented in Table 6.7; these should be reinforced at regular intervals.
- *Exclusion of other causes of neuropathy* – alternative causes of neuropathy, notably chronic excessive alcohol consumption, should be identified. A detailed history and simple biochemistry and haematology tests will identify most alternatives. Discontinuation or avoidance of drugs with neurotoxic potential is important. Uraemia due to advanced nephropathy may exacerbate diabetic neuropathy.
- *Glycaemic control* – should be optimized; the United Kingdom Prospective Diabetes Study (UKPDS 33) also showed that better glycaemic control was associated with less deterioration in vibration sense at 15 years. However, the effects of improving glycaemic control have not been substantiated in controlled trials in symptomatic patients. Studies of the effect of hyperglycaemia on pain thresholds have produced conflicting results.
- *Analgesia* – therapeutic options are limited for painful neuropathic syndromes. Analgesia appropriate to the degree of pain must be provided; paracetamol is usually inadequate; opiates may be required. Start with codeine or dihydrocodeine. Beware the nephrotoxic potential of non-steroidal anti-inflammatory drugs in patients with renal impairment (in fact these drugs are often

not very effective for neuropathic symptoms). The centrally acting opioid-like non-narcotic agent tramadol may be useful for short-term therapy.

- *Antidepressants* – tricyclic antidepressants (imipramine 25–50 mg before bed or, as a second choice with a higher risk of side-effects, amitryptiline) may be useful adjuncts to simple analgesics; their antidepressant effects may also be useful, but these drugs block noradrenaline (norepinephrine) reuptake thereby reducing pain. Their hypnotic effect may also aid sleep, but response is variable. Venlafaxine has been reported as helpful.

- *Anticonvulsants* – carbamazepine (starting at 100 mg/day) or phenytoin (100 mg/day) can sometimes alleviate shooting pains. Gabapentin has recently been licensed for painful neuropathic syndromes and may be effective when other approaches have failed. Its safety profile appears to be superior to that of the tricyclics, but transient dizziness and somnolence are reported in up to 25% of patients.

- *Other therapies* – reported benefits for aldose reductase inhibitors (page 70) have been unimpressive to date and these drugs are not licensed in the UK. Capsaicin (0.075% cream), a recently introduced topical alkaloid derived from capsicum peppers, depletes levels of a peptide neurotransmitter, substance P, in nociceptive C fibre nerve terminals. Clinical experience to date is limited; transient stinging pain and erythema have been reported; the cream must be applied three to four times daily. Duloxetine can now be used to treat diabetic neuropathic pain in the USA. Sheathing painful limbs with surgical adhesive may help to alleviate allodynia, but a bed-cradle to avoid contact with bedclothes is more practical. Implantable spinal cord stimulators are occasionally of reported benefit in patients with severe, intractable pain. Quinine has long been used for night cramps. The role of complementary therapies, such as acupuncture, is uncertain.

- *Psychological support* – its importance should not be underestimated and it should always be underpinned by explanation of the prospect of improvement in acute neuropathies.

c) Acute painful sensory neuropathy

This uncommon syndrome presents as acute severe distal neuropathy, usually following the institution of insulin therapy. Recovery can be expected, but may be incomplete. Histological studies have shown regenerating nerve fibres; these are thought to be the origin of the symptoms. Treatment is symptomatic – good long-term glycaemic control should be maintained.

d) Motor neuropathies

Motor neuropathies include classic diabetic amyotrophy which may cause constitutional disturbance and weight loss (neuropathic cachexia of Ellenberg). The patient is typically a middle-aged male with type 2 diabetes in whom recent antecedent glycaemic control may have been surprisingly satisfactory. The presentation – pain (possibly severe) and weakness in the quadriceps – is abrupt. Muscle wasting follows rapidly. The weakness may be profound, leading to falls and immobility and painful hypersensitivity of the skin over the anterior aspect of the thigh is also characteristic. The symptoms lead to insomnia, anorexia, weight loss and depression. The knee jerk is characteristically absent and the plantar response reportedly may be extensor. While the nature of the responsible lesion remains uncertain, some features point to spinal cord or nerve root damage. An acute vasculopathy of the vasa nervorum is a popular explanation, but the predilection for the femoral nerve roots is unexplained. Other motor neuropathies are recognized (usually painful with hyperaesthesia; localized muscle weakness may occur), but truncal neuropathies affecting the abdomen are rare.

In classic amyotrophy few, if any, investigations are required. The major differential diagnoses are a nerve root or cauda equina lesion. Radiographs of the lumbar spine are usually unhelpful; magnetic resonance imaging may sometimes be indicated. Cerebrospinal fluid protein concentrations can be elevated and nerve conduction studies may show a localized femoral neuropathy – although evidence of spinal lesions is also recognized. Treatment is symptomatic and supportive with adequate analgesia and physiotherapy. Maintenance of good glycaemic control is recommended, although there is no clear relationship to recovery. Recovery (sometimes incomplete) usually occurs within a few months. Ipsilateral recurrence is uncommon.

e) Autonomic neuropathy

Diabetes-associated autonomic dysfunction usually remains asymptomatic. The most common clinical manifestation in men is probably erectile dysfunction (estimated to affect around 30%), although factors other than diabetic neuropathy are often contributory. Subclinical abnormalities of autonomic function are also relatively common and can be detected by simple bedside tests of cardiovascular reflex integrity, including:

- *Heart rate variability* – mainly assesses parasympathetic (vagal) function during deep breathing over 1 minute. The mean ratio of the electrocardiographic R-R interval in expiration to inspiration is calculated; less than 1.20 is considered abnormal (ie heart rate shows reduced variability).

- *Orthostatic blood pressure response* – this is a test of sympathetic integrity. Many variations, including the heart rate response to standing (the ratio at 30 and 15 seconds), or the Valsalva manoeuvre, for example, have been described. More sophisticated computer-aided systems are now available to provide comprehensive assessments of autonomic function.

- *Other specialized techniques* – such as the acetylcholine sweat spot test and measurement of pupillary adaptation to dark are chiefly used for research purposes.

Studies of spectral analysis of heart rate variability and baroreceptor reflex sensitivity may reveal even more subtle abnormalities of autonomic function, the long-term clinical implications of which are uncertain.

Patients with clinically overt autonomic neuropathy have been found to have a relatively high mortality rate in some follow-up studies. Autonomic dysfunction has been implicated in the sudden perioperative death of some diabetic patients. The electrocardiographic QT interval may be prolonged in diabetic patients; another measure, QTc dispersion, predicted death in a recent prospective study of patients with newly diagnosed type 2 diabetes. Improvements in glycaemic control have little beneficial effect on symptomatic autonomic neuropathy since advanced histological changes within nerves (axonal loss, demyelination, obliteration of vasa nervorum) are only partially, if at all, reversible. The United Kingdom Prospective Diabetes Study (page 60) was unable to demonstrate any benefits of improved glycaemic control, but the multifactorial Steno type 2 diabetes intervention study showed a 62% reduction in the risk of progression of measurements of autonomic neuropathy (page 89).

Erectile dysfunction is probably the most common manifestation of diabetic autonomic neuropathy in men, particularly with advancing age and use of antihypertensive drugs – notably the β-blockers and thiazide diuretics. Psychological factors are often present, making the distinction between primary organic and psychogenic impotence difficult. Devices enabling detection of nocturnal tumescence may sometimes be helpful, but many clinicians adopt a more pragmatic approach. Physical examination concentrates on genital anatomy (phimosis, Peyronie's disease) and evidence of peripheral neuropathy or peripheral vascular disease. Hormonal investigations (plasma testosterone, prolactin, gonadotrophins) are indicated if there is loss of libido or other features suggesting hypogonadism. The therapeutic options include:

- *Counselling* – by a clinician or specialist nurse. Should include demonstration of therapeutic options.

- *Mechanical devices* – vacuum tumescence devices, very occasionally surgical penile implants.

- *Vasoactive drugs* – prostaglandin E_1 administered intracorporeally or intraurethrally by the patient before intercourse; also α-blockers such as phenoxybenzamine.

- *PDE-5 inhibitors* (sildenafil, tadalafil and vardenafil) – these recently introduced oral agents appear to improve sexual function in 50–60% of diabetic men. Each is taken approximately one hour before intercourse, and the duration of action varies between agents. Diabetic patients generally require a higher dose than non-diabetic individuals. PDE-5 (phosphodiesterase) inhibitors inhibit the breakdown of cyclic guanosine monophosphate (cGMP) by a specific type 5 phosphodiesterase. This does not induce an erection; appropriate visual, psychological or physical stimuli are necessary. The agents are generally well-tolerated and no major problems such as priapism (which occasionally complicates injection therapy) have been reported. One major contraindication has emerged: concomitant use of nitrate drugs (or possibly nicorandil) may cause a precipitous fall in blood pressure which has been implicated in some deaths. The drugs may be contraindicated in approximately 10% of men.

In general, care should be exercised by men with cardiovascular disease – particularly severe angina or major impairment of left ventricular function – for whom sexual activity may be hazardous. Note that erectile dysfunction may be a marker for subclinical cardiovascular disease.

PDE-5 inhibitors are contraindicated in patients taking nitrate drugs

---

Orthostatic hypotension is defined arbitrarily as an otherwise unexplained fall in systolic blood pressure of 25–30 mmHg or more in a volume-replete patient on standing for two minutes. In fact, blood pressure may continue to fall for up to 15 minutes. This rare complication can be very disabling and difficult to manage. The differential diagnoses include other causes of autonomic failure in middle-aged or elderly patients (eg Shy-Drager syndrome), Addison's disease (uncommon) and hypopituitarism (uncommon). Antihypertensive agents and tricyclics may aggravate orthostatic hypotension and should be avoided. Support stockings may help to prevent venous pooling. Careful use of fluorocortisone may be beneficial but higher doses carry a risk of supine hypertension, oedema and hypokalaemia. Another alternative is midodrine, an α-adrenergic agonist.

Gastroparesis and diabetic diarrhoea rarely affect patients with type 2 diabetes. The motility agent cisapride, which had been used for gastroparesis, was withdrawn in 2000 following reports of serious cardiac arrhythmias, mainly in patients on concomitant therapy or with contraindications. Recent animal research suggests a pathophysiological role for diminished nitric oxide generation raising the possibility of novel forms of therapy. However, metformin (chapter 10) and acarbose (chapter 9) are much more common iatrogenic causes of gastrointestinal symptoms in patients with type 2 diabetes. On rare occasions, bladder paresis may produce hesitancy and retention and predispose to urinary infection. Prostatic disease should be excluded, but self-catheterization may be necessary in a few patients.

Also very rarely, patients with diabetic autonomic neuropathy may suffer drenching sweats of the head and upper torso while eating. This is known as gustatory sweating and is unrelated to hypoglycaemia. Anticholinergic drugs have been tried, but their side-effects are often intolerable. Peripheral oedema is another rare consequence of autonomic neuropathy. Ephedrine may be helpful and exacerbation of lower limb oedema avoided through use of drugs such as nifedipine, amlodipine and the thiazolidinediones.

Diabetic foot disease

Diabetic patients have an approximately 15-fold increased risk of non-traumatic lower-limb amputation compared with the non-diabetic population. In elderly patients with type 2 diabetes, there is a significant mortality rate associated with such major amputation; this largely reflects serious co-morbidity in this group. In the UK, foot complications remain a common reason for the hospitalization of diabetic patients. All health districts should establish a specialist foot clinic to which patients can be referred, or self-refer, for urgent assessment of serious lesions. Combined foot clinics with input from a podiatrist, vascular surgeon and diabetologist have been shown to reduce amputation rates. A coordinated approach is recommended.

> Diabetic patients with foot disease are at greatly increased risk of surgical amputation

The syndrome of diabetic foot disease includes elements of:

- *Peripheral neuropathy* – this is the major factor, manifest as insensitivity, motor imbalance with abnormal pressure distribution, and the consequences of local sympathetic denervation.
- *Peripheral arterial disease* – this leads to impaired tissue perfusion and is present in more than half of all cases; in combination with peripheral neuropathy, this comprises the neuro-ischaemic foot.
- *Tissue infection* – this occurs secondary to trauma or neuropathic ulceration.

The neuropathic foot

The neuropathic foot is insensitive (due to sensory neuropathy), dry (due to sympathetic denervation) and warm (well perfused in the

absence of co-existing peripheral vascular disease; page 102). Note that peripheral arterial disease may modify these features. Areas of high pressure develop with weight bearing due to alterations in foot anatomy. The latter, in turn, is a consequence of denervation of intrinsic foot muscles and tearing of the plantar fascia at the distal insertions. The resulting 'clawing' of toes exposes the metatarsal heads to abnormally high local pressures during normal gait. Calluses develop over these areas in response to the high pressure. Neuropathic toes may be compressed (painlessly) by ill-fitting or inappropriate footwear. Patients with 'at-risk' feet should receive verbal instruction about foot care, supplemented, where appropriate, by a written leaflet (Table 6.3); advice should be reinforced by regular contact with a podiatrist.

> **Table 6.3**
> Basic rules for care of the neuropathic foot.
>
> - Inspect feet daily (or have someone else inspect them)
> - Check footwear for foreign objects before use
> - Have feet measured carefully when purchasing shoes
> - Buy lace-up shoes with plenty of toe-room
> - Attend for regular podiatry
> - Keep feet away from heaters, hot water bottles, and other hot objects
> - Check temperature of bath water before entry
> - Avoid walking barefoot, especially outdoors
> - Use moisturizing cream for dry, fissured skin
> - Avoid unaccustomed lengthy walks, eg on holiday

> Callus formation indicates chronic local high pressure with risk of ulceration

Shearing forces during normal walking can disrupt the tissues under a callus which may lead to local haemorrhage. In fact, haemorrhage under a callus is a sign of imminent ulceration, secondary infection and, ultimately, gangrene due to septic arterial thrombosis. The major risk

Diabetic foot disease

Table 6.4
Indicators of feet at increased risk of ulceration.

- Neuropathy – especially with callus, blisters or fissures
- Ischaemia
- Previous ulceration
- Previous amputation
- Anatomical abnormalities, eg hallux valgus
- Impaired mobility due to age or co-morbidity
- Social isolation or low socioeconomic status

factors for ulceration are listed in Table 6.4. Previous ulceration is particularly important, as recurrence is common. The elderly, socially isolated patient who cannot inspect or perhaps even reach his or her feet is also a high-risk case. Oedema from congestive cardiac failure, nephropathy or immobility renders feet vulnerable as does the chronic deformity associated with Charcot neuropathy (page 85).

Haemorrhage within a plantar callus is a warning sign of impending ulceration

Referral

Patients should be referred to the podiatry service if they have any of the indications presented in Table 6.5. Regular callus debridement is required to reduce the risk of ulceration. Amateur treatment by the patient directed against lesions such as corns or deformed toenails should be discouraged. For established ulcers, particularly indolent or recurrent ulcers, three innovative therapies have recently become available:

Table 6.5
Indications for referral to a podiatrist.

- Patients with peripheral neuropathy
- Patients with significant ischaemia
- Patients with other foot lesions (eg callus, corns, ingrowing toenails)
- Patients requiring detailed foot assessments for other indications

- *Platelet-derived growth factor* – alongside good wound care, becaplermin (0.01% gel) has been shown to improve healing of chronic, uninfected ulcers compared with placebo. Further studies are required.
- *Cultured dermis* – this preparation is akin to a skin graft constructed from neonatal fibroblasts embedded in a synthetic matrix (supplied deep frozen). Studies to date suggest that more ulcers can be healed if this treatment is applied, but, again, infection must be controlled before application.
- *Fibrinogen adsorption* – this represents a major departure from conventional topical treatments. The process requires extracorporeal passage of plasma through a sepharose matrix. Evidence of efficacy and safety is presently inadequate.

Healthcare professionals such as district and general practice nurses and appropriately trained community podiatrists should be able to refer urgently to the local (hospital) specialist foot clinic. Patients should also be able to self-refer, if necessary. Indications for referral are listed in Table 6.6.

Table 6.6
Criteria for referral to a specialist diabetes foot clinic.

- Patients with neuropathic ulceration which has not responded to treatment within four weeks
- Patients with a foot infection not responding to antibiotics
- Acute or chronic Charcot neuroarthropathy
- Patients requiring special shoes or insoles
- Patients requiring weight-relieving casts

Infection

Infection with spreading cellulitis and/or deep infection represents an immediate threat to the viability of the foot, and sometimes even to the patient's life. However, signs of infection can be difficult to detect in a neuropathic, ischaemic foot. Unless there is a prompt and convincing response to initial outpatient treatment the following actions are required:

- *Hospital admission* – bed rest to facilitate ulcer healing. An ulcer will not heal if the patient continues to walk and pressure-relief is essential; failure to rest is usually responsible for recurrence. Provided the infection is controlled, a removable or lightweight plaster cast can be applied to allow healing; a window is left in the plaster to enable inspection. Simultaneous care must be taken to avoid the consequences of immobility, notably decubitus neuro-ischaemic heel ulcers in debilitated patients. Action should also be directed towards relevant co-morbidity such as peripheral oedema, which is common in diabetic patients with multiple co-morbidities.

- *Assessment of the extent of the infection and state of the peripheral vasculature.* Radiographs will exclude chronic osteomyelitis in deep infections. They may, however, appear normal in the earliest stages of osteomyelitis. Neuropathy in the absence of bone infection may produce translucency of the metatarsal heads. Arterial calcification is asymptomatic but may also be visible on radiographs of feet exhibiting extensive diabetic neuropathy. Vascular calcification needs to be documented, because the results of Doppler studies of the peripheral vasculature may be misleading. Chronic, deep-seated infection has a general debilitating effect and hypoalbuminaemia (a negative acute-phase reactant), a mild normochromic normocytic anaemia, is common. Additionally, erythrocyte sedimentation rate and C-reactive peptide concentrations are usually elevated during active infection and tissue repair.

> Radiographs of feet with deep or chronic infection should be taken to exclude osteomyelitis

- *Bacterial treatment.* A mixed bacterial growth is common, usually containing *Streptococcus pyogenes*, *Staphylococcus aureus* and anaerobic species, such as the bacteroides (notable for their odour). Radiographs should be checked for tissue gas formation; gram-negative bacilli may contribute to deep infections. Deep wound swabs will guide the choice of antibiotic, but action against all the organisms listed above will be required in cases of serious infection. Initially, antibiotic therapy may be required, particularly if peripheral arterial supply is impaired. Subsequently, oral treatment may need to be continued for several weeks in cases of deep tissue infection or osteomyelitis. Examples of commonly used antibiotic regimens are presented in Table 6.7. If, after 12 weeks of appropriate therapy, an ulcer can be probed down to underlying bone, surgical resection of the osteomyelitic bone may be indicated.

> Radiographs should be taken to exclude gas formation by *Clostridium* spp

- *Surgery.* Judicious debridement, digit amputation and deep abscess drainage (beware the patient with neuropathy who has severe foot discomfort) can all be performed by a trained podiatrist or surgeon. The aim is always to preserve the limb but life-threatening infection may demand major intervention such as mid-foot or, as a last resort, below-knee amputation.

> Severe discomfort in an infected neuropathic foot raises the possibility of abscess formation

- *Amputation* may be required for non-healing lesions (eg through an inadequate peripheral blood supply), gangrene, osteomyelitis, or recurrent lesions at a single site. 'Ray' amputation of the second,

Table 6.7
Examples of antibiotic regimens for diabetic foot infections.

Superficial infections
- Oral ampicillin + flucloxacillin
- Oral amoxycillin/clavulanate
- Azithromycin (if penicillin allergy)

Deep-tissue infections
- Intravenous ampicillin + flucloxacillin + oral metronidazole
- Intravenous amoxycillin–clavulanate
- Intravenous ciprofloxacin + clindamycin

Osteomyelitis
- Fusidic acid
- Trimethoprim
- Clindamycin
- Rifampicin

Methicillin-resistant Staphylococcus aureus
- Fusidic acid
- Trimethoprim
- Rifampicin
- Vancomycin (requires monitoring of blood levels)
- Teicoplanin

Notes: Liaison with the local microbiology service is recommended. Appropriate safety monitoring is required with some agents. Complications (eg pseudomembranous colitis) may develop during or after antibiotic therapy. Infection with methicillin-resistant *S. aureus* (MRSA) is an increasing problem in many units. Debridement and local antiseptic measures may be useful. Linezolid may also help with infections that are resistant to other antibacterials.

third or fourth toes, taking the associated metatarsal, can result in a highly satisfactory outcome (although healing will take some weeks), but major amputation is usually a devastating event. The prospects for successful rehabilitation are often remote. Walking using a below-knee prosthesis increases energy expenditure by 50%, which is an impossible target for many elderly or debilitated patients. Further, the risk of ulceration in the contralateral foot tends to increase due to compensatory weight-bearing. Confinement to a wheelchair may be the unfortunate consequence.

- *Prevention of recurrence.* Education of patient and carer, provision of special

footwear, home help, and careful follow-up in the foot clinic will all help to prevent recurrence. Orthotist assessment is essential in patients with severe deformity. Ready-to-wear boots may be helpful in the short term, but are unaesthetic, so compliance is poor. Shoes may need to be made to order to accommodate special insoles. Technology can now be used to identify local high-pressure sites, aiding insole and shoe design. Sports training shoes are worn by some patients, being a relatively inexpensive and acceptable alternative.

Charcot neuroarthropathy

Increased blood flow through the foot, secondary to local autonomic denervation together with abnormal pressure loading, may lead to unsuspected fractures resulting from minimal normal daily trauma. Patients often present acutely with a foot that is warm, tender and oedematous – palpable pedal pulses are characteristic. While these features strongly suggest an acute Charcot neuroarthropathy, (Figures 6.6 and 6.7), erroneous diagnoses of infection, inflammatory arthritis or even deep venous thrombosis are not uncommon. A penetrating ulcer that can be probed down to bone is probably the most reliable single sign of osteomyelitis; if there is doubt, antibiotics should be given. Contrary to common belief, some degree of discomfort is often present in the acute Charcot foot. However, the onset of pain in a neuropathic foot may signal the development of a deep infection.

Radiographs will usually confirm the diagnosis, except in the earliest phases, when they may appear normal. Initially fractures (of a metatarsal, for example) may be apparent, but these progress rapidly to extensive subluxation, fragmentation and disorganization with remodelling. Isotope bone scans are often unhelpful in distinguishing acute neuroarthropathy from infection, since local uptake of tracer occurs in both circumstances. Magnetic resonance imaging and computed tomography are more helpful. Plasma levels of bone-specific alkaline phosphatase are often elevated. Once remodelling is complete, the patient is left with a deformed neuroarthropathic foot at high risk of ulceration (Figure 6.6). A 'rocker bottom' deformity is characteristic and bilateral changes are often evident on radiographs (Figure 6.7), even in the absence of clinical evidence of bone destruction.

> Radiographs must be taken if a patient with neuropathy presents with an acutely swollen hot foot

Management

Treatment during the acute stages of Charcot neuroarthropathy is controversial; no adequate randomized controlled trials have been performed. The ultimate aim is to minimize the degree of deformity in the quiescent phase:

- *Immobilization* – a walking plaster or removable cast is usually favoured, taking care to avoid trauma and ulceration from the cast itself. It is recommended that weight-bearing be recommenced very gradually over a period of weeks.
- *Intravenous bisphosphonates* – these drugs inhibit osteoblast activity and have been used in the hope of suppressing bone remodelling.
- *Custom-made footwear* – will help to prevent subsequent ulceration – if worn! (Ask the patient and inspect footwear.)
- *Reconstructive orthopaedic techniques* – realignment techniques have been described, especially to help patients with unstable hind feet, but surgical intervention should be considered only as a last resort.

> Charcot neuroarthropathy is associated with high risk of recurrent foot ulceration

Diabetic nephropathy

It is estimated that approximately 25–30% of patients with type 2 diabetes develop some degree of nephropathy. Certain ethnic groups, eg African–Americans, South Asians and Native Americans, appear to be at higher risk. Diabetic nephropathy is currently the single largest cause of end-stage renal failure in Western countries and the rapidly increasing global incidence of type 2 diabetes seems set to ensure that it continues to be a major consumer of healthcare resources. Diabetes is now responsible for more than one-third of all patients starting renal replacement therapy.

> Diabetes is the single largest cause of end-stage renal failure in developed countries

Diabetic nephropathy does not only result in progressive renal failure; it is also closely associated with increased morbidity and mortality from coronary heart disease, cerebrovascular disease and peripheral arterial disease. In fact, most patients with type 2 diabetes die from atherosclerotic disease before they develop end-stage renal failure. Renal replacement therapy does not diminish this risk. Thus, diabetic nephropathy, in common with other causes of chronic renal failure, may be regarded as a state of greatly accelerated atherosclerosis.

> Diabetic nephropathy is associated with a greatly increased incidence of atherosclerosis

Natural history

Several distinct (if somewhat arbitrary) phases are recognized in the natural history of nephropathy. The earliest are asymptomatic. The important prognostic implications of this condition necessitate regular (annual) testing of urine for albumin – its presence being the earliest clinical indicator of nephropathy. While distinct stages in the development of nephropathy are recognized, the pathogenic process is actually a continuum (Table 6.8).

Table 6.8
Natural history of diabetic nephropathy.

- *Stage 1: Functional changes*
  These include an increased glomerular filtration rate and filtration fraction at diagnosis; such subclinical changes are fairly common in type 2 diabetes, demonstrable in approximately 30% of patients. Glycaemic control reduces glomerular filtration rate, but the abnormalities persist in some patients.

- *Stage 2: Renal structural lesions*
  Early structural (subclinical) changes may be present even at diagnosis in some patients with type 2 diabetes.

- *Stage 3: Microalbuminuria*
  Blood pressure starts to rise (although remaining within the normotensive range); otherwise asymptomatic. Glomerular filtration rate tends to be stable up to this point.

- *Stage 4: Overt clinical nephropathy*
  Dipstick tests for protein become positive, initially intermittently then persistently. Nephrotic syndrome may develop. Glomerular filtration rate starts to decline and plasma creatinine starts to rise. Hypertension is usually well established by this stage (if not present at an earlier stage).

- *Stage 5: Progression to end-stage renal failure*
  Plasma creatinine rises above 500 μmol/l, usually at a constant rate for individuals who have had clinical nephropathy for seven to 10 years, but with considerable inter-individual variation. Once plasma creatinine has exceeded 200 μmol/l, the point at which dialysis will be required can be predicted using a plot of the reciprocal of the plasma creatinine concentration. Blood pressure is usually difficult to control by this time. The rate of decline in glomerular filtration rate is closely associated with elevated systolic blood pressure in patients with type 2 diabetes. Intercurrent illnesses, eg urinary tract infection or pharmacological over-diuresis, may cause a temporarily rapid decline in renal function. Fluid retention may result in pulmonary or peripheral oedema, which may be misinterpreted as cardiac decompensation. The incidence of macrovascular events (myocardial infarction, stroke, peripheral vascular disease) is dramatically increased by this stage.

Note: these stages have been identified mainly through studies in patients with type 1 diabetes.

Proteinuria is the clinical hallmark of diabetic nephropathy

Considerable emphasis has been placed on pharmacological intervention in the early stages of nephropathy, particularly with angiotensin converting enzyme (ACE) inhibitors. These are advocated even in the absence of overt hypertension, reflecting an apparent renoprotective effect that is held to be independent of changes in systemic blood pressure. However, the methodology used for screening for early nephropathy and the timing and type of pharmacological intervention are all areas of controversy; the debate reflects the absence of long-term outcome data, but studies are seriously hampered by the long natural history of this complication. Most interventional studies to date have been relatively small and short-term. Moreover, they have tended to rely on surrogate endpoints such as transition from microalbuminuria to clinical grade proteinuria. Finally, they have mostly been performed in patients with type 1 diabetes. To complicate the picture further, microalbuminuria is recognized as a less specific predictor of nephropathy in type 2 diabetes – progression in only about 25% of cases compared to 50–70% of those in patients with type 1 diabetes. Thus, although progression, defined as the crossing of arbitrary proteinuria thresholds, may suggest renoprotection, extrapolation to the long-term outcome is fraught with difficulties. Despite all this, evidence has accumulated to suggest that it may be possible to delay the progression of diabetic nephropathy, at least in some patients.

Annual testing for proteinuria is recommended in order to detect the development of diabetic nephropathy

Diagnosis

Microalbuminuria

The concept of 'microalbuminuria' was introduced in the 1960s. In the earliest clinically detectable stage, urinary albumin excretion is increased to 30–300 mg/day. Sensitive assays are required to measure albuminuria accurately, and these are best performed as a timed overnight collection. An albumin concentration <20 mg/l is regarded as normal. A urinary albumin:creatinine ratio, measured in the first-voided sample of the morning is a more practical alternative: 2.5 mg/mmol in adult men and 3.5 mg/mmol in adult women are diagnostic of microalbuminuria (assuming exclusion of confounding factors and alternative possibilities). Cross-sectional studies in patients with type 2 diabetes have suggested a prevalence of microalbuminuria ranging from 15% to >50%, depending on ethnicity. Microalbuminuria is also a marker for cardiovascular risk and overall mortality. It is typically associated with a constellation of risk factors for cardiovascular disease: insulin resistance, poor glycaemic control, dyslipidaemia, left ventricular hypertrophy, endothelial dysfunction and abnormalities of blood pressure regulation (impaired nocturnal 'dipping').

Microalbuminuria: 30–300 mg/day
Proteinuria: >300 mg/day

Proteinuria

When albumin excretion exceeds 300 mg/day, the Albustix (or equivalent) dipstick test becomes positive, marking the development of clinical nephropathy. Nephrotic syndrome may occasionally develop, with distinctive symptoms including urinary protein excretion >5 g/day, hypoalbuminaemia and peripheral oedema. However, urinary protein excretion may be influenced by several factors, including:

- *Hyperglycaemia* – tests for microalbuminuria at diagnosis and during periods of poor glycaemic control may be misleading

because of transient increases in urinary protein excretion.

- *Intercurrent illness* – especially urinary tract infection, is common. It may be asymptomatic and therefore must be excluded.

- *Posture* – an upright posture increases protein excretion. Testing the first-voided sample of the day avoids this effect.

- *Exercise* – also increases urinary protein excretion.

- *Congestive cardiac failure* – is a prominent cause of proteinuria.

- *Ageing* – urinary creatinine declines in old age, resulting in a relative increase in the albumin:creatinine ratio.

- *Other renal pathology* – such as glomerulonephritis and drug-induced renal disease (eg penicillamine). Renal vein thrombosis is closely associated with the nephrotic syndrome.

Thus, care must be exercised before concluding that proteinuria is attributable to diabetic nephropathy. Rather, microalbuminuria or a positive Albustix test result should prompt exclusion of these alternatives. Albuminuria should be confirmed with at least one additional sample, especially if treatment is being considered and for levels within the microalbuminuria range. The following screening strategy has been suggested by expert groups:

- Once diabetes has been stabilized, the albumin:creatinine ratio should be checked at least annually up to the age of 70 years.

- A positive result should prompt re-testing and exclusion of alternative possibilities.

- Timed overnight urine samples are regarded as the gold standard test, but repeat early morning albumin:creatinine ratios are also acceptable and far more practical.

- Persistently positive results should lead to careful assessment of glycaemic control, blood pressure, plasma lipids, plasma creatinine and to a careful search for other micro- and macrovascular complications.

Further investigations

Renal biopsy is usually unnecessary unless there are atypical features, such as rapid (and otherwise unexplained) deterioration in renal function, absence of significant diabetic retinopathy, development of nephrotic syndrome, and features suggesting alternative pathology such as haematuria, or evidence of autoimmune disease. Once diabetic nephropathy is well advanced, microscopic haematuria may be detectable on dipstick testing, but alternative renal tract pathology should be excluded. Macroscopic haematuria is not a feature of diabetic nephropathy and should prompt careful examination of the renal tract.

Co-morbidity

By the time dialysis is required, most patients will have significant multiple diabetic complications. In particular, retinopathy will have resulted in severe visual impairment in some patients. Indeed, the association between retinopathy and nephropathy is so strong that the absence of the former should prompt consideration of alternative reasons for renal failure. Patients are also likely to have advanced neuropathy, not infrequently with features of autonomic dysfunction (page 80). The risk of neuropathic ulceration is high and may be exacerbated by pedal oedema. Postural hypotension may occasionally pose management difficulties, particularly in relation to haemodialysis (page 92). The incidence of major ischaemia of the peripheries is greatly increased with chronic renal failure – with concomitant risk of gangrene in the upper and lower limbs.

Management

Glycaemic control

The United Kingdom Prospective Diabetes Study (page 60) showed a 30% reduction in the risk of microalbuminuria at 15 years' follow-up with intensive therapy. Care should be taken to avoid oral antidiabetic agents that may be hazardous in the presence of renal impairment, notably long-acting sulphonylureas such as glibenclamide (glyburide) (page 140) and metformin (page 154). Insulin is often the treatment of choice, but doses may have to be reduced in patients with renal impairment since a proportion of insulin is cleared via the kidney. Anorexia may also require a reduction in insulin dose. On the other hand, insulin resistance associated with microalbuminuria and renal failure and intercurrent illnesses may make glycaemic control difficult to attain. The key points of the Steno type 2 diabetes study, in which multiple risk factors including hyperglycaemia were targeted in high-risk patients with microalbuminuria, are presented in Table 6.9 and Figure 6.8.

Table 6.9
The Steno-2 study. Intensified multifactorial intervention in patients with type 2 diabetes and microalbuminuria. Sourced from the *N Engl J Med* 2003; **348**: 383-93.

Study design
Randomized, unblinded trial comparing intensive multifactorial therapy (low-fat diet and exercise, smoking cessation, ACE inhibitors, vitamins C and E, aspirin and stepwise therapy directed against hyperglycaemia, dyslipidaemia and hypertension) in a specialized hospital diabetes centre ($n=80$) with standard treatment by general practitioners ($n=80$). Mean age of patients 55 years; mean follow-up 7.8 years.

Results
Compared with patients in the standard treatment group, those in the intensive group had reduced risks for clinical nephropathy (56% relative risk reduction; $p=0.01$), progression of retinopathy (40%; $p=0.04$), blindness in one eye (85%; $p=0.03$), progression of autonomic neuropathy (62%; $p=0.01$) and the combined endpoint of death and macrovascular events (37%; $p=0.03$).

Interpretation
Multifactorial intervention reduced the development of nephropathy and other complications. However, the relative contribution of each intervention to outcomes was unclear.

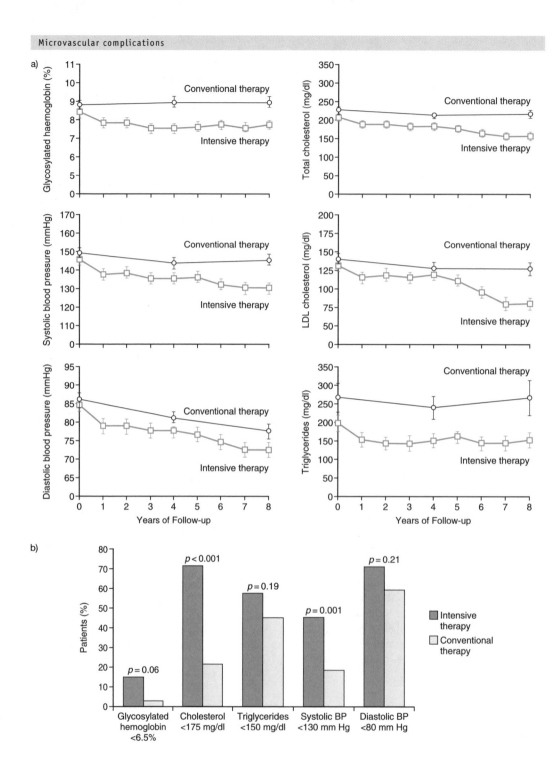

Figure 6.8
Key results of Steno-2 study. *N Engl J Med* 2003; **348**: 383–93.

Control of hypertension

Blood pressure gradually rises as urinary albumin excretion increases. It may remain within the normotensive range in the initial stages, but will still be elevated for the individual patient concerned. Glomerular filtration declines with progression to end-stage renal failure (over about a decade but with considerable inter-individual variation). Polymorphisms of the ACE gene may have prognostic and therapeutic implications for patients with diabetic nephropathy. However, the impact of these polymorphisms on diabetic nephropathy and implications for ACE inhibitor therapy remain unclear.

> Genetic factors that may increase susceptibility to nephropathy in diabetic patients have been identified

Control of hypertension is essential. Tight blood pressure targets have been proposed by expert groups. Table 6.10 presents current guidelines for blood pressure targets in diabetes. Recently the British Hypertension Society, European Society of Hypertension and the American Diabetes Association suggested an optimal target of <130/80 mmHg for type 2 diabetic patients. This is gaining widespread acceptance (see page 120). To add confusion, the UK suggests audit standards of <140/80, or 70% of diabetic hypertensive patients <145/80 mmHg. The various targets have been derived from studies showing that tight control of blood pressure is associated with a slower decline in glomerular filtration rate. While blood pressure control may be more important than the type of drug used to achieve it, differences between classes of antihypertensive agent have been noted, particularly in terms of reducing proteinuria. Although a firm evidence-base for the use of ACE inhibitors has been amassed, their superiority in this specific subgroup remains uncertain – in animal models, they have been shown to have renoprotective effects independent of their effects on systemic blood pressure. Combination therapy will usually be required in the pursuit of target blood pressures (page 104). There is some evidence that non-dihydropyridine calcium antagonists (eg diltiazem) have greater antiproteinuric effects than dihydropyridines (eg nifedipine). Recent short-term data suggest that combining an ACE inhibitor with an angiotensin II receptor antagonist may be advantageous in providing superior blood pressure control. This approach is currently not recommended. Further studies are required. Care is required to avoid the development of hyperkalaemia in patients with overt nephropathy. Care must also be taken with ACE inhibitors and angiotensin II receptor blockers in women of childbearing age.

> Hyperkalaemia is a hazard with potassium-retaining drugs in patients with nephropathy

The potential dangers posed by bilateral renal artery stenosis in patients with type 2 diabetes are discussed in chapter 7. A combination of

Table 6.10
Current guidelines for blood pressure targets in diabetes.

	Type 1 diabetes (mmHg)	Type 2 diabetes (mmHg)
JNC VI	<130/85	<130/85
National Kidney Foundation	<125/75*	<125/75*
British Hypertension Society	<140/80[†]	<140/80[‡]
– Optimal[†]	<130/80	<130/80
Scottish Intercollegiate Guidelines Network	<140/80	<140/80
National Institute for Clinical Excellence	<140/80	<135/75*
American Diabetes Association	<130/80	<130/80

*if nephropathy; [†]optimal target <130/80 mmHg; [‡]<120/75 mmHg if ambulatory blood pressure monitoring (ABPM) or home measurements.

antihypertensive drugs is often required, particularly in patients with type 2 diabetes and clinical nephropathy. Use of loop diuretics, β-blockers, long-acting calcium antagonists and centrally acting drugs may all be necessary. In particular, the early addition of a loop diuretic such as frusemide is helpful; as plasma creatinine concentrations rise, large doses of the latter agent may be required.

> Combinations of antihypertensive agents are usually required for patients with clinical nephropathy

Blood pressure and renal function should be assessed at least every three months, more frequently in some patients.

Treatment of dyslipidaemia

The high toll from accelerated macrovascular disease suggests that routine use of statins is indicated in nephropathy, but there are presently no outcome data from randomized controlled trials to confirm the benefits. Unfavourable alterations in lipid profiles – increased low-density lipoprotein (LDL)-cholesterol, increased triglycerides, reduced high-density lipoprotein (HDL)-cholesterol – can be detected before creatinine levels rise; increases in plasma levels of atherogenic lipoprotein(a) may also contribute. The risk of myositis is increased when statins are co-prescribed with cyclosporin following renal transplantation. Fibrates are contraindicated in patients with renal impairment because of the increased risk of myositis. Statins may have renoprotective effects in addition to their beneficial actions on blood lipids.

Cigarette smoking

Cigarette smoking should be avoided completely.

Protein restriction

A modest restriction in diet to 0.6–0.7 g/kg/day is often recommended for patients with clinical

nephropathy, but the benefits remain controversial.

Dialysis

Survival rates have improved for patients with diabetic nephropathy on dialysis. If a patient is considered unsuitable for renal transplantation, dialysis is used as the sole long-term therapy. Because of a greater tendency to fluid retention, dialysis may have to be introduced at an earlier stage in some diabetic patients. By the time that plasma creatinine level has reached 500 µmol/l, dialysis should be a serious consideration. Specialist referral is suggested when creatinine rises above 150–200 µmol/l.

> Dialysis should be considered once plasma creatinine levels have reached 500 µmol/l

Continuous ambulatory peritoneal dialysis is now the favoured form of therapy: it is relatively inexpensive compared with haemodialysis, avoids rapid fluctuations in intravascular volume and is therefore better suited to patients with cardiovascular disease or autonomic neuropathy. No vascular access is required and insulin may be delivered into the peritoneal cavity by injection into the dialysate; its pharmacokinetics are altered by factors including the volume of dialysate and the tonicity (ie isotonic vs hypertonic), approximately 50% is systemically absorbed. Reported survival rates remain less favourable for diabetic patients but also similar to those achieved on haemodialysis. Peritonitis is the principal complication.

Haemodialysis requires the construction of vascular access, either an arteriovenous fistula or an artificial graft. These not only tend to fail more rapidly in diabetic patients, but distal necrosis of digits may occur. Autonomic neuropathy-related hypotension may make removal of excess fluid problematic and blood glucose concentrations may be erratic. Survival is generally worse in elderly patients. Oxidative stress may contribute to cardiovascular risks in patients on dialysis.

Renal transplantation

Renal transplantation is usually cadaveric but sometimes from a living related donor and the treatment of choice in patients with end-stage diabetic nephropathy. Patient and graft survival rates remain inferior to those of non-diabetic recipients but, otherwise, rehabilitation is usually satisfactory. Several key selection criteria must usually be fulfilled for renal transplantation in the UK (Table 6.11).

Table 6.11
Criteria for renal transplantation in diabetic patients.

- Absence of severe cardiovascular or cerebrovascular disease
- Absence of significant sepsis
- Absence of life-limiting co-morbidity

Assessment of the coronary vasculature is routine; coronary angiography is required by most centres. The diabetogenic effects of immunosuppressive agents (corticosteroids, cyclosporin and tacrolimus) may necessitate increased insulin doses post-transplantation. Dyslipidaemia may also be exacerbated by immunosuppressive therapy. The main causes of death post-transplantation are atheromatous cardiovascular disease and sepsis, but autonomic neuropathy (page 80) may also be a factor. There is an increase in the risk of neoplastic disease with long-term immunosuppressive therapy.

Further reading

Aiello LP. Perspectives on diabetic retinopathy. *Am J Ophthalmol* 2003; **136**: 122-35.

Anon. Drug treatment of neuropathic pain. *Drug Ther Bull* 2000; **12**: 89-93.

Backonja M, Beydoun A, Edwards KR et al. Gabapentin for the symptomatic treatment of painful neuropathy in patients with diabetes mellitus. *JAMA* 1998; **280**: 1831-6.

Barnett AH, Bain SC, Bouter P et al. Angiotensin-receptor blockade versus converting-enzyme inhibition in type 2 diabetes and nephropathy. *N Engl J Med* 2004; **351**: 1952-61.

Clark CM Jr, Lee DA. Prevention and treatment of the complications of diabetes mellitus. *N Engl J Med* 1995; **332**: 1210-7.

Cooper ME. Pathogenesis, prevention and treatment of diabetic nephropathy. *Lancet* 1998; **352**: 213-9.

Edmonds ME. Progress in the care of the diabetic foot. *Lancet* 1999; **354**: 270-2.

Embil JM. The management of diabetic foot osteomyelitis. *Diabetic Foot* 2000; **3**: 76-84.

Ferris FL III, Davis MD, Aiello LM. Treatment of diabetic retinopathy. *N Engl J Med* 1999; **341**: 667-78.

Gaede P, Vedel P, Parving H-H, Pedersen O. Intensified multifactorial intervention in patients with type 2 diabetes mellitus and microalbuminuria: the Steno type 2 randomized study. *Lancet* 1999; **353**: 617-22.

Kohner E, Allwinkle J, Andrews J et al. Saint Vincent and improving diabetes care. Report of the visual handicap group. *Diabetic Med* 1996; **13**: S13-26.

Locatelli F, Pozzoni P, Del Vecchio L. Renal replacement therapy in patients with diabetes and end-stage renal failure. *J Am Soc Nephrol* 2004; **15 (suppl 1)**: S25-S29.

Marshall SM. Recent advances in diabetic nephropathy. *Clin Med* 2004; **4**: 277-82.

Mason J, O'Keeffe C, McIntosh A et al. A systematic review of foot ulcer in patients with type 2 diabetes mellitus. 1: prevention. *Diabetic Med* 1999; **16**: 801-12.

Mayfield JA, Reiber GE, Sanders LJ et al. Preventive foot care in people with diabetes (technical review). *Diabetes Care* 1998; **21**: 2161-77.

Stratton IM, Adler AI, Neil HAW et al. Association of glycaemia with macrovascular and microvascular complications of type 2 diabetes (UKPDS 35): prospective observational study. *Br Med J* 2000; **321**: 405-12.

Thomas S, Viberti G-C. Proteinuria in diabetes. *J R Col Physicians Lond* 2000; **34**: 336-9.

Tuomilheto J. Controlling glucose and blood pressure in type 2 diabetes. *Br Med J* 2000; **321**: 394-5.

UK Prospective Diabetes Study Group. Tight blood pressure control and risk of macrovascular and microvascular complications in type 2 diabetes (UKPDS 38). *Br Med J* 1998; **317**: 703-13.

UK Prospective Diabetes Study Group. Efficacy of atenolol and captopril in reducing risk of macrovascular and microvascular complications in type 2 diabetes (UKPDS 39). *Br Med J* 1998; **317**: 713-20.

Viberti G-C, Marshall S, Beech R et al. Saint Vincent and improving diabetes care. Report on renal disease in diabetes. *Diabetic Med* 1996; **13**: S6-12.

Wieman TJ, Smiell JM, Su Y. Efficacy and safety of a topical gel formulation of recombinant human platelet-derived growth factor-BB (becaplermin) in patients with chronic neuropathic diabetic ulcers. *Diabetes Care* 1998; **21**: 822-7.

7. Macrovascular disease

Risk factors for atherosclerosis
Coronary heart disease
Acute myocardial infarction
Peripheral arterial disease
Cerebrovascular disease
Hypertension
Dyslipidaemia

Type 2 diabetes is a strong risk factor for cardiovascular disease in both men and women. Longitudinal studies indicate that the risk of atherosclerotic cardiovascular disease is two to four times higher in patients with type 2 diabetes than in non-diabetic individuals. The annual rate of fatal and non-fatal cardiovascular disease among people with type 2 diabetes is 2–5%. This risk is greater than that explained by classic risk factors for atherosclerosis. Further, it is operative in many different populations with dissimilar background rates of cardiovascular disease. The prevalence of some cardiovascular risk factors, including glucose intolerance, however, does differ between ethnic groups (page 2).

> Coronary heart disease is the principal cause of premature mortality in patients with diabetes

Patients with proteinuria (microalbuminuria or clinical proteinuria) are at significantly increased risk of atheromatous cardiovascular disease; the reasons remain only partially understood. Cardiovascular event risk is increased nearly two-fold by the presence of microalbuminuria and it has been hypothesized that microalbuminuria reflects generalized endothelial dysfunction which predisposes to

atheroma. The vascular endothelium has a complex structure and disturbances of endothelial function have been reported in patients with type 2 diabetes. However, this should not detract from the fact that type 2 diabetes *per se* is a major risk factor for coronary heart disease, amply demonstrated by the observation that the normal protection from coronary heart disease afforded to pre-menopausal women is negated by diabetes. Some studies indicate that rates of atherosclerotic cardiovascular disease are higher in diabetic women than diabetic men, relative to their non-diabetic counterparts.

> The normal protection from cardiovascular disease afforded to pre-menopausal women is negated by diabetes

Risk factors for atherosclerosis

Both longitudinal and interventional studies have indicated that glycaemia is an independent risk factor for atherosclerotic cardiovascular disease. Current evidence suggests that there is a linear association between glycated haemoglobin (HbA_{1c}) levels and cardiovascular risk in patients with type 2 diabetes. This was demonstrated by prospective population-based studies in Finland (Figure 7.1) and Sweden in which cardiovascular mortality was linearly associated with glycaemia, independent of mode of treatment. In a second Finnish study, elevated HbA_{1c} was significantly associated with coronary heart disease mortality after adjustment for other cardiovascular risk factors. In the United Kingdom Prospective Diabetes Study (UKPDS 23), increased baseline HbA_{1c} and fasting plasma glucose concentrations were associated with coronary heart disease. Other predictive risk factors included an increased LDL-cholesterol concentration, a decreased HDL-cholesterol concentration and an increased fasting triglyceride concentration (but triglycerides were no longer independently predictive when other risk factors were included in the analysis). The estimated hazard ratio for smokers compared with non-smokers was 1.41. The multicentre European DECODE Study showed that elevated two-hour plasma glucose concentrations correlated more strongly with cardiovascular mortality than fasting hyperglycaemia.

> Elevated fasting plasma glucose concentrations and elevated HbA$_{1c}$ levels are associated with an increased risk of coronary heart disease

The main modifiable risk factors for atherosclerosis in diabetic patients are identical to those in non-diabetic individuals, ie:

- hypertension
- dyslipidaemia
- cigarette smoking.

The adverse effects of hypertension and dyslipidaemia also seem to be amplified by the presence of diabetes. Lipid levels and blood pressures that might be regarded as acceptable in non-diabetic subjects are not acceptable in diabetic patients.

When a multiplicity of risk factors is present, the risk of macrovascular disease is greatly enhanced (Figure 7.2). Chronic inflammation, detectable using high-sensitivity assays for C-reactive protein, is a feature of the metabolic syndrome that is thought to contribute to atherogenesis. The impact of other cardiovascular risk factors, such as fibrinogen, plasminogen activator inhibitor-1, lipoprotein(a) and homocysteine, has yet to be fully elucidated. The extent of coronary calcification, detectable using electron

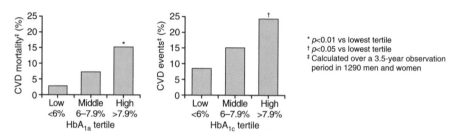

* $p<0.01$ vs lowest tertile
† $p<0.05$ vs lowest tertile
‡ Calculated over a 3.5-year observation period in 1290 men and women

Figure 7.1
Glycated haemoglobin (HbA$_{1c}$) at baseline as a predictor of cardiovascular disease in nearly 1300 Finnish men and women (aged 65–74 years). Reproduced with permission from Kuusisto *et al.* Diabetes 1994; **43**: 960-7.

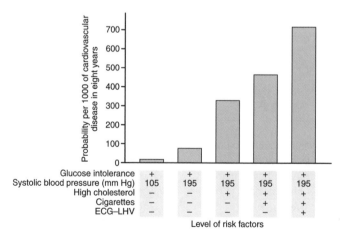

Figure 7.2
Effect of multiple risk factors for coronary heart disease. Reproduced with permission from Kannel WB, McGee DL. *Diabetes Care* 1979; **2**: 120-6.

beam computed tomography (EBCT), tends to be greater in diabetes.

> The coronary risk associated with dyslipidaemia, hypertension or cigarette smoking is amplified by the presence of diabetes

Coronary heart disease

Coronary heart disease is the most common cause of mortality among patients with type 2 diabetes. The magnitude of the increased risk in diabetic patients was forcefully demonstrated in a population-based study. During a seven-year follow-up, Finnish patients with type 2 diabetes who had no overt coronary heart disease at entry were found to be at as high a risk of myocardial infarction and cardiovascular death as non-diabetic individuals who had already sustained a myocardial infarction (Figure 7.3). Recent expert guidelines suggest that patients with type 2 diabetes should still be regarded as candidates for therapeutic measures hitherto reserved for patients with established coronary heart disease – eg judicious use of aspirin, statins and antihypertensive drugs. A decision to intervene pharmacologically as primary prevention should be based on calculation of

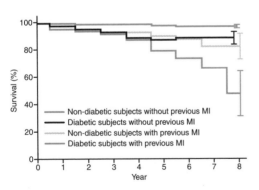

Figure 7.3
Kaplan–Meier estimates of the probability of death from coronary heart disease in subjects who had not had a previous myocardial infarction. 1059 type 2 diabetic vs 1378 non-diabetic subjects. Reproduced with permission from Haffner SM et al. N Engl J Med 1998; **339**: 229-34.

the absolute risk of cardiovascular events for the individual concerned. However, the latest (2004) revision of the British Hypertension Society guidelines (available at www.bhsoc.org) provides no chart for patients with type 2 diabetes. The rationale for this change is the aforementioned high risk which the majority of patients (especially those aged >50 years or with disease duration >10 years) with type 2 diabetes will generally have. Thus, this group is automatically placed in the secondary prevention category.

> Patients with type 2 diabetes should be regarded as candidates for therapeutic measures used in patients with established coronary heart disease

Acute myocardial infarction

The prognosis for patients with type 2 diabetes who survive a myocardial infarction is poor and the incidence of recurrent coronary events high. In the 4S study, approximately half of all placebo-treated patients with diabetes who had had a myocardial infarction had sustained a major coronary event at five years. Mortality (both immediate in-hospital, and late) is also high. Even with the use of thrombolysis, the mortality rate of patients with diabetes after a myocardial infarction is approximately twice as high as that of their non-diabetic counterparts. Left ventricular failure and cardiogenic shock are the principal causes of death, but while various plausible hypotheses have been proposed, the continuing dismal prognosis of patients with diabetes has not been satisfactorily explained. For example, there is no conclusive evidence that infarct size is larger or that the histology of coronary heart disease differs appreciably in diabetic patients. However, it is recognized that coronary artery disease may progress more rapidly in those with diabetes and the existence of a specific diabetic cardiomyopathy has been postulated which may contribute to the development of cardiac failure (page 101) in some people.

Silent infarcts

> Immediate and later mortality rates following myocardial infarction are high in patients with type 2 diabetes

The symptoms of myocardial infarction may also be modified by diabetes. So-called clinically 'silent' infarcts are more common – neuropathy in the autonomic fibres that transmit pain sensation from the myocardium is held to be responsible. Since angina pectoris may also be less prominent, acute coronary ischaemia may present atypically with symptoms such as dyspnoea, syncope and, in the elderly, confusion. Electrocardiograms suggestive of ischaemia are more common in asymptomatic diabetic than non-diabetic patients.

Subclinical myocardial ischaemia

Using specialized techniques, subclinical myocardial ischaemia can be detected in a significant proportion of patients with type 2 diabetes, however, the precise excess compared to non-diabetics is uncertain.

> Acute myocardial infarction may present with minimal or atypical symptoms in diabetic patients

Management

There is no evidence for diminished therapeutic efficacy of accepted cardiovascular interventions in patients with diabetes. The acute effect of aspirin, for example, is similar in subjects with and without diabetes. Due to their higher absolute risk, however, diabetic patients may derive even greater benefit from interventions such as thrombolysis and β-blockers, and there is evidence that these drugs are underused in this high-risk group.

> The benefits of thrombolysis and β-blockers may be greater in diabetic patients, as a result of their higher absolute risk

Thus, in addition to measures such as analgesia, the management of acute myocardial infarction in diabetic patients should include, as appropriate:

- *Aspirin* – to be given at presentation and in the long term if no contraindications exist (75 mg/day, enteric-coated).
- *Thrombolysis* – as for non-diabetics. The small risk of vitreous haemorrhage from streptokinase or tissue plasminogen activator (tPA) in patients with advanced retinopathy should not deter use of these agents. The beneficial effects outweigh any potential detrimental retinal effects.
- *Angiotensin converting enzyme (ACE) inhibitors* – these are indicated primarily for cardiac failure or impaired left ventricular function revealed on echocardiogram. The results of the MICRO-HOPE study (page 109) extended the indications for these agents.
- *β-blockers* – subgroup analyses have suggested that these agents may be particularly beneficial in diabetic patients. So-called 'third generation' agents may have metabolic advantages over more traditional β-blockers.

> The small risk of retinopathic intraocular haemorrhage should not deter use of streptokinase and tPA in diabetic patients who have suffered a myocardial infarction

Meticulous control of the metabolic disturbances associated with acute myocardial infarction may also help to reduce mortality in diabetic patients. The associated hormonal stress response, for example, includes a massive release of catecholamines, and has several potentially adverse metabolic consequences:

- Acute exacerbation of insulin resistance.
- Acute hyperglycaemia.
- Increased lipolysis – fatty acids increase infarct size and may be pro-arrhythmic. Decreased insulin secretion and elevated

fatty acid levels conspire to increase myocardial oxygen requirements, which may be detrimental in the acutely ischaemic myocardium.

- Suppression of insulin secretion – this exacerbates the direct adverse effects of catecholamines and other stress hormones on carbohydrate and lipid metabolism.

A proportion of non-diabetic patients with acute myocardial infarction will develop transient hyperglycaemia as a consequence of this hormonal stress response. Acute left ventricular failure is particularly likely to lead to acute hyperglycaemia. Glycated proteins may be of some diagnostic use in this situation. However, they are relatively insensitive for diagnostic purposes, particularly of minor degrees of glucose intolerance (chapter 4), if there is any continuing doubt, a 75 g oral glucose tolerance test (pages 43 and 190) performed approximately six weeks after infarct recovery will provide a definitive answer.

In a recent study from Sweden, after excluding patients known to have diabetes, only about one-third of patients with acute myocardial infarction had normal glucose tolerance at follow-up three months later.

Glucose–insulin infusion

Even in the absence of diabetes, intravenous infusions of glucose/insulin/potassium reduce myocardial infarct size in experimental animal models. Convincing evidence for benefit in hyperglycaemic patients was also provided by a multicentre, randomized study from Sweden, the Diabetes Mellitus Insulin Glucose Infusion in Acute Myocardial Infarction (DIGAMI) study (Tables 7.1 and 7.2, Figure 7.4).

As a secondary prevention measure, and in cost-effectiveness terms, the glucose–insulin protocol used in the DIGAMI study compares favourably with established interventions such as thrombolysis. For the cohort as a whole, 11 patients were treated to save one life at 3.5 years. A second DIGAMI study has been designed to separate the effects of the early insulin–glucose infusion from subsequent subcutaneous insulin administration. The mechanism responsible for the improvement in survival remains unclear, but acute insulin-mediated suppression of plasma fatty acid levels (page 23) may be relevant. Another intriguing, but largely theoretical, possibility is that the reduced mortality in the intensively treated patients might at least partly have resulted from sulphonylurea withdrawal. The impressive results of the subgroup analysis may reflect the higher intrinsic cardiovascular risk of patients previously treated with oral antidiabetic agents.

Table 7.1
The Diabetes Mellitus Insulin Glucose Infusion in Acute Myocardial Infarction (DIGAMI) study.

Study design
620 subjects, more than 80% of whom were considered to have type 2 diabetes, were randomly assigned to (a) intensive treatment with an intravenous insulin–glucose infusion on the coronary care unit followed by multiple daily insulin injections (n=306), or (b) to a control group who received insulin only if clinically indicated (n=314). Approximately 13% were previously undiagnosed. Thrombolysis, aspirin, ACE inhibitor and β-blocker use was similar between the groups. At discharge, 87% of the intensive treatment group, compared with 43% of the control group, were taking insulin. Although 15% of the intensive treatment group experienced hypoglycaemia, this was not associated with any adverse events.

Study results
HbA$_{1c}$ decreased significantly in both groups during follow-up, the reduction was greatest in the intensively treated group at three and 12 months.
- A relative reduction in mortality of 30% was observed in the intensively treated group during the first year of follow-up.
- A significant ($p<0.05$) reduction in absolute mortality of 11% was still evident after nearly 3.5 years. This was most pronounced in a pre-defined subgroup of patients who had not previously received insulin treatment and who had a lower predicted cardiovascular risk because they were younger (<70 years) with no previous history of myocardial infarction or congestive cardiac failure.

Table 7.2
Protocol used on coronary care units during the DIGAMI study.

Infusion = 500 ml 5% glucose with 80 units of short-acting insulin, ie ~1 unit insulin per 6 ml infusate. Initial infusion rate 30 ml/hour. Blood glucose should be checked after 1 hour. Infusion rate adjusted, aiming for 7–10 mmol/l. Glucose checked every two hours, or every one hour after infusion rate altered. If initial decrease in glucose is >30% and blood glucose is >11 mmol/l, infusion rate should be left unchanged. It should be reduced by 6 ml/hour if blood glucose is 7–10.9 mmol/l. It should be reduced by 50% during the night, if blood glucose is stable at <11 mmol/l after 2200 hours, and intermittent monitoring continued.

Blood glucose (mmol/l)	Action
>15	Give 8 units insulin as iv bolus and increase infusion rate by 6 ml/hour.
11–14.9	Increase infusion rate by 3 ml/hour.
7–10.9	Leave infusion rate unchanged.
4–6.9	Decrease infusion rate by 6 ml/hour.
<4	Stop infusion for 15 minutes. Test blood glucose every 15 minutes until ≥7 mmol/l. If symptoms of hypoglycaemia are present, administer 20 ml of 30% glucose iv. Restart infusion with the rate decreased by 6 ml/hour when blood glucose is ≥7 mmol/l.

NB: careful monitoring by trained staff is required for safe protocol implementation.

Concerns about the cardiovascular safety of sulphonylureas were initially raised by the findings of the University Group Diabetes Program in the US in the 1970s. Although this controversial study has since been strongly criticised, it reported an increased risk of cardiovascular mortality in patients randomized to tolbutamide. More recently, the United Kingdom Prospective Diabetes Study did not demonstrate any difference in risk of coronary heart disease between patients treated with sulphonylureas and those treated with insulin. While the cardiovascular safety of sulphonylureas has been requestioned from time to time, there is no clear evidence to deter sulphonylurea use in the pursuit of metabolic control in type 2 patients. Sulphonylureas are considered further in chapter 9.

> Intravenous infusion of insulin and glucose followed by subcutaneous insulin injection reduces mortality in diabetic patients who have had a myocardial infarction

> In the DIGAMI study, patients with type 2 diabetes considered to be at relatively low risk of cardiovascular death showed the greatest benefit from insulin therapy

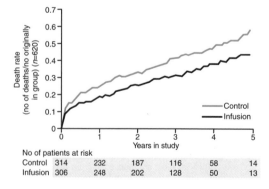

No of patients at risk

Control	314	232	187	116	58	14
Infusion	306	248	202	128	50	13

Figure 7.4
Actuarial mortality curves during long-term follow-up in patients receiving insulin–glucose infusion followed by subcutaneous insulin, and controls. Reproduced with permission from Malmberg K et al. Br Med J 1997; **314**: 1512-5.

The intravenous insulin–glucose infusion should be continued for 24 hours, at which stage the patient should be moved on to small doses of subcutaneous insulin. Whether twice-daily insulin is as effective as multiple daily injections is not yet known, but it is almost certainly more acceptable to most patients. Long-term therapy may not be feasible in some – recurrent hypoglycaemia with small daily doses may necessitate withdrawal, for example – but, otherwise, insulin should probably be continued as long as possible. Metformin should be withdrawn in patients with acute ischaemic heart disease because of the potential for lactic acidosis in the setting of tissue hypoxia (page 154).

The recently announced results of the DIGAMI 2 study have unfortunately not clarified the relative contributions of early versus long-term intensive insulin therapy as had been hoped. Nonetheless, the DIGAMI 2 study confirmed hyperglycaemia to be a strong independent risk factor for mortality after myocardial infarction.

Revascularization procedures

In general, revascularization procedures (angioplasty, coronary artery bypass grafting) seem to be less effective in patients with type 2 diabetes – both graft and patient survival rates are lower. Restenosis following angioplasty seems to be more common in diabetic patients. In an analysis of the Bypass Angiography Revascularization Investigation (BARI), survival was better in diabetic subjects after a myocardial infarction if they had previously undergone coronary artery bypass grafting rather than coronary angioplasty. Therapeutic developments, such as increasing use of intracoronary stents and new agents directed against platelet aggregation, are increasingly being used. The pace of change has been such that it is now difficult to interpret earlier studies, which were performed mainly in the 1980s. Ongoing studies include the BARI-2D trial which is examining the impact of insulin-sensitizing thiazolidinedione treatment versus provision of insulin after angioplasty or bypass surgery.

Cardiac failure

Studies in diabetic animals and humans provide support for a specific defect in myocardial function independent of atheroma of the coronary vasculature. Subclinical echocardiographic abnormalities of left ventricular function have been reported in diabetic patients. Measurement of natuiretic peptides may be helpful in diagnosing early heart failure. Subclinical cardiac dysfunction can be detected in a proportion of patients who might benefit from treatment with ACE inhibitors. Microangiopathy and fibrosis of the myocardium are histological features to which systemic hypertension may contribute. These abnormalities may help to explain the well documented excess incidence of cardiac failure in diabetic patients – up to five times higher than in non-diabetic individuals. The Hypertension in Diabetes Study (page 106) documented a significant reduction in the incidence of cardiac failure with tight blood pressure control. Insulin resistance is a feature of cardiac failure and its role is being examined with respect to possible novel therapeutic strategies. Obesity may make an independent contribution to heart failure.

> Type 2 diabetes is associated with an increased risk of cardiac failure

Peripheral arterial disease

Together with neuropathy and infection, peripheral arterial disease contributes to foot disease in diabetic patients (page 82). The incidence of peripheral arterial disease is about twice as high in diabetic patients. Abnormalities of circulating lipids, hypertension and smoking are all recognized risk factors for peripheral arterial disease.

> The prevalence of peripheral arterial disease is approximately doubled in diabetic patients

Clinical features

In people with type 2 diabetes, atherosclerosis has a predilection for the distal vessels, ie those below the popliteal fossa. The typical presentation is a palpable femoral pulse, but there may be no pulse below this level. The condition is asymptomatic until significant arterial stenoses develop. Symptoms, which depend on site and degree of stenosis, may then include:

- *Intermittent claudication* – classic calf claudication on walking, which is rapidly relieved by rest
- *Rest pain* – this denotes critical ischaemia, usually distal disease
- *Leriche syndrome* – buttock and leg claudication, and erectile dysfunction due

to major stenosis of the aortofemoral vessels

- *Ischaemic foot lesions* – in isolation, ischaemia accounts for <10% of diabetic foot ulcers, but it is a significant co-pathology in the neuroischaemic lesions that accompany about 50% of all ulcers
- *Impaired functional capacity* – this is less well defined but may also occur.

Co-existing vascular disease may impede the healing of ulcers that are predominantly neuropathic in origin, particularly when there is deeper infection in soft tissues or bone. This combination of pathologies is particularly common in elderly people with type 2 diabetes. Occasionally, atherosclerosis may also lead to functional renal artery stenosis, which is relevant to the pathogenesis and treatment of hypertension.

> Atherosclerosis has a predilection for vessels below the popliteal fossa in diabetes

Assessment of peripheral vasculature

Clinical evaluation

The history should enquire about: claudication, rest pain in limbs, features of Leriche syndrome, past or present foot ulcers, smoking history, family history of premature atherosclerosis, and personal history of atherosclerosis including history of myocardial infarction, transient ischaemic attacks, stroke and lipid status, if known.

Physical examination

Physical examination should include manual palpation of peripheral pulses and auscultation for bruits. Trophic changes in the skin should be sought and limb temperature assessed. While a limb will be pale and cold in the presence of significant ischaemia, limbs may also appear red where blood flow is critically impaired ('sunset foot'). Buerger's sign may be positive: ie the limb blanches on being raised from the horizontal, but assumes a dusky red

colour when dependent (over the edge of the bed). Evidence of additional risk factors for atherosclerosis, including corneal arcus, xanthelasma and hypertension, should be sought, as should aggravating disorders such as anaemia.

Doppler studies

Doppler studies are readily performed at the bedside with a hand-held probe, but interpretation will require experience; there is potential for misinterpretation in patients with diabetes. The ratio of the Doppler-measured ankle pressure to the Doppler-measured brachial artery pressure is normally 1.0, values less than 0.5 indicate severe disease. It should be noted that the ratio may be falsely elevated by arterial calcification in subjects with chronic neuropathy, which renders the vessels resistant to compression by the ankle pressure cuff. The quality of the Doppler signal may be a helpful pointer: normally three components are discerned and the signal is said to be triphasic, but arterial calcification may lead to a bi- or monophasic signal instead. Further assessment is then indicated.

Duplex scanning

Duplex scanning is a non-invasive technique that combines ultrasound imaging with Doppler assessment to provide information about the haemodynamic significance of a lesion. Once again, calcification may limit the quality of the information obtained. Duplex scanning is usually a prelude to angiography when contemplating surgery.

Oxygen tension

Oxygen tension can be measured transcutaneously on the dorsum of the foot using a laser Doppler probe to confirm critical ischaemia. The technique is not widely available.

Angiography

Angiography is used to delineate the site and extent of the lesions which often affect the distal arterial tree. Digital subtraction of bone improves the quality of the imaging of below-knee vessels. There is also the major advantage of being able to perform angioplasty or give thrombolytic agents simultaneously. Care should be taken to ensure adequate hydration of patients with renal impairment. Metformin should be omitted on the day of angiography (assuming normal renal function). Since iodinated radiographic contrast can sometimes cause acute renal impairment, it should only be reinstated when normal renal function has been confirmed.

Management

The management options for peripheral vascular disease include aspirin, foot care, vasodilating agents, surgical sympathectomy, reconstructive surgery or angioplasty, amputation and rehabilitation. It should be remembered that patients with peripheral arterial disease are at high risk of cardiovascular events; this reflects generalized atheroma.

- *Aspirin* – reduces mortality from cardiovascular disease and should be given where there are no contraindications. Always control blood pressure first in patients with severe hypertension.
- *Clopidogrel* – in the CAPRIE study this drug was superior to aspirin in reducing vascular events in patients with arterial disease.
- *Foot care* – is of great importance and patients should receive appropriate instruction. Regular inspection by a trained professional and timely podiatry may avert the development of more serious lesions.
- *Vasodilators* – Oral agents are usually ineffective.
- *Cilotazol* – this recently introduced oral phosphodiesterase type 3 inhibitor can improve 'pain-free walking distance'.
- *Surgical sympathectomy* – in the lumbar region is ineffective for intermittent claudication. Patients with severe co-existing neuropathy will often already have clinical features suggestive of sympathetic denervation.

- *Reconstructive surgery or angioplasty* – may preserve limbs and avoid major amputation. Where there is proximal disease – patients with weak femoral pulses, and absent pulses more distally – angioplasty (localized short stenoses are most suitable) or arterial bypass grafting (aortofemoral and femoropopliteal) may help. Distal disease – normal femoral and popliteal pulses with absent foot pulses – is, however, more commonly encountered in diabetes and much more difficult to treat by either route, particularly when there is diffuse disease below the level of the popliteal fossa.
- *Amputation* – may need to be radical, ie below knee, if it is required for major arterial occlusion. Above-knee is avoided where possible because rehabilitation is more difficult.
- *Rehabilitation* – prospects after major amputation are often overestimated and old age and serious co-morbidity are major limiting factors. The aim must be to preserve a functionally useful limb wherever possible.

Patients with peripheral arterial disease are also at high risk of coronary events. Thus, measures aimed at reducing cardiovascular risk, including statins, antihypertensive therapy and aspirin, should be considered.

> Patients with peripheral vascular disease are at high risk of coronary heart disease

Cerebrovascular disease

Stroke is the second most common cause of death among people with type 2 diabetes. The incidence of cerebrovascular disease is roughly doubled in diabetic patients. A role for the central nervous system in the regulation of glucose metabolism has long been recognized: Claude Bernard described *piqûre* diabetes – glycosuria following transfixion of the medulla oblongata – in rabbits as long ago as the 19th century. Transient hyperglycaemia may be observed after an acute stroke in much the same way that it is observed after acute myocardial infarction, but limited observational studies suggest that hyperglycaemia at presentation with acute stroke is an independent marker of adverse clinical outcome, principally mortality, within the first month.

> Cerebrovascular disease is the second most common cause of death in subjects with type 2 diabetes

Transient defects associated with acute metabolic derangements

Hemiplegia

In addition to atheromatous cerebrovascular disease, transient hemiplegia has a recognized but rare association with hypoglycaemia in insulin-treated diabetic patients.

Other focal neurological deficits

Reversible focal neurological lesions are also recognized in patients presenting with non-ketotic, hyperosmolar pre-coma or coma.

Convulsions

Epilepsy may occasionally be triggered in susceptible patients by hyperglycaemia, especially if there is hyperosmolarity.

Cognitive dysfunction

Atherosclerotic dementia may contribute to impaired psychomotor performance, learning and memory in older diabetic individuals. Correlations between psychological dysfunction and hyperglycaemia have been reported in elderly subjects – hypertension and other factors are also implicated. There is some evidence suggesting that better glycaemic control may improve cognition, but further studies are required.

Atrial fibrillation

Diabetes is regarded as an additional risk factor for stroke (along with hypertension and advancing age) in individuals with atrial fibrillation. In the United Kingdom Prospective Diabetes Study, atrial fibrillation was identified as a major risk factor for stroke in subjects with type 2 diabetes.

Dyslipidaemia

Some statins, eg pravastatin and simvastatin, are licensed for the prevention of stroke in subjects who have already sustained a myocardial infarction, but there are no data specifically relating to diabetes.

> Atrial fibrillation is a major risk factor for stroke in patients with type 2 diabetes

Hypertension

Hypertension is a common, important and modifiable risk factor for both the micro- and macrovascular complications of diabetes. Although prevalence rates are highly dependent on specific definitions, numerous studies have shown that hypertension is more common in diabetic than in non-diabetic individuals; it is present in 50–80% of patients with type 2 diabetes, according to modern definitions (ie ≥140/90 mmHg). It is well recognized that obesity increases blood pressure; the effect attributable to gender is less clear – some studies suggest that women are at higher risk. While hypertension is more common in patients with type 2 diabetes, the prevalence essentially reflects the general background of the population concerned; black patients, for example, are at particular risk. Hypertension is closely associated with insulin resistance (page 26) in type 2 diabetes patients, but the strength and nature of the association is still unclear.

> Hypertension is an important modifiable risk factor for several micro- and macrovascular complications of type 2 diabetes

There is considerable evidence that hypertension is both underdiagnosed and inadequately treated in patients with diabetes. Regular and accurate monitoring of blood pressure is an important and undervalued aspect of diabetes care.

Haemodynamic abnormalities in diabetes

Abnormal haemodynamics in patients with type 2 diabetes may increase the risk of tissue damage attributable to hypertension. The implication is that, for any level of systemic blood pressure, patients with diabetes are more susceptible to tissue damage. Postulated mechanisms include:

- *Autoregulation* – when this is interrupted (through hyperglycaemia) in vulnerable vascular beds such as those of the retina and renal glomeruli, systemic blood pressure is transmitted directly to the microvasculature.

- *Decreased vascular compliance* – of major vessels such as the aorta, perhaps resulting from non-enzymatic glycation (page 69), may lead to the transmission of higher pressures to distal vascular beds. This abnormality may also contribute to isolated systolic hypertension in patients with type 2 diabetes.

- *Increased blood pressure variability* – has been reported during 24-hour ambulatory recordings.

- *Reduced decline in nocturnal blood pressure* – failure of the nocturnal decline in blood pressure (during sleep) is a reported early feature associated with microalbuminuria. 24-hour blood pressure exposure of vulnerable tissues is increased as a result.

Assessment of the diabetic patient with hypertension

Secondary hypertension should be excluded, target organ damage identified and other cardiovascular risk factors otherwise assessed in all diabetic patients with hypertension. A history and physical examination will usually reveal any endocrine or other cause of hypertension (Table 7.3). Most endocrine causes, with the exception of thyrotoxicosis, are uncommon. Signs of target organ damage include left ventricular hypertrophy, arterial bruits, absent pedal pulses (increased risk of renal artery stenosis) and hypertensive retinal changes.

Table 7.3
Endocrine causes of hypertension.

- Thyrotoxicosis – common and usually clinically evident.
- Acromegaly – uncommon, with characteristic appearance.
- Cushing's syndrome – uncommon, with typical clinical features.
- Conn's syndrome – may be asymptomatic hypokalaemia, often unrecognized.
- Phaeochromocytoma – uncommon, with typical clinical features.
- Primary hyperparathyroidism – common, associated with insulin resistance and hypertension.

Note that these disorders may be accompanied by glucose intolerance or type 2 diabetes.

Investigations

For most patients these should include:

- *Urinalysis* – to identify microalbuminuria or clinical grade proteinuria.

- *Renal function and electrolytes* – for renal impairment, hypokalaemia (usually due to diuretic use), Conn's syndrome (due to aldosterone excess) and hyperkalaemia (renal impairment and type III renal tubular acidosis).

- *Electrocardiogram* – for evidence of left ventricular hypertrophy (which indicates an adverse prognosis; echocardiography is more sensitive), ischaemia (may be subclinical), and atrial fibrillation (relatively common; suggests increased risk of stroke).

- *Plasma lipids*.

- *Ambulatory blood pressure monitoring* – the role of home measurements has not been delineated clearly, but ambulatory measurements may be useful if there is unusual variability in clinic pressures, hypertension apparently resistant to three or more drugs, symptoms suggestive of hypotension, or a suspicion of 'white coat hypertension'. The 1999 British Hypertension Society guidelines suggest an optimal mean daytime ambulatory pressure or home measurement of <130/75 in diabetic subjects.

Other investigations such as exercise testing and isotope studies (eg captopril renogram) to exclude renal artery stenosis may be indicated in some.

> Hypertension in type 2 diabetes is regarded as a component of the insulin resistance syndrome

Hypertension in Diabetes Study

In 1987, a randomized study of blood pressure control, the Hypertension in Diabetes Study, was embedded within the main United Kingdom Prospective Diabetes Study using a factorial design (UKPDS 38 and 39). The study provided important confirmation of the adverse effect of hypertension in patients with type 2 diabetes and Table 7.4 summarizes its key points. Whether any particular class of antihypertensive drug is associated with advantages or disadvantages for diabetic patients remains unclear, but considerable evidence suggests that the most important consideration is the level of blood pressure attained, rather than the agent used. Atenolol and captopril were shown to have similar efficacy in the Hypertension in Diabetes Study. The study did not have sufficient statistical power to identify real differences between these two classes.

> In type 2 diabetes, the blood pressure level attained appears to be more important than the type of antihypertensive drug used to attain it

Metabolic effects of antihypertensive drugs

Much debate has surrounded the influence of antihypertensive agents on the risk factors for cardiovascular disease. While the clinical significance of such effects remains unclear, it is obvious that antihypertensive treatment with β-blockers and thiazides has not led to the reductions in mortality from coronary heart disease that were expected. It has been

suggested that adverse metabolic effects might have offset the beneficial effects of these two classes of drug in the trials concerned.

Insulin action

β-blockers (particularly non-selective agents) and high-dose thiazide diuretics aggravate insulin resistance (in contrast, ACE inhibitors and α-blockers may improve insulin action). Interestingly, during the first few years of the Hypertension in Diabetes Study, HbA_{1c} levels were significantly higher in the atenolol-treated group than in the captopril-treated group – accordingly, more antihyperglycaemic therapy was required in the atenolol-treated patients. In longitudinal studies, both β-blockers and thiazides, particularly in combination, have been implicated in the pathogenesis of type 2 diabetes in patients with essential hypertension, but the nature of the association remains uncertain.

Dihydropyridine calcium antagonists with a short duration of action, such as nifedipine, may impair insulin action, while longer-acting drugs (eg amlodipine) and modified-release preparations, together with non-dihydropyridine drugs (eg diltiazem and verapamil) appear to have neutral effects. In contrast, several classes of more recently introduced antihypertensive agent may have beneficial effects of insulin sensitivity:

- *ACE inhibitors* – are either neutral or may improve insulin sensitivity in non-diabetic and diabetic patients. ACE gene polymorphisms may have implications for insulin action (chapter 2) as well as the blood pressure response to ACE inhibitors.
- *Angiotensin II$_1$ receptor antagonists* – improved insulin action has been reported with use of these agents.
- *α$_1$-receptor blockers* – doxazosin can improve insulin sensitivity and plasma lipid profiles, but was withdrawn from the multicentre comparative Antihypertensive and Lipid Lowering treatment to prevent Heart Attack Trial (ALLHAT) because it was

Table 7.4
The Hypertension in Diabetes Study (UKPDS 38 and 39).

Methodology
This prospective, randomized, multicentre, double-blinded study of type 2 diabetic patients compared (a) tight control of blood pressure (target <150/85, *n*=758) either with the ACE inhibitor captopril (25–50 mg bid, *n*=400) or atenolol (50–100 mg/day, *n*=358) plus additional agents as necessary (suggested sequence: frusemide, slow-release nifedipine, methyldopa and prazocin) with (b) less tight (<180/105, *n*=390) control.

Results (UKPDS 38)
- Mean blood pressure was reduced to 144/82 vs 154/87 mmHg (a difference of 10/5 mmHg) for the tight and less tight control groups, respectively (*p*<0.0001).
- Multiple drug therapy (three or more agents) was required more often in the tight control group (29% vs 11%, respectively). However, at nine years only 56% of patients in the tight control group had attained the target blood pressure of <150/85.
- Tight control reduced diabetes-related endpoints (fatal or non-fatal) by 24% (*p*=0.0046; Figure 7.5), diabetes-related deaths by 32% (*p*=0.019), stroke by 44% (*p*=0.013) and microvascular disease by 37% (*p*=0.0092).
- The reduction in microvascular complications was predominantly attributable to a reduced risk of photocoagulation for retinopathy; there were associated reductions in the progression of retinopathy (34%, *p*=0.0004). In addition, a measure of visual loss (equivalent of a reduction from 6/6 to 6/12 or 6/9 to 6/18 on the Snellen chart) was reduced, suggesting prevention of maculopathy, the main cause of visual impairment in type 2 diabetes (47%, *p*=0.004).
- A transient reduction in microalbuminuria (*p*=0.009) at six years in the tight control group was not sustained at nine years; there was no difference in clinical grade proteinuria or serum creatinine between the groups by the end of the study.
- All-cause mortality was not significantly reduced (18%, *p*=0.17) by tight blood pressure control. However, there was a 34% reduction in combined macrovascular endpoints (ie myocardial infarction, sudden death, stroke and peripheral vascular disease, *p*=0.019).
- Although the reduction in myocardial infarction (21%) was not statistically significant ECG Q-wave abnormalities were reduced by 48% (*p*=0.007). In addition, the risk of cardiac failure was reduced by 56% (*p*=0.0043).

Results (UKPDS 39: Atenolol vs captopril for hypertension)
- Captopril and atenolol were equally effective in reducing the incidence of diabetic complications (although study not adequately powered to detect small differences).
- The mean weight gain was higher in the atenolol group (3.4 vs 1.6 kg) while glycated HbA_{1c} concentrations were slightly higher over the first four years. No difference in the rate of severe hypoglycaemia was observed between the drugs.
- Captopril was better tolerated than atenolol with 78% vs 65% of patients still taking their allocated drug at their last clinic visit (*p*<0.0001).

Post-study monitoring
When the UKPDS ended, all surviving patients returned to routine care according to clinical need, with follow-up for 5 years (1997–2002).
- Mean blood pressure in patients originally randomized to tight control rose after 2 years to converge with those patients originally randomized to less tight control.

less effective in preventing cardiac failure than diuretic-based therapy.

- *Selective imidazoline-receptor agonists –* moxonidine improves insulin action in animal models and in obese hypertensive patients. Rilmenidine has also been reported to improve glucose metabolism in animals and humans and to have minor effects on lipid metabolism.

Lipids

The adverse effects of β-blockers and thiazide diuretics on plasma lipid levels (increased very low-density lipoproteins and

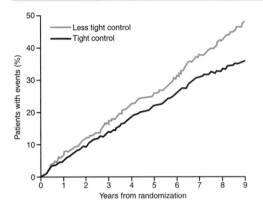

Figure 7.5
The Hypertension in Diabetes Study: effect of tight control of blood pressure on diabetes-related endpoints (fatal and non-fatal). Reproduced with permission from *Br Med J* 1998; **317**: 703-17.

hypercholesterolaemia, respectively) have also received attention.

Associated haemostatic abnormalities such as increased fibrinogen, factor VII levels and plasminogen activator inhibitor-1 activity may contribute to atherogenesis.

Hypokalaemia

There have been reports of an increased risk of sudden death in diabetic and non-diabetic patients with electrocardiographic abnormalities who have been treated with thiazide diuretics. The metabolic effects of thiazides can be minimized by the use of lower doses (eg bendrofluazide ≤2.5 mg/day). Higher doses have limited additional antihypertensive effects and carry greatly increased risks of adverse effects.

Other considerations

Several other large, randomized studies (Table 7.5) have demonstrated substantial benefits from treating hypertension in type 2 diabetes. These trials have used regimens based on thiazide diuretics and long-acting calcium antagonists and suggested that therapeutic

benefit was greater in diabetic than non-diabetic subgroups, reflecting the higher absolute risk associated with diabetes. Reductions in both systolic and diastolic blood pressure are important. The difference between systolic and diastolic pressures (ie the pulse) is a superior indicator of vascular events than either systolic or diastolic pressure alone.

There have been reports of higher cardiovascular event rates in patients treated with calcium antagonists than other agents, but a lack of placebo comparisons and use of secondary endpoints complicate the interpretation of such findings. The Nordic Diltiazem (NORDIL) study and the International Nifedipine Study: Intervention as a Goal in Hypertension Treatment (INSIGHT) confirmed that the efficacy of these two agents was similar to that of diuretic- or β-blocker-based therapy.

Concerns about another long-running controversy, the 'J-shaped curve' (ie the suggestion that very low blood pressure is associated with adverse effects), have also been largely allayed. We may now conclude that the lower the blood pressure attained, the greater the clinical benefit (UKPDS 36). Studies in non-diabetic individuals have not suggested any significant differences between the major classes of antihypertensive agent to date and the 1999 World Health Organization International Society for Hypertension guidelines stated that any of the main classes of antihypertensive drug are suitable as first-line therapy. However, the MICRO-HOPE study (Table 7.5) showed benefits for ramipril on microvascular and macrovascular events in (type 2) diabetic patients. In this – and the main HOPE study – the benefits were disproportionate to the observed reductions in blood pressure, and raised the possibility of an endothelial protective effect for this drug (ramipril). More recently, the EUROPA study of perindopril versus placebo reported similar results. In a diabetic subgroup the relative risk reductions were similar to those observed overall (the PERSUADE substudy). The incidence of self-reported new cases of diabetes was reduced in the main HOPE

Table 7.5

Other randomized clinical trials of antihypertensive therapy in patients with type 2 diabetes.

1. SHEP (Systolic Hypertension in the Elderly Program)
JAMA 1996; **276**: 1886-92.
Total *n*=4736; diabetic *n*=583. Duration: 5 years.
Chlorthalidone ± atenolol or reserpine vs placebo.
Findings:
34% reduction in major cardiovascular events (cerebral and cardiac) with active treatment vs placebo. Greater benefit in diabetic subgroup reflecting higher absolute risk of these patients.

2. HOT (Hypertension Optimal Treatment)
Lancet 1998; **351**: 1755-62.
Total *n*=18790; diabetic *n*=1501. Duration: 3.8 years.
Felodipine + other agents (vs placebo) as required to attain diastolic blood pressure targets.
Findings:
Reduction (by 50%) in major cardiovascular events with target diastolic of 80 mmHg vs 90 mmHg in diabetic patients. Additional benefit of aspirin.

3. SYST-EUR (Systolic Hypertension in Europe)
Lancet 1997; **350**: 757-64 and *N Engl J Med* 1999; **340**: 677-84.
Total *n*=4695; diabetic *n*=492. Duration: 2 years (median).
Nitrendipine + enalapril or thiazide vs placebo.
Findings:
Excess risk of diabetes almost completely eliminated by antihypertensive therapy with major reductions (approx 70%) in cardiovascular mortality and all cardiovascular endpoints. Similar results to the Chinese study SYS-CHINA.

4. HOPE (Heart Outcomes Prevention Evaluation)
N Engl J Med 2000; **342**: 145-53.
Total with pre-existing coronary heart disease, stroke or peripheral vascular disease *n*=9297; 38% had diabetes.
Duration: 4.5 years.
Ramipril (as well as other agents) vs placebo.
Findings:
Overall, 25% reduction in risk of cardiovascular death, 20% for myocardial infarction and 32% for stroke with ramipril vs placebo. For diabetic subgroup, 17% risk reduction in diabetic complications. New cases of diabetes reduced by 32%. This was not a treat-to-target (blood pressure) study; other agents were permitted as required.

5. MICRO-HOPE (Microalbuminuria, Cardiovascular, and Renal Outcomes) Lancet 2000; **355**: 253-59.
n= 3577 patients with diabetes (subgroup of HOPE) aged >55 years, with a previous cardiovascular event or one other cardiovascular risk factor (hypertension, raised cholesterol, low HDL-cholesterol, smoking or microalbuminuria).
Duration: 4.5 years.
Ramipril (in addition to other agents) vs placebo.
Findings:
Ramipril reduced the primary combined outcome (myocardial infarction, stroke, cardiovascular death) by 25%, myocardial infarction by 22%, stroke by 33%, cardiovascular death by 37% and overt nephropathy by 24%. Risk reduction was in excess of that anticipated for reduction in blood pressure (2.4/1.0 mmHg).

6. ALLHAT (Antihypertensive and Lipid Lowering Treatment to Prevent Heart Attack Trial) JAMA 2002; **288**: 2981-97.
Total 33 357 hypertensive patients aged >55 years, of whom 15 297 had diabetes as an additional risk factor.
Mean follow-up: 4.9 years.
Chlorthalidone, amlodipine or lisinopril (doxazosin arm discontinued because of increased risk of heart failure relative to diuretic).
Findings:
No major differences between groups in the primary end point of fatal coronary artery disease or non-fatal myocardial infarction.

cohort, as it was in the Captopril Prevention Project (CAPPP) and INSIGHT study. Several trials have now shown that both ACE inhibitors and angiotensin II receptor blockers are associated with a lower risk of new-onset diabetes compared to diuretics and β-blockers.

> The lower the blood pressure, the greater the benefit in patients with type 2 diabetes

Cautions and contraindications

Diabetic patients are at risk of developing long-term tissue complications which may render certain antihypertensive drugs unsuitable (Table 7.6). Initially, the most appropriate drug should be selected (Table 7.7).

Table 7.6
Cautions and contraindications to antihypertensive therapy in diabetic patients.

Caution or contraindication	Drugs to avoid
Dyslipidaemia	β-blockers, thiazide diuretics (high doses)
Erectile dysfunction	β-blockers, thiazide diuretics
Gout	Thiazide diuretics
Peripheral vascular disease	β-blockers
Renal artery stenosis	ACE inhibitors, AII$_1$ receptor antagonists

Table 7.7
Indications for particular antihypertensive drugs in type 2 diabetic patients.

Indication	Drugs of choice
Nephropathy	ACE inhibitors (+ loop diuretics), non-dihydropyridine calcium antagonists
Ischaemic heart disease	β-blockers, long-acting calcium antagonists
Cardiac failure	ACE inhibitors, AII$_1$ receptor antagonists, loop diuretics, β-blockers (certain agents in selected patients)

Risk of hypoglycaemia

Problems of impaired recognition of warning symptoms of and recovery from hypoglycaemia with β-blockers are uncommon with the cardioselective drugs such as atenolol. Insulin treatment should not generally be regarded as a contraindication to the use of cardioselective β-blockers, which are of proven benefit in diabetic patients. Reports of an increased risk of hypoglycaemia with ACE inhibitors in insulin-treated patients remain unsubstantiated: the United Kingdom Prospective Diabetes Study showed no difference in risk of severe hypoglycaemia between atenolol- and captopril-treated groups.

Renal artery stenosis

A minority of patients with type 2 diabetes, mainly those with evidence of peripheral vascular disease, have clinically significant renal artery stenosis. Certain drugs, such as the ACE inhibitors and angiotensin II receptor antagonists should be used with caution in such patients because of the risk of precipitating an acute deterioration in renal function. This occurs as a consequence of the effects of these drugs on intraglomerular haemodynamics. Where there are significant functional stenoses of both renal arteries, glomerular filtration is maintained by the vasoconstrictor effect of angiotensin II on efferent glomerular arterioles. Removal of this effect may lead to major reductions in the capacity for glomerular filtration. Under certain circumstances (patients with congestive cardiac failure with generalized atherosclerosis) unilateral renal artery stenosis may also lead to deterioration in renal function. The risk may be somewhat overstated, but it is prudent to remeasure plasma creatinine and electrolytes within a week of starting ACE inhibitor or angiotensin II$_1$ receptor antagonist therapy.

Effect of ethnicity on response to treatment

Hypertensive patients of African ethnicity, who tend to have low plasma renin levels, respond better to β-blockers and calcium antagonists than to ACE inhibitors. Similarly, it makes sense to select metabolically neutral or advantageous drugs (page 106) as first-line agents in South Asian patients with multiple components of the insulin resistance syndrome. The British Hypertension Society advises against the use of thiazide diuretics with β-blockers in non-diabetic patients because of the adverse effects of this combination on insulin action and glucose tolerance. It may be particularly important to use drugs shown to decrease the risk of diabetes relative to diuretics and β-blockers in high-risk groups, such as South Asians.

Strategies for the management of hypertension in diabetes

Non-pharmacological strategies include attainment of ideal body weight, reduced dietary salt intake, and appropriate duration and severity of aerobic physical exercise (chapter 8). When blood pressure targets are not being achieved, start with the most appropriate drug for the particular patient. Add or substitute drugs in logical combinations (for example, ACE inhibitor plus diuretic, or long-acting calcium channel antagonist plus β-blocker) and use low doses of each agent to minimize the unwanted effects. Avoid potentially hazardous combinations such as ACE inhibitor and spironolactone (risk of hyperkalaemia), or diltiazem with a β-blocker. Diuretics are often useful, since hypertension in diabetic patients is associated with an expanded plasma volume. Loop diuretics are often necessary for patients with renal impairment (in whom hypertension may be particularly difficult to control).

Patients with diabetes will often require a multiplicity of drugs – for example, oral antidiabetic agents, lipid-lowering agents and aspirin – and since hypertension is largely asymptomatic, once-daily dosing and use of well-tolerated drugs are likely to improve compliance (which is recognized to be fairly poor). The angiotensin II$_1$ receptor antagonists appear to be particularly well tolerated; they do not lead to the cough that is induced in a

proportion of patients treated with ACE inhibitors.

> British Hypertension Society guidelines
> (*BMJ* 2004; **328**: 634–40): *AB/CD* approach.
> *A* = ACEi or AIIRA. *B* = β-blocker.
> *C* = Calcium channel antagonist. *D* = Diuretic.
> Start: *A* or *D*, or *A* + *D*, or *B* + *C*
> Continue: (*A* or *B*) + (*C* or *D*)
>   or (*A* or *B*) + *C* + *D*

Dyslipidaemia

Quantitative and qualitative alterations in plasma lipid levels alter the risk of atheromatous complications in patients with type 2 diabetes. The impact of dyslipidaemia is also magnified by the presence of diabetes and the development of microvascular complications. Thus, diabetic nephropathy is associated with additional disturbances of plasma lipids that exacerbate any existing risk. Common genetic dyslipidaemias, such as familial combined hyperlipidaemia, are just as common among diabetic as non-diabetic individuals. The rare syndromes of lipodystrophic diabetes are associated with marked hyperlipidaemia, but the most common plasma lipid abnormalities encountered in type 2 diabetes patients are hypertriglyceridaemia and a reduced HDL-cholesterol level. Hypertriglyceridaemia is associated with tissue insulin resistance (page 26). Elevations in total and LDL-cholesterol levels are not as prevalent, with total cholesterol, in general, being similar to that in the non-diabetic population.

Antidiabetic drugs may improve lipid metabolism through several mechanisms, all of which reflect improved insulin action in target tissues involved in the regulation of lipid metabolism:

- the stimulatory effect of insulin on the endothelial lipoprotein lipase hydrolyses circulating triglycerides in very low-density lipoproteins (VLDL) and chylomicrons, leading to a secondary reduction in LDL-cholesterol levels
- the suppression of adipocyte lipolysis (via hormone-sensitive lipase) reduces the release of non-esterified fatty acids for metabolism by the liver and muscle

- the direct suppression of hepatic VLDL-lipoprotein production.

In type 2 diabetes, reduced breakdown of VLDL (consequent to insulin deficiency or insulin resistance) increases the circulating concentration of atherogenic triglyceride-rich particles. Low HDL-cholesterol levels are closely associated with hypertriglyceridaemia because of increased transfer of cholesteryl ester from HDL to VLDL and chylomicrons by cholesteryl ester transfer protein. LDL-cholesterol particle size is reduced by increased activity of hepatic lipase, which produces smaller, more dense, apoprotein-rich LDL particles (the so-called pattern B on electrophoresis) regarded as having enhanced atherogenicity. These abnormalities seem to be about twice as prevalent in subjects with type 2 diabetes.

However, any specified level of cholesterol has a greater impact on coronary risk in the presence of diabetes, and epidemiological data indicate that the risk of a coronary event is particularly high when all of the following are present: low HDL-cholesterol, a high ratio (>5.0) of total cholesterol to HDL cholesterol, and hypertriglyceridaemia. While this profile is also associated with a disproportionately increased risk of cardiovascular disease in non-diabetic individuals, it is suggested that the atherogenicity of disordered lipid metabolism in diabetes may be further increased by:

- *Glycation of lipoproteins* – apoprotein B, the major protein component of LDL, is susceptible to non-enzymatic glycation, which reduces the affinity of LDL for its tissue receptors, thereby reducing LDL clearance from plasma.
- *Oxidative modification* – the uptake of LDL by scavenger pathways which lead to atherosclerosis may be increased by oxidation, which may, in turn, be increased by glycation.

> Any level of cholesterol has a greater impact on coronary risk in the presence of diabetes

As already mentioned, nephropathy has a major impact on lipids. The development of diabetic nephropathy leads to an aggravated dyslipidaemia with elevated levels of total cholesterol, LDL-cholesterol and triglycerides combined with a reduced level of cardioprotective HDL-cholesterol. In addition, the plasma concentration of lipoprotein(a), an independent risk factor for coronary heart disease, will increase as a result of impaired renal catabolism.

Management

The greatly increased risk of atherosclerotic disease in patients with type 2 diabetes has led to an increased awareness of the importance of detecting and treating dyslipidaemia. This should be done in the context of total risk factor management, and based on a calculation of absolute cardiovascular risk. Although fasting plasma lipids are usually measured (in order to include triglycerides and HDL-cholesterol) there are practical difficulties involved in patients on insulin and increasing research attention is being focused on post-prandial lipid status. In patients with type 2 diabetes, post-prandial clearance of lipoproteins from the circulation is impaired and it is hypothesized that this post-prandial hyperlipidaemia contributes to atheroma development. Although many subtle alterations in plasma lipid levels have been described, therapeutic decisions rest on measurement of some or all of: total cholesterol, triglycerides (fasting), LDL-cholesterol (calculated with reasonable accuracy using the Friedewald formula when triglycerides are <4.5 mmol/l), and HDL-cholesterol (which also allows calculation of the ratio of total cholesterol:HDL cholesterol).

Friedewald formula (mmol/l)
$$\text{LDL-chol} = \text{Total-chol} - (\text{HDL-chol} + \frac{TG}{2.2})$$

Therapeutic targets in diabetic dyslipidaemia

Although observational studies suggest that low HDL-cholesterol and hypertriglyceridaemia may be more predictive than elevated LDL-cholesterol levels, the results of interventional clinical trials using statins strongly favour LDL-cholesterol lowering as the primary therapeutic aim (Table 7.8). Other markers, such as apoprotein B and lipoprotein(a), are not routinely available in most institutions.

> Reduction of LDL-cholesterol concentrations is currently regarded as the primary therapeutic aim of lipid-lowering therapy

Both the 4S and CARE studies (Table 7.8) contained relatively small diabetic subgroups. In 2004 CARDS was published – the first statin trial exclusively conducted in patients with type 2 diabetes (see Table 7.9). Current guidelines for secondary prevention with lipid-modifying drugs should be followed in diabetic patients with established cardiovascular disease, but primary prevention is less clearcut and differences in recommendations between expert groups have generated confusion.

The magnitude of benefit derived from well-tolerated drugs such as the hydroxymethyl glutaryl coenzyme A (HMG-CoA) reductase inhibitors (statins) depends on the absolute cardiovascular risk. The available data suggest that diabetic patients should be considered at high risk.

Non-pharmacological approaches to treatment

Dietary measures

Dietary measures include attainment of ideal body weight and reduction in total fat consumption to around 30% of total calorie intake, and in saturated fat to <10% of total calorie intake. Excessive alcohol must also be curbed – alcohol can exacerbate hypertriglyceridaemia. The United Kingdom Prospective Diabetes Study (UKPDS 45) showed that three months' dietary therapy (hypocaloric for overweight patients, total maximum fat intake <35% with substitution of polyunsaturated for saturated fats) in newly diagnosed patients reduced mean plasma triglyceride levels (17% in men, 10% in women)

Table 7.8
Trials demonstrating benefits of lowering LDL-cholesterol concentrations in patients with diabetes.

1. *The Scandinavian Simvastatin Survival Study (4S)*
Significant (55%) reduction in the incidence of major coronary events in diabetic men with high LDL-cholesterol levels (5.5–8.0 mmol/l) and previous coronary heart disease. Mean follow-up duration: 4.5 years. *Diabetes Care* 1997; **20**: 614-20.

2. *The Cholesterol and Recurrent Events (CARE) study*
Pravastatin significantly reduced the incidence of coronary heart disease events in diabetic patients with average LDL-cholesterol levels and previous coronary disease over 5 years. *Circulation* 1998; **98**: 2513-9.

3. *Heart Protection Study (HPS)*. Of 20 536 patients randomized to simvastatin 40 mg daily or placebo, 5963 had diabetes with or without evidence of cardiovascular disease. In the subgroup with diabetes, 2912 patients had no previous history of arterial disease. Among the patients with diabetes, over a mean follow-up period of 4.8 years, there was a 27% reduction in major coronary events ($p<0.0001$), a 20% reduction in coronary mortality ($p=0.02$) and a 24% reduction in stroke ($p=0.0002$). Benefit was seen in primary and secondary prevention groups, in all age groups and in those with a pretreatment low-density lipoprotein cholesterol <3 mmol/l. *Lancet* 2002; **360 (9326)**: 7–22.

4. *The Antihypertensive and Lipid Lowering Treatment to Prevent Heart Attack Trial (ALLHAT)*. The lipid-lowering arm of ALLHAT comprised a subset of hypertensive patients, 35% of whom had type 2 diabetes. Coronary event rates were not significantly different between pravastatin and usual care groups possibly due to the small differences in cholesterol that were seen. *JAMA* 2002; **288 (23)**: 2998–3007.

5. *The Anglo-Scandinavian Cardiac Outcomes Trial-Lipid Lowering Arm (ASCOT-LLA)*. This comprised a subgroup of 10 305 patients from the main trial, which is comparing antihypertensive therapies. Patients were randomly assigned additional atorvastatin 10 mg or placebo. Treatment was stopped after a median follow-up of 3.3 years due to earlier than expected beneficial effects of the statin. *Lancet* 2003; **360 (9364)**: 1149–58.

Note: results are derived from analyses of diabetic subgroups in each trial. The AFCAPS/TEXCAPS and LIPID studies also included diabetic subgroups.

Table 7.9
The Collaborative Atorvastatin Diabetes Study (CARDS)

This was the first primary prevention study of statin therapy conducted exclusively in patients with type 2 diabetes, and in which 2838 patients with no history of cardiovascular disease aged 40–75 years were randomized to placebo (n=1410) or atorvastatin (n=1428). Patients had a low-density lipoprotein cholesterol concentration of 4.14 mmol/l or lower, a fasting triglyceride amount of 6.78 mmol/l or less, and one or more of the following: retinopathy, albuminuria, being a current smoker, hypertension. The pre-specified early stopping rule for efficacy was met 2 years earlier than planned; median follow-up was at 3.9 years. During this period 127 patients allocated placebo (2.46 per 100 person-years at risk) and 83 allocated atorvastatin (1.54 per 100 person-years at risk) had at least one major cardiovascular event (rate reduction 37%, $p=0.001$).

Treatment would be expected to prevent at least 37 major vascular events per 1000 such people treated for 4 years. Assessed separately, acute coronary arterial disease events were reduced by 36%, coronary revascularization procedures by 31% and rate of stroke by 48%. Atorvastatin reduced the death rate by 27% (-48 to 1, $p=0.059$). No excess of adverse events was noted in the atorvastatin group.

Lancet 2004; **364**: 685–96.

and led to marginal improvements in total cholesterol and cholesterol subfractions. Body weight was reduced by a mean of 5% and fasting plasma glucose by 3 mmol/l over the three-month period. A Mediterranean diet has been shown to be beneficial after myocardial infarction.

Aerobic physical exercise

Aerobic physical exercise can sometimes be useful in reducing hypertriglyceridaemia and LDL-cholesterol and raising HDL-cholesterol levels.

Optimization of metabolic control

Hepatic LDL receptors, the major regulators of plasma LDL level, are dependent on insulin, and total and LDL-cholesterol levels may therefore decline with improved glycaemia. Elevated triglyceride levels may respond even more to the use of insulin to attain good glycaemic control.

Avoidance of drugs that exacerbate dyslipidaemia

β-blockers as well as higher doses of thiazide diuretics exacerbate dyslipidaemia, but clinical indications such as angina pectoris and post-myocardial infarction should take precedence. Moreover, the Hypertension in Diabetes Study found no consistent trends in lipid levels between the atenolol- and captopril-based treatments. Post-menopausally, low-dose oestrogen replacement therapy tends to improve the plasma lipid profile.

The role of hormone replacement therapy for postmenopausal women has recently come under intense scrutiny. Hormone replacement therapy can improve endothelial function, reduce low-density lipoprotein concentrations and raise high-density lipoprotein cholesterol concentrations. However, oestrogen can increase C-reactive protein levels, a potentially detrimental effect. Two major US trials, which used a combination of conjugated equine oestrogen (0.625 mg) and medroxyprogesterone acetate (2.5 mg) did not confirm observation studies suggesting a protective effect. In the *Heart and Estrogen/progestin Replacement Study (HERS)* there was no overall cardiovascular benefit and a pattern of early increase in risk of coronary events during the first year in women who had a history of coronary artery disease. The *Women's Health Initiative (WHI)* was designed to study primary prevention of cardiovascular disease. Increased risks of stroke and pulmonary emboli were observed. Outcomes between diabetic and non-diabetic women in these trials were similar. The adverse effects associated with this combination has moved medical thinking away from using HRT for the prevention of cardiovascular disease.

Exclusion of other factors

Hepatic dysfunction, renal impairment and hypothyroidism may all cause or exacerbate dyslipidaemias and should be excluded.

The effects of post-menopausal oestrogen and progestogen replacement therapy on the lipid profile are variable

Therapeutic targets

The results of interventional clinical trials using statins strongly favour lowering the concentration of low-density lipoprotein (LDL) cholesterol as the principal aim of therapy. The Heart Protection Study extended this approach to patients with pre-treatment cholesterol levels previously regarded as targets for intervention, rather than thresholds for treatment. Thus, if pre-treatment total LDL cholesterol concentration is >3.5 mmol/l, the level should be reduced with a statin if the cardiovascular risk is sufficiently high, as pertains to most patients with type 2 diabetes. In such circumstances, the 2004 British guidelines suggest lowering total cholesterol by 25% or LDL cholesterol by 30%, or to <4.0 mmol/l or <2.0 mmol/l respectively, whichever is greater. A recent update of the US National Cholesterol Education Program guidelines includes the option of even more intensive therapy for those at highest risk, eg in diabetic patients with cardiovascular disease, a target of <1.8 mmol/l is proposed. Apolipoprotein B levels are regarded as being near optimal at this concentration of LDL cholesterol. This view has generated debate. Some of the evidence for this new low target level comes from studies in patients with acute coronary syndromes who have shown benefits from high-dose atorvastatin. The high toll among patients with diabetes and stable cardiovascular disease provides a rationale for intensive statin therapy. It should be noted that current strategies still leave many patients at risk of recurrent vascular events. The issue of titrating to target levels of lipids is likely to be further fuelled by the results of ongoing studies in which more aggressive lipid goals are being studied.

Pharmacological approaches to treatment

Lipid-lowering drugs will be indicated for many patients in light of the evidence of their efficacy and safety.

Statins

The HMG-CoA reductase inhibitors (statins) reduce intracellular cholesterol synthesis, thereby upregulating the expression of hepatic LDL receptors and leading to increased clearance of LDL-cholesterol from the circulation. LDL-cholesterol and apoprotein B concentration then decline by about 25–30%. The statins are generally very well-tolerated drugs with an excellent safety record and large clinical trials have clearly demonstrated their beneficial effect on LDL-cholesterol levels. Reductions of approximately 25% have generally been observed in coronary events. Higher-dose statins, in particular, may also reduce elevated plasma triglyceride levels, and other effects, such as improved endothelial function and stabilization of atheromatous plaques may also be important. Improvements (ie increases) in low HDL-cholesterol concentrations are less marked, but current clinical trial evidence favours statins as first-line drugs for patients with established coronary heart disease. Although their effects on insulin resistance remain unclear, there is some evidence suggesting improvements in carbohydrate metabolism. Recent data from the West of Scotland study showing that pravastatin reduced the risk of new cases of type 2 diabetes by 30% have not been confirmed in other studies, however.

Statins are currently regarded as first-line drugs for diabetic patients with established coronary heart disease or raised LDL-cholesterol concentrations

Fibric acid derivatives

The fibrates represent a logical alternative, particularly for mixed dyslipidaemia treatment, although the current evidence from clinical trials is less convincing than that for the statins. These drugs reduce triglyceride levels and increase HDL-cholesterol levels, but to a lesser extent. Glycaemic control may be slightly improved by lowering plasma fatty acid levels and reducing the activity of the glucose–fatty acid (Randle) cycle, but this is rarely clinically apparent. However, some fibrates also seem to decrease plasma fibrinogen levels, an independent risk factor for atherosclerosis, and several trials have reported variable rates of reduction in coronary events in non-diabetic and diabetic patients (Table 7.10). It is worth noting that LDL-cholesterol concentrations were not altered by gemfibrozil in the Veterans Administration HDL Intervention Trial (VA-HIT), suggesting there may be another mechanism of action for these drugs. In fact, the benefit in VA-HIT was largely confined to patients with insulin resistance. The Diabetes Atherosclerosis Intervention Study (DAIS) was performed exclusively in men and women with type 2 diabetes who had the typical lipid phenotype discussed above. This angiographic study showed a significant reduction in the progression of focal coronary lesions with fenofibrate, but was not powered to demonstrate a reduction in clinical events.

The choice between statins and fibrates in diabetic patients is the topic of several large comparative clinical trials currently in progress. Further information on efficacy and safety will emerge in the next few years. Combination therapy using statins and fibrates together is presently not generally recommended since the risk of myositis may be increased (although clinically evident myositis is uncommon).

Cerivastatin was withdrawn in 2001 due to a high incidence of severe myositis, especially when combined with gemfibrozil.

Other pharmacological options include:

Ezetimibe – This is a promising inhibitor of intestinal cholesterol absorption. It can be used as monotherapy or in combination with a statin to potentiate the action of the latter. Ezetimibe was launched in the UK in 2003. A combination preparation containing ezetimibe and

---

Table 7.10
Placebo-controlled trials of effects of fibrates on coronary events. Sourced from *N Engl J Med* 1987; **317**: 1237-45, *Diabetes Care* 1992; **15**: 820-5, *N Engl J Med* 1999; **341**: 410-8 and data presented at the European Society of Cardiology meeting, 1998 and the XIIth International Symposium on Atherosclerosis, 2000.

1. Helsinki Heart Study
n=4081 men; n=135 diabetic men.
Non-significant reduction in coronary heart disease in diabetics with gemfibrozil *vs* placebo. *N Engl J Med* 1987; **317**: 1237-45; *Diabetes Care* 1992; **15**: 820-5.

2. Veterans Administration HDL Intervention Trial (VA-HIT)
n=2531 men with coronary heart disease; 25% diabetic. Mean HDL-cholesterol at entry 0.8 mmol/l. Reduction in combined non-fatal and fatal coronary events (22%, p=0.006) and stroke (27%, p=0.05) with gemfibrozil *vs* placebo. Median follow-up 5.1 years. *N Eng J Med* 1999; **341**: 410-8.

3. Bezafibrate Infarction Prevention Study (BIP)
3090 patients, mean age 60 years.
Patients with diabetes largely excluded, duration 5+ years. Benefits for subgroup with hypertriglyceridaemia, ie 40% reduction in combined coronary endpoints (p=0.02) with bezafibrate *vs* placebo. No significant reduction in events for the total cohort. *Circulation* 2000; **102**: 21-7.

4. Diabetes Atherosclerosis Intervention Study (DAIS)
n=418 men and women with type 2 diabetes and dyslipidaemia. Fenofibrate 200 mg/day *vs* placebo. Mean duration of follow-up 38 months. Angiographic measurement of progression of coronary atherosclerosis. Significant 40% reduction in progression of focal lesions. Non-significant 23% reduction in clinical events. *Lancet* 2001; **357**: 905-10.

---

simvastatin in doses ranging from 10:10 mg to 10:80 mg is available in the USA.

Nicotinic acid (niacin) preparations – These are effective in elevating high-density lipoprotein (HDL) cholesterol and reducing triglyceride levels. With some preparations, deterioration of glycaemic control is a concern in patients with diabetes or glucose intolerance. A once daily, extended-release formulation was launched recently in the UK. To date, clinical experience has been limited; the problem of facial flushing has not been eliminated. Acipimox, an analogue of nicotinic acid, has not been extensively used in the UK – there are reports of improved insulin sensitivity with this agent.

Omega-3 fatty acids – Recent clinical trial data, including studies using a concentrated omega-3 fatty acid preparation (Omacor) indicate that omega-3 fatty acids can prevent sudden death following myocardial infarction. This preparation is also useful in the treatment of hypertriglyceridaemia, both as monotherapy and in combination with statins.

Plant sterols – These have a modest effect on LDL-cholesterol levels; the commercial preparations are relatively expensive.

Resins – The use of these agents has declined as the statins and fibrates have gained ground.

Antioxidants – Large clinical trials that have included high doses of vitamin E have generally shown no benefit in terms of preventing cardiovascular events.

Specialist advice should be sought in the management of major or resistant dyslipidaemias. Apparent drug intolerance is frequently encountered.

Emerging therapies for dyslipidaemia

Over the next few years it seems likely that in addition to a continuing debate about optimal levels of LDL cholesterol, attention will also be turned to raising HDL cholesterol. This is a logical target, particularly in patients with type 2 diabetes. Currently, of the available drugs, nicotinic acid (niacin) preparations are regarded as being most effective (see above). A new approach to raising HDL levels is the inhibition of cholesteryl ester transfer protein – trials are in progress. The emerging cannabinoid receptor antagonists also have favourable effects on HDL cholesterol levels.

Further reading

Adler AI, Stratton IM, Neil HAW *et al*. Association of systolic blood pressure with macrovascular and microvascular complications of type 2 diabetes (UKPDS 36): prospective observational study. *Br Med J* 2000; 321: 412-19.

American Diabetes Association. Aspirin therapy in diabetes. *Diabetes Care* 2004; **27 (suppl 1)**: S72–S73.

American Diabetes Association. Dyslipidaemia management in adults with diabetes. *Diabetes Care* 2004; **27 (suppl 1)**: S68–S71.

American Diabetes Association. Hypertension management in adults with diabetes. *Diabetes Care* 2004; **27 (suppl 1)**: S65–S67.

Barrett-Connor E, Giardina EG, Gitt AK *et al*. Women and heart disease: the role of diabetes and hyperglycaemia. *Arch Intern Med* 2004; **164**: 934–42.

Capes SE, Hunt D, Malmberg K, Gerstein HC. Stress hyperglycaemia and increased risk of death after myocardial infarction in patients with and without diabetes: a systematic overview. *Lancet* 2000; **355**: 773-8.

Curb JD, Pressel SL, Cutler JA *et al* for the systolic hypertension in the elderly program cooperative research group. Effect of diuretic-based antihypertensive treatment on cardiovascular disease risk in older patients with systolic hypertension. *JAMA* 1996; **276**: 1886-92.

Detre KM, Lombardero PHMS, Brooks MM *et al*. The effect of previous coronary artery bypass surgery on the prognosis of patients with diabetes who have acute myocardial infarction. *N Engl J Med* 2000; **342**: 989-97.

Frick MH, Elo O, Haapa K *et al*. Helsinki heart study: primary prevention trial with gemfibrozil in middle-aged men with dyslipidemia. *N Engl J Med* 1987; **317**: 1237-45.

Gaede P, Vedel P, Parving H-H, Pedersen O. Intensified multifactorial intervention in patients with type 2 diabetes mellitus and microalbuminuria: the Steno type 2 randomized study. *Lancet* 1999; **353**: 617-22.

Gerstein HC, Yusuf S. Dysglycaemia and risk of cardiovascular disease. *Lancet* 1996; **347**: 949-50.

Goldberg RB, Mellies MJ, Sacks FM *et al*. Cardiovascular events and their reduction with pravastatin in diabetic and glucose intolerant myocardial infarction survivors with average cholesterol levels: subgroup analyses in the cholesterol and recurrent events (CARE) trial. *Circulation* 1998; 2513-9.

Gress TW, Nieto FJ, Shaha E *et al*. Hypertension and antihypertensive therapy as risk factors for type 2 diabetes mellitus. *N Engl J Med* 2000; **342**: 905-12.

Groeneveld Y, Petri H, Hermans J, Springer MP. Relationship between blood glucose level and mortality in type 2 diabetes mellitus: a systematic review. *Diabetic Med* 1999; **16**: 2-13.

Guidelines subcommittee. 1999 World Health Organization - International Society for Hypertension guidelines for the management of hypertension. *J Hypertens* 1999; **17**: 151-83.

Haffner SM, Lehto S, Ronnemaa T, Pyörälä K, Laasko M. Mortality from coronary heart disease in subjects with type 2 diabetes and in non-diabetic subjects with and without prior myocardial infarction. *N Engl J Med* 1998; **339**: 229-34.

Hansson L, Zanchetti A, Carruthers SG et al for the HOT study group. Effects of intensive blood-pressure lowering and low-dose aspirin in patients with hypertension: principal results of the hypertension optimal treatment (HOT) randomized trial. Lancet 1998; 351: 1755-62.

Joint British recommendations on prevention of coronary heart disease in clinical practice. Heart 1998; 80(2): S1-29.

Kannel WB, McGee DL. Diabetes and glucose tolerance as risk factors for cardiovascular disease: the Framingham study. Diabetes Care 1979; 2: 120-6.

Koskinen P, Manttari M, Manninen V et al. Coronary heart disease incidence in NIDDM patients in the Helsinki heart study. Diabetes Care 1992; 15: 820-5.

Krentz AJ. Lipoprotein abnormalities and their consequences for patients with type 2 diabetes. Diabetes Obes Metab 2003; 5 (suppl 1): S19–S27.

Laakso M. Glycemic control and the risk for coronary heart disease in patients with non-insulin-dependent diabetes mellitus. The Finnish studies. Ann Intern Med 1996; 124: 127-30.

Lithell HO. Effect of antihypertensive drugs on insulin, glucose, and lipid metabolism. Diabetes Care 1991; 14: 203-9.

Malmberg K for the DIGAMI (Diabetes Mellitus, Insulin Glucose Infusion in Acute Myocardial Infarction) Study Group. Prospective randomized study of intensive insulin treatment on long term survival in patients with diabetes mellitus. Br Med J 1997; 314: 1512-5.

Nesto RW. Correlation between cardiovascular disease and diabetes mellitus: current concepts. Am J Med 2004; 116 (suppl 5): 11S–22S.

Rubins HB, Robins SJ, Collins D et al. Gemfibrozil for the secondary prevention of coronary heart disease in men with low levels of high-density lipoprotein cholesterol. N Eng J Med 1999; 341: 410-8.

Scheen AJ. Prevention of type 2 diabetes through inhibition of the renin–angiotensin system. Drugs 2004; 64: 2537–65.

Sowers JR. Treatment of hypertension in patients with diabetes. Arch Intern Med 2004; 164: 1850-7.

Staessen JA, Fagard R, Lutgarde T et al for the systolic hypertension in Europe (Sys-Eur) trial investigators. Randomized double-blind comparison of placebo and active treatment for older patients with isolated systolic hypertension. Lancet 1997; 350: 757-64.

Tuomilheto J, Rastenyte D, Birkenhäger WH et al for the systolic hypertension in europe trial investigators. Effects of calcium-channel blockade in older patients with diabetes and systolic hypertension. N Engl J Med 1999; 340: 677-84.

Turner RC, Millins H, Neil HAW et al. Risk factors for coronary artery disease in non-insulin dependent diabetes mellitus: United Kingdom prospective diabetes study (UKPDS: 23). Br Med J 1998; 316: 823-8.

UK Prospective Diabetes Study Group. Tight blood pressure control and risk of macrovascular and microvascular complications in type 2 diabetes (UKPDS 38). Br Med J 1998; 317: 703-13.

UK Prospective Diabetes Study Group. Efficacy of atenolol and captopril in reducing risk of macrovascular and microvascular complications in type 2 diabetes (UKPDS 39). Br Med J 1998; 317: 713-20.

UK Prospective Diabetes Study (UKPDS) Group. Effects of three months' diet after diagnosis of type 2 diabetes on plasma lipids and lipoproteins (UKPDS 45). Diabetic Med 2000; 17: 518-23.

Williams B, Poulter NR, Brown MJ et al. British Hypertension Society guidelines for hypertension management 2004 (BHS-IV): summary. BMJ 2004; 328: 634–40.

Yudkin JS. Which diabetic patients should be taking aspirin? Br Med J 1995; 311: 641-2.

8. Non-pharmacological treatment

Treatment targets
Treatment algorithm
Diet
Exercise
Body weight control

Treatment targets

The importance of controlling metabolic and other risk factors is central to the reduction of diabetic complications. Treating with the aim of achieving the best possible targets (ie with the lowest risk of complications) is now emerging as an important part of most diabetes care plans.

Glycaemic control

Any decrease in hyperglycaemia will decrease the risk and severity of diabetic complications (chapters 6 and 7). Benefits will continue to accrue until blood glucose concentrations are returned to within normal limits. The United Kingdom Prospective Diabetes Study has demonstrated that each 1% decrease in HbA_{1c} over 10 years reduces the risk of a myocardial infarction by about 14% and the risk of a microvascular complication by about 25%.

> Decreasing hyperglycaemia prevents or delays the onset and reduces the severity of diabetic complications

The European Diabetes Policy Group has recommended a graded system of glycaemic targets based on vascular risk (Table 8.1a), while the American Diabetes Association has essentially defined its goal as a return to a value within the normal glucose range (Table 8.1b). Their messages are more consistent than they sound: glycaemic control should attempt to achieve glucose values as near normal as possible, given the circumstances of the individual patient. A fasting plasma glucose (FPG) level <7.0 mmol/l (126 mg/dl) and an HbA_{1c} level <7.5% would be acceptable, but, ideally, where appropriate, attempts should be made to achieve an FPG <6.0 mmol/l (110 mg/dl) and an HbA_{1c} <6.5%.

Over-rigorous efforts to achieve ideal targets may lead to hypoglycaemic episodes in some patients, despite careful attention to the treatment regimen and all reasonable precautions. In these patients less-than-ideal may have to suffice.

Blood lipid profile

The blood lipid profile provides a well-recognized link with cardiovascular disease. Raised circulating concentrations of total cholesterol, low-density lipoprotein (LDL)-cholesterol and triglyceride are all associated with increased cardiovascular risk, as is a lowered circulating concentration of high-density lipoprotein (HDL)-cholesterol. In line with its approach to targets for glycaemic control, the European Diabetes Policy Group has recommended a graded system of lipid targets based on the extent of vascular risk (Table 8.2a). A similar approach has been taken by the American Diabetes Association (Table 8.2b). Several authorities have, however, produced more complicated guidelines based on the ratios of total cholesterol to HDL-cholesterol, or LDL-cholesterol to HDL-cholesterol. The Joint British Societies provided a graduated assessment for risk of coronary heart disease, taking into account gender, age, smoking, total cholesterol to HDL-cholesterol ratio, and systolic blood pressure. However, as discussed in chapter 7, the latest guidelines do not include tables for risk calculations in patients with type 2 diabetes; this reflects the high risk of cardiovascular disease, which merits secondary prevention measures in the great majority of these patients.

Table 8.1
Targets for glycaemic control suggested by (a) the European Diabetes Policy Group and (b) the American Diabetes Association.

(a) European targets (*Diabetic Med* 1999; **16**: 716-30)

	Low risk	Arterial risk	Microvascular risk
HbA$_{1c}$ %	≤6.5	>6.5	>7.5
Venous plasma glucose			
Fasting/pre-prandial			
mmol/l	≤6.0	>6.0	≥7.0
mg/dl	<110	≥110	≥126
*Self-monitored blood glucose**			
Fasting/pre-prandial			
mmol/l	≤5.5	>5.5	>6.0
mg/dl	<100	≥100	≥110
Post-prandial or peak			
mmol/l	<7.5	≥7.5	>9.0
mg/dl	<135	≥135	>160

*Fasting capillary blood glucose is about 1.0 mmol/l (18 mg/dl) lower than venous plasma blood glucose. Post-prandial capillary blood glucose is about the same as venous plasma blood glucose.

(b) American targets (*Diabetes Care* 2004; **27**: S15-35)

	Non-diabetic (mg/dl)	Non-diabetic (mmol/l)	Goal (mg/dl)	Goal (mmol/l)	Additional action suggested (mg/dl)	Additional action suggested (mmol/l)
Pre-prandial plasma glucose	<110	<6.0	90–130	5.0–7.2	<90/>150	<5.0/>8.3
Post-prandial plasma glucose	<140	<7.8	<180	<10.0	>180	>10.0
Bedtime glucose	<120	<6.6	110–150	6.0–8.3	<110/>180	<6.0/>10.0
HbA$_{1c}$ (%)	<6		<7		>8	

These values are guidelines for non-pregnant individuals and may need modification in the light of factors such as age, co-morbidity, etc. Subsequent action will depend on individual patient circumstances. HbA$_{1c}$ is referenced to a non-diabetic range of 4.0–6.0% (mean 5.0%, SD 0.5%). To convert mg/dl to mmol/l, divide by 18.

> Treatment should be intensified to achieve targets for glucose, lipids and blood pressure that confer low risk for the development of diabetic complications

The British Hypertension Society guidelines and targets are considered in chapter 7. Possible benefits of even tighter targets for glycaemia are being tested in the ACCORD study (Action to Control Cardiovascular Risk in Diabetes).

> Cardiovascular risk is increased by raised LDL-cholesterol, raised triglyceride, or reduced HDL-cholesterol, and particularly by all three in combination

Blood pressure

The United Kingdom Prospective Diabetes Study demonstrated the substantial benefits of blood pressure control in type 2 diabetic patients, and recognized that these benefits increased in line with blood pressure reduction until a normal blood pressure had been achieved. The benefits were reflected in both macrovascular and microvascular complications, and diabetes-related deaths were reduced by about 30% for every 10 mmHg decrease in systolic blood pressure over a nine-year period.

The British Hypertension Society, European Society of Hypertension and American Diabetes Association have each recommended an ideal blood pressure target of <130/80 mmHg for

Table 8.2
Targets for blood lipids control suggested by (a) the European Diabetes Policy Group, and (b) the American Diabetes Association (2004).

(a) European target: risk of macrovascular disease			
	Low risk	At risk	High risk
Serum total cholesterol			
mmol/l	<4.8	4.8–6.0	>6.0
mg/dl	<185	184–230	>230
Serum LDL-cholesterol			
mmol/l	<3.0	3.0–4.0	>4.0
mg/dl	<115	115–155	>155
Serum HDL-cholesterol			
mmol/l	>1.2	1.0–1.2	<1.0
mg/dl	>46	39–46	<39
Serum triglycerides			
mmol/l	<1.7	1.7–2.2	>2.2
mg/dl	<150	150–200	>200

(b) For patients with diabetes and no cardiovascular disease		
	Target/low risk	Action level*
Plasma LDL-cholesterol	<100 (2.6)	≥130 (3.35)
Plasma HDL-cholesterol	>40 (1.0)†	<40 (1.0)
Plasma triglycerides	<150 (1.7)	>400 (4.5)‡

Units are mg/dl (mmol/l)
*Action level = threshold for starting pharmacological therapy
†For women, a higher level (+10 mg/dl) may be appropriate, ie >50 mg/dl (1.29 mmol/l)
‡Between 200–400 mg/dl (2.3–4.5 mmol/l), physicians discretion should be applied

type 2 diabetic patients (page 91). Antihypertensive drug therapy is recommended for patients with a blood pressure >140/90 mmHg, although some authorities would suggest starting drug therapy below this.

Reducing hypertension reduces morbidity and mortality in type 2 diabetes

Body weight

It is well-recognized that excess abdominal adiposity is a risk factor for type 2 diabetes and other components of the insulin resistance or metabolic syndrome. There is also a wealth of evidence to suggest that reducing adiposity in overweight and frankly obese patients will improve both metabolic control and life expectancy. Any reduction in adiposity down towards the normal weight range is strongly recommended.

Excess visceral adiposity is an important cardiovascular risk factor

Obesity is usually defined as a body mass index (BMI) >30. (BMI is calculated by dividing weight in kg by height in m², ie kg/m².) Overweight has been defined by the World Health Organization (WHO) as a BMI between 25 and 30 kg/m² (lower values apply to Asian peoples), and 'normal' as a BMI within the range 18.5–25 kg/m². However, BMI provides an estimate of whole-body size and does not take account of fat distribution. Since visceral (intra-abdominal) obesity rather than generalized or lower body subcutaneous obesity has been recognized as an important cardiovascular risk factor, it has been suggested that girth measurements at the waist and hip (enabling calculation of the waist:hip ratio) may be more useful. Waist-to-hip ratio should be:

* <0.95 for men
* <0.80 for women.

Alternatively, waist circumference alone may be used – >102 cm (40 in) for men and >88 cm (35 in) for women is considered indicative of abdominal adiposity.

Other targets

Ideal goals for glycaemic control, lipid profile, blood pressure and body weight offer helpful benchmarks, even if they are neither realistically attainable nor sustainable in many patients. In such cases it may be appropriate to lay greater emphasis on the means employed to work towards these goals – reducing snacking, walking a defined distance each day, or even re-doubling efforts to take all medication and attend all clinic appointments – than the goals themselves. It cannot be overstated that progression towards these targets, however modest, will reap rewards in terms of offsetting both the onset and severity of long-term vascular and neuropathic complications.

Treatment algorithm

The standard procedure for treatment of type 2 diabetes follows a stepwise progression starting with non-pharmacological measures, ie diet, exercise, weight control and health education. If these do not achieve or sustain targets for metabolic control, an oral antidiabetic agent is then introduced. If targets are still not achieved a second (and possibly a third) differently acting oral agent is introduced. Patients who still fail to achieve and maintain targets should be switched to insulin – an oral agent may be added back if appropriate. Alternatively, the most suitable oral agent may be continued and insulin added-in, initially as a single injection before bed. This algorithm is summarized in Figure 8.1.

> Rapid progression through a treatment algorithm may be necessary to achieve optimal glycaemic control

This treatment algorithm can be adapted readily to suit particular groups of patients (eg the obese or elderly) through the choice of therapeutic agent(s). The targets can also be adjusted to accommodate individual circumstances. The presence of diabetic complications and the concurrent use of other medications will inevitably restrict the choice of antidiabetic agent, potentially reducing the scope for achieving targets.

Type 2 diabetes is highly variable in its presentation and usually progressive, presenting different problems at different stages of its natural history. The fundamental features of insulin resistance and defective insulin secretion, and the metabolic disturbances created in muscle, liver and adipose tissue will gradually change. Accordingly, type 2 diabetes constitutes a moving target that requires a selection of different agents to treat different aspects at different stages of the disease process.

> Type 2 diabetes presents a therapeutic 'moving target' due to the progressive course of its natural history

Given the proven advantages of effective metabolic control, it is important not to delay movement through the treatment algorithm if control at any particular step is clearly unsatisfactory. Non-pharmacological (lifestyle) measures should be reinforced at every opportunity – they are seldom fully exploited. For patients who present with severe hyperglycaemia and/or severe symptoms it may be necessary to proceed very rapidly through the algorithm – even beginning with oral combination or insulin therapy in some cases. Some patients require insulin initially but may subsequently be satisfactorily controlled using oral agents.

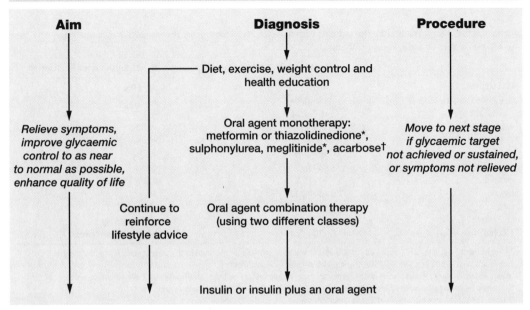

Figure 8.1

An algorithm for the treatment of type 2 diabetes mellitus. The progressive hyperglycaemia of type 2 diabetes requires a stepped care approach with treatment being modified and added to over time. Rapid progression to the next stage is recommended if glycaemic target is not achieved or sustained. Late introduction of combinations of oral agents is often a prelude to insulin treatment.

*Note that in Europe thiazolidinediones are presently recommended as monotherapy only when metformin is not appropriate. Also, in Europe thiazolidinediones are not recommended for use with insulin.

†Other alpha-glucosidase inhibitors are available in some countries.

> Controlling body weight, blood pressure, lipids and glycaemia retards the onset and severity of diabetic complications

Diet

Diet is the cornerstone of treatment for type 2 diabetes. Every patient should receive detailed advice from a dietician, explaining the types and amounts of food that will enable dietary compliance. Dietary recommendations should be reinforced by all members of the care team whenever the opportunity arises. In fact, the 'diabetic' diet is nothing more than a normal balanced diet – ie rich in complex high-fibre carbohydrates and low in saturated fats and cholesterol. Meals should be taken regularly, and the total energy content adjusted in an effort to maintain body weight within the normal range. Ideally >55% of the total energy content will come from complex carbohydrate, while <30% will come from fat (Table 8.3).

> Diet is the cornerstone of treatment for type 2 diabetes

It seems that visualizing meal structures in terms of a 'healthy eating pyramid' (Figure 8.2) can help some patients translate these dietary recommendations into eating habits. The pyramid emphasizes that fatty foods and sugars should be reduced or eliminated from the diet wherever possible, and that snacking between main meals is discouraged unless required to alleviate symptoms or prevent an anticipated episode of hypoglycaemia. Lean meats and fish are encouraged in moderation so that total daily protein intake (about 0.8 g/kg body weight; typically about 50–70 g) is responsible for

Table 8.3

Recommended dietary composition for patients with diabetes. Major nutrients are given in terms of their percentage contribution to the total energy content of the diet.*

	European Diabetes Policy Group[+]	American Diabetes Association
Carbohydrate[a]	>55%	55–60%
– added sugar	<25 g/day	–
– total sugar	<50 g/day	–
Fat	<30%	<30%
– saturated	<10%	<10%
– mono-unsaturated	10–15%	<12%
– polyunsaturated	<10%	6–8%
Protein	10–15%	0.8 g/kg body weight
Fibre	>30 g/day	40 g/day[e]
Salt	<6 g/day[b]	<3 g/day
Cholesterol[c]	<300 mg/day	<300 mg/day
Alcohol[d]	<30 g/day	<4 equivalents/week

*A typical daily diet might comprise about 2000 kcal (8400 kJ) – more for active individuals, slightly less for highly sedentary individuals, and <1500 kcal (6300 kJ) for those on an energy-restricted diet.

[+]Where explicit values are not stated in the recommendations, appropriate values from Diabetes UK have been inserted.

[a]Carbohydrates should be mainly fibre-rich and complex, with little (<50 g/day) as simple sugars.

[b]Salt intake should be <3 g/day if patient is hypertensive.

[c]Cholesterol should be substantially less than 250 mg/day if patient is dyslipidaemic.

[d]Alcohol intake should be <20 g/day in women and only taken with meals. Equivalents are 1 fl oz spirit, 4 fl oz wine, and 12 fl oz beer.

[e]Fibre intake should be about 25 g/day on a low-energy diet.

about 10–15% of the total energy content of the diet. The current mainstay of every meal is food rich in complex carbohydrate, although these foods should not be eaten in excess.

An example of the implementation of the healthy eating pyramid is given in Figure 8.3 and further represented as a daily meal plan in Table 8.4. It often proves necessary to illustrate physically to patients the amount that constitutes a serving, and to introduce some patients to a greater variety of vegetables, fruits, beans, etc, which they might otherwise ignore. Equally, it can be helpful to point out the increasing range of 'low-fat' products available and to practise devising balanced but varied and appetizing menus that comply with the general dietary recommendations.

If food intake is spread out into three or four discrete meals a day, it can often be combined more effectively with drug treatment regimens and help to facilitate control of day-time hyperglycaemia. Furthermore, introducing this

kind of routine will assist compliance and highlight any variance from the expected norm. Most people seem to consume most of their energy in their evening meal at the end of the day, but the use of some drug treatments is facilitated if energy intake is more evenly distributed among the three or four main meals.

Reducing fat

Avoiding fatty foods, confectionery and snacking are key messages to include from the outset in any programme of dietary advice. Recognizing fatty foods and finding alternatives are useful skills in the conversion to a starch-based diet. The importance of reducing fat (including cholesterol) intake is usually expressed in terms of reducing the overall risk of macrovascular complications, but significant improvements in insulin sensitivity can also result. Since fat is more than twice as energy-dense as carbohydrate or protein (Table 8.5), reducing fat intake is an effective approach to

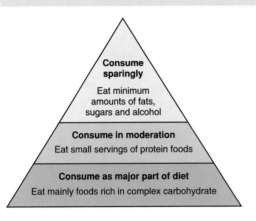

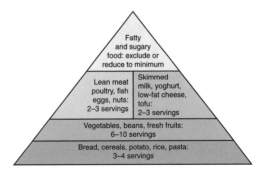

Table 8.4
An example of a daily meal plan, based on healthy eating pyramid use.

Meal	Food	Amount/Type
Breakfast	Egg	1
	Bread	2 slices
	Milk	200 ml
	Fruit	Peach
Lunch	Lean meat	2 oz
	Rice	4 oz
	Vegetables	3 oz
	Beans	3 oz
	Yoghurt	150 ml
Snack	Fruit	Apple
Dinner	Salad	Green
	Fish	2 oz
	Potato	4 oz
	Vegetables	2 x 3 oz
	Fruit	Pear
Supper	Cereal	2 oz

Please cross-refer to Figures 8.2 and 8.3. 1 oz = 28.3 g.
NB some ethnic groups will require modified advice, but the relevant teaching materials should be available in the appropriate languages.

Figure 8.2
Healthy eating pyramid for a diabetic diet.
Foods rich in fat and sugar should be consumed very sparingly. Lean meat, fish and other foods rich in protein, as well as low-fat dairy produce, should be eaten in moderation. Foods with a high complex carbohydrate content such as bread, rice, pasta, potatoes and other garden vegetables can be eaten liberally, along with ample amounts of fresh fruit.

Figure 8.3
An example of a healthy eating pyramid, reflected in numbers of servings daily.
An approximate guide to servings sizes is: meat, poultry, fish about 2 oz (50 g) after cooking; 1 egg; nuts about 1.5 oz (40 g); milk, yoghurt, tofu about 200 ml or 200 g; cheese 1–2 oz (25–50 g); fresh vegetables, fruit and beans about 2–4 oz (50–100 g); bread 1–2 slices; cereals about 1–2 oz (25–50 g); potatoes, rice, pasta about 3–5 oz (80–130 g).

Table 8.5

The energy content of foods – illustrating that fats are more than twice as energy-dense as carbohydrates and proteins – and recommended daily intake of each for an average diabetic patient

	Energy content		Recommended daily intake*			
	kcal/g	kJ/g	g	kcal	kJ	% total energy
Carbohydrate	4	17	285	1140	4790	57
Fat	9	38	65	580	2440	29
Protein	4	17	70	280	1170	14

*total energy content 2000 kcal (8,400 kJ).

weight-control. It is always worth clarifying the energy content of different food types: an individual striving to achieve a total daily intake of 2,000 calories (kcal) (8,400 kJ) might try to consume about 280–320 g carbohydrate, 50–65 g fat, and 50–70 g protein (Table 8.5).

Saturated fatty acids

Saturated fatty acids, eg palmitic acid, contain no double-bonds and are the predominant components of animal fat. Their intake should be minimized, certainly to <10% of the total daily energy intake. This reduction will also facilitate a reduction in serum cholesterol, especially in patients with raised cholesterol levels.

Polyunsaturated fatty acids

Polyunsaturated fatty acids, eg linoleic acid, contain two or more double-bonds, and are mainly derived from plant sources (especially vegetable oil). Their intake should be restricted, although small quantities of some polyunsaturates are essential (they cannot be synthesized by the human body). γ-linolenic acid, derived from evening primrose oil, is said to be helpful in the treatment of neuropathy. Small amounts of polyunsaturated fish oils can reduce triglyceride concentrations and decrease platelet aggregability, but large quantities may impair glycaemic control.

Monounsaturated fatty acids

Monounsaturated fatty acids, eg oleic acid, contain one double-bond and are also derived from vegetable sources (eg olive oil). These fats can assist in the reduction of saturated fats and there is tentative evidence that modest amounts of monounsaturated fatty acids can reduce the risk of macrovascular disease (whether or not this is largely due to their replacement of dietary saturated fats is not clear).

Complex carbohydrate and fibre intake

The rationale for consuming complex carbohydrate is mainly the time taken to digest this food type into absorbable sugar. It slows digestion which, in turn, slows the rate at which sugars, principally glucose, enter the circulation. Although glucose uptake by the liver and peripheral tissues is always outpaced by glucose absorption after a meal, the slower the latter, the greater the reduction in post-prandial hyperglycaemia. The different types of carbohydrate and the presence of other nutrients and fibre within the food ingested will each impact on overall rate of digestion and subsequent hyperglycaemic effect. The hyperglycaemic potential of different foods is sometimes expressed as the 'glycaemic index', a measure of the area under the blood glucose curve for up to three hours after ingestion of 50 g of the foodstuff compared with 50 g of glucose (some calculations are alternatively based on 50 g of white bread):

$$\text{Glycaemic index (\%)} = \frac{\text{Area under glycaemic curve of foodstuff}}{\text{Area under glycaemic curve of glucose}}$$

Use of the glycaemic index has been limited by variations in composition of different varieties and different sources of the same foodstuff, but the similarly low glycaemic indices of cereals, rice, pasta and potatoes, provide the basis for recommending a large amount of complex carbohydrate in the diet. Views vary widely concerning the usefulness of this concept in clinical practice.

> Soluble fibres are particularly effective in reducing post-prandial hyperglycaemia

Dietary fibre further slows the digestion of carbohydrate and absorption of sugars. Fibre traps carbohydrates within its matrix and forms a diffusional barrier which impedes access by digestive enzymes and slows the release of sugars. Most dietary fibres are non-digestible plant polysaccharides. Some of these are soluble and form viscous gels, others are insoluble. Soluble fibres such as gums, pectins, hemicellulose and mucilages are generally more effective in reducing post-prandial hyperglycaemia than insoluble fibres such as celluloses and wheat bran.

The fibre content of a diabetic diet (>30 g/day, Table 8.3) is usually achieved by the patient eating a good selection of vegetables and pulses, in addition to the main sources of complex carbohydrate. Fibre supplements such as guar gum (a galactomannan from the Indian cluster bean *Cyamopsis tetragonoloba*) have a modest additional antihyperglycaemic effect in some patients and can improve the lipid profile, but they can also cause abdominal discomfort and flatulence, and interfere with the absorption of other micronutrients and drugs. A diet naturally rich in fibre from vegetables, fruit and cereals is most appropriate.

Low carbohydrate diets

Although these diets are currently very popular and apparently of some benefit (albeit with high drop-out rates), no randomized trials lasting longer than a year have been published.

Reductions in triglycerides and elevations in high-density lipoproteins may be offset by increases in low-density lipoprotein concentrations. Limited data suggest that low-density lipoproteins may become less atherogenic. It is unclear whether the changes in lipids are sustained during weight maintenance. Further research is required before such diets can be recommended.

For patients with diabetes the implications of these diets include the potential for hypoglycaemia if insulin or secretagogoues are being used. The supposed ketogenic effect of these diets has not raised any serious concerns. However, the impacts of a higher protein intake in patients with nephropathy merit consideration if such diets are to be adopted on a long-term basis.

Artificial sweeteners

Non-nutritive sweeteners are already widely used in food and drink. To avoid consuming extra sugars, non-nutritive sweeteners such as aspartame, saccharin and acesulphame K provide a valuable alternative in beverages, particularly in 'diet' soft drinks for thirst-quenching. Previous concerns in the US about the putative carcinogenicity of saccharin seem to have been misplaced, and this sweetener is no longer scorned.

Diabetic speciality foods

'Diabetic foods' typically contain fructose or sorbitol for sweetening and bulking. They are generally *not* recommended, because large quantities can have unwanted effects. For example, excess fructose can cause hypertriglyceridaemia and diarrhoea.

Salt

Sodium consumption should be restricted to reduce the risk of hypertension. A daily salt consumption of <3 g is strongly recommended in hypertensive patients. Potassium chloride may be an appropriate substitute, but care must be taken in patients using potassium-sparing antihypertensive agents and in those with renal impairment.

Alcohol

Diabetic patients are advised to consume alcohol strictly in moderation and preferably with food. This is especially pertinent for those on antidiabetic drug treatment, because alcohol can cause hypoglycaemia. Alcohol is also a significant energy (calorie) source. Alcohol abuse is unacceptable and dangerous, because hypoglycaemia can pass undiagnosed in inebriated patients. In Europe, <30 g/day in men and <20 g/day in women are the recommended maxima; the US recommendation is less than four 'equivalents'/week (one 'equivalent' is approximately 1 fl oz spirit, 4 fl oz wine, or 12 fl oz beer). There is evidence that *low* but regular alcohol intake (eg one glass of wine a day) may reduce cardiovascular risk in diabetic and non-diabetic individuals.

Vitamins and minerals

Vitamin deficiencies are not a recognized problem in diabetes, but this condition may be associated with reduced concentrations of water-soluble vitamins. It has been tentatively claimed that supplements of the antioxidant vitamins (C, E and β-carotene) might combat insulin resistance, reduce glycation and atherogenesis, but this has not been established.

Deficiencies of some of the minerals required for glucose metabolism have been noted in type 2 diabetic patients and appropriate supplementation is usually beneficial. Hypomagnesaemia (plasma levels more than 2 SD below normal), usually due to increased magnesium excretion, is found in about 25% of diabetic patients, and magnesium supplementation (≥350 mg/day) in this subgroup can help to improve insulin sensitivity and glycaemic control and thus, possibly, cardiovascular prognosis.

Chromium levels are often reduced in diabetic patients, especially the elderly, probably as a result of poor diet. Supplements of trivalent chromium (≥200 µg/day) in such patients have been shown to improve glycaemic control and reduce total cholesterol concentration.

Reduced zinc levels are not uncommon in diabetic patients. Absolute zinc deficiency is rare, but supplementation has proven helpful in some patients with liver disease.

Vanadium is not known to be deficient in type 2 diabetic patients, but preliminary trials have shown that vanadium supplements improve glycaemic control without stimulating insulin secretion. The potential toxicity of vanadium salts has stimulated research into more potent vanadium compounds which can be used at much lower dosages and carry less risk. Several other trace elements (eg molybdenum and selenium) produce insulin-like effects or enhance insulin action, and general mineral supplements which contain the recommended daily allowances of these substances may be helpful in those with poor nutrition.

Exercise

Physical exercise, particularly aerobic exertion, improves insulin sensitivity and glycaemic control in type 2 diabetes. Regular exercise also helps to maintain muscle mass, reduce adiposity and improve the blood lipid profile. Clearly, exercise can be a valuable therapeutic approach, provided that the patient is willing and able to participate (Table 8.6). Recommendations must, however, be based on a thorough clinical assessment to evaluate potential contraindications. Activities can then be selected that are appropriate for the individual's medical circumstances, age, ability and interest. Even very modest amounts of exercise can benefit a previously sedentary individual, and even apparently trivial activities may be usefully introduced in some cases.

> Aerobic exercise improves insulin sensitivity and glycaemic control

Table 8.6
Establishment of an exercise programme for a type 2 diabetic patient.

- Assess contraindications and gauge suitability.
- Design a realistic programme with the patient – jointly select type, duration and intensity of exercise. Aerobic exercise, for example, might involve walking briskly for >15 minutes once or twice a day (which should raise heart rate to more than halfway between basal and maximum levels).
- Provide general advice – that intensity and duration should be built up gradually, that it is important to warm-up and warm-down, and that exercise should be timed to fit in with drug treatment and eating patterns.
- Identify risks and explain precautions – hypoglycaemia and the need for good foot care, the dangers of isometric exercise, the special considerations that apply to cardiovascular diseases, and the need to avoid strenuous exercise during times of peak insulin absorption.
- Remind the patient that they should always carry glucose and identification with them, quench thirst appropriately, and avoid overexertion.

Since subclinical cardiovascular disease is not uncommon in patients with type 2 diabetes, a cautious approach to starting an exercise programme is warranted. High-risk patients might be considered for exercise treadmill testing. Once on a programme, patients should build up the intensity and duration of their exercise gradually. Examples of commonly enjoyed exercise types are brisk walking once or twice daily for more than 15 minutes, swimming, cycling, and gentle jogging. If there is any prospect of inducing hypoglycaemia, however, exercise should be carefully integrated with both dietary intake and drug therapies. It may also be advisable, particularly during the escalation of exercise, to check blood glucose levels both before and after the workout. The patient should always carry glucose and fluid replacement with them, drink regularly, wear suitable clothing, especially comfortable footwear, and warm-up and warm-down slowly. Normal warnings for insulin-treated patients

should always be reinforced – notably that exercise can increase the absorption of insulin injected close to muscle, so it is better not to take strenuous exercise soon after an insulin injection or at the time of peak absorption. Likewise, advice on the timing of exercise in relation to dietary intake and on the need to carry identification and glucose and to be aware of hypoglycaemic symptoms should be given.

Isometric exercises that increase intrathoracic pressure should be avoided, especially where there is hypertension or retinopathy. Pulse rate can be checked by the patient and exercise intensity then adjusted so that heart rate is ideally raised to between 50 and 70% of the range between basal and maximum (maximum estimated as 220 minus age). Appropriate precautions must be taken for patients with hypertension, any evidence of heart disease and a potentially high susceptibility to stroke. The risk of foot damage, delayed hypoglycaemia and dehydration must also be appreciated, in order to ensure that exercise does not do more harm than good in high-risk patients.

$$\text{Maximum heart rate for aerobic exercise} = 220 - \text{age}$$

Body weight control

When body weight either falls rapidly without active intervention or declines to the lower end of the normal range, it is often a sign of uncontrolled hyperglycaemia, and may warrant insulin therapy. Body weight usually increases when insulin therapy is introduced, and total energy intake should then be adjusted to achieve and consolidate body weight within the normal range. A low body weight may indicate over-obsessive dietary management, sometimes poor diet (particularly in the elderly), an undiagnosed concurrent illness (such as tuberculosis), or a malabsorption syndrome.

Excess adiposity, especially visceral adiposity, is commonplace among type 2 diabetic patients – more than 70% are obese on diagnosis in the

US. Combining a low-energy diet and exercise can be very effective in obese patients and patients with lesser degrees of overweight (ie BMI 25–30 kg/m²) or a high waist:hip ratio (>0.95 in men and >0.80 in women).

Low-energy diets

Energy-restricted diets can usually be designed by cutting out snacks, reducing the sizes of servings and altering the selection of foods within the normal balanced diet. A moderate energy deficit about 500–1,000 kcal (2,100–4,200 kJ) less than the estimated energy requirement for the individual concerned is usually sufficient to improve glycaemic control rapidly and weight loss more gradually. However, it must be appreciated that weight loss will usually be accompanied by increased metabolic efficiency, so that body weight will tend to level out, despite adherence to a low-energy diet. (The compensation is due to reduced resting energy expenditure, typically consequent to loss of lean tissue.) Energy-restricted diets should reduce fat content whenever possible and ensure adequate consumption of vitamins, minerals, fibre and protein.

Very low calorie diets ('VLCDs'), typically providing about 400–800 kcal/day (1,680–3,360 kJ/day), are available as formula-based preparations including vitamin and mineral supplementation. While a very low energy intake is generally correlated with faster and greater weight loss, it must be ensured that lean body mass (including cardiac muscle) is not decreased. Patients with heart disease must approach these diets with extra caution, and thyroid hormones should not be used as a means of weight loss for the same reason. Non-nutritive 'bulking' agents are occasionally helpful in energy-reduced diets.

Reducing the energy content of a normal diet by 500–1,000 kcal (2,100–4,200 kJ) will usually cause weight loss of about 2 kg (4.5 pounds) in the first week, diminishing thereafter to level out at one to three months when 5–15 kg (about 11–33 pounds) have been lost (corresponding to

5–10% of initial body weight). Sustained weight loss of this magnitude is likely to reduce HbA_{1c} by about 0.5%, and lower serum triglyceride and total cholesterol levels by 10%. Greater weight loss is usually associated with greater improvement in metabolic control. In fact, each kg of sustained weight loss increases average life expectancy by three to four months. Weight loss through diet and exercise provides a fundamental treatment strategy for every overweight or obese type 2 diabetic patient.

> Reinforce dietary and exercise advice to optimize weight loss before considering antiobesity drugs

Antiobesity drugs

One of the most widely used antidiabetic drugs, metformin, does not cause weight gain, and may assist with modest weight loss. α-glucosidase inhibitor drugs used in the treatment of post-prandial hyperglycaemia are also unlikely to cause weight gain. However, this is not the case with other antidiabetic agents, further complicating treatment for the obese type 2 diabetic patient. Antiobesity drugs have not generally been included in most algorithms for diabetes treatment, due mainly to safety concerns. However, safer agents are emerging, and these may have a place in the treatment of some overweight patients, such as those who have already responded to an energy-reduced diet but require further weight control (and who are not contraindicated). Current antiobesity agents include orlistat and sibutramine, but the latter is not presently available in all European countries. Given the benefits that can be realized with sustained weight reduction in obese and overweight type 2 diabetic patients (and overweight IGT subjects, see page 10), it is appropriate to consider these agents.

> The antidiabetic drugs metformin and the α-glucosidase inhibitors do *not* promote weight gain

Orlistat

Orlistat is a gastrointestinal lipase inhibitor which slows the rate of triglyceride digestion by binding to the active site of intestinal lipases. This can reduce the amount of fat absorbed from the intestine by up to 30% and increase weight loss by about 2–4 kg more than is achieved by energy restriction alone. Trials with orlistat in obese type 2 diabetic patients found that more patients achieved a significant reduction in body weight than without this agent, and that those who maintained a weight loss of >6 kg also showed a decrease in HbA_{1c} of >0.5%. Orlistat may inadvertently provide a means of assisting dietary compliance due to the inevitable problem of excess fat passing through to the faeces. More frequent defaecation, loose oily stools, diarrhoea and even faecal incontinence may become a problem, especially if the fat content of the diet is not maintained at a low level. The possibility of impaired absorption of fat-soluble vitamins and concomitant medications should be borne in mind.

In the UK orlistat is considered suitable for most obese persons or overweight adults (BMI >28 kg/m²) who have comorbid risk factors such as type 2 diabetes. It is taken in conjunction with a reduced calorie diet (particularly reduced fat intake) starting with a dose of 120 mg with the main meal and titrating up to a maximum of 120 mg with each of three meals per day. Compliance may be limited by the gastrointestinal side-effects and continued use is normally dependent on >5% weight loss by 3 months and >10% weight loss by 6 months. Treatment is not indicated beyond 2 years. In the XENDOS trial, orlistat reduced the rate of progression to type 2 diabetes in obese subjects who had impaired glucose tolerance (see chapter 1).

Sibutramine

Sibutramine enhances the satiety response by acting centrally as a serotonin and noradrenaline (norepinephrine) reuptake inhibitor. It may also increase energy expenditure by increasing sympathetic stimulation of thermogenesis. In obese type 2 diabetic patients, sibutramine, like orlistat, enhances weight reduction with a low-energy diet by an extra 2–4 kg. A corresponding improvement in HbA_{1c} is also observed. In a recent multicentre trial, sibutramine, used as an adjunct to weight maintenance after weight loss, increased HDL-cholesterol levels and reduced triglycerides in non-diabetic subjects.

Sibutramine may cause a small rise in pulse rate and blood pressure in some individuals, but this effect is usually more than countered by the decreased adiposity. However, sibutramine is not recommended for patients whose hypertension is not controlled. Unlike some previous satiety inducers, sibutramine is not a serotonin releaser, is not addictive and has no known effects on heart valves or pulmonary vascular function.

In the UK sibutramine (10–15 mg daily) can be used in obese or overweight adults (BMI >27 kg/m²) with type 2 diabetes or hypercholesterolaemia. For the use of sibutramine to be continued, a serious prior attempt to lose weight by dieting and overall weight loss >5% is required by 3 months of treatment. Pulse rate and blood pressure should be checked regularly (every 2 weeks for the first 3 months) and treatment is not indicated beyond 1 year.

Cannabinoid receptor antagonists

There is intense interest in this new class of drugs as aids to weight reduction.

Further reading

American Diabetes Association. Position statement. Standards of medical care in diabetes mellitus. *Diabetes Care* 2004; **27 (suppl 1)**: S15-S35.

American Diabetes Association. Position statement. Nutrition principles and recommendations in diabetes. *Diabetes Care* 2004; **27 (suppl 1)**: S36-S46.

American Diabetes Association. Position statement. Physical activity/exercise and diabetes. *Diabetes Care* 2004; **27 (suppl 1)**: S58-S62.

Astrup A, Larsen TM, Harper A. Atkins and other low-carbohydrate diets: hoax or an effective tool for weight loss? *Lancet* 2004; **364**: 897-9.

European Diabetes Policy Group 1998-1999. Guidelines for diabetes care. A desktop guide to type 2 diabetes mellitus. *Diabetic Med* 1999; **16**: 716-30.

James WP, Astrup A, Finer N *et al*. Effect of sibutramine on weight maintenance after weight loss: a randomized trial. *Lancet* 2000; **356**: 2119-25.

Scheen AJ, Lefèvre PJ. Management of the obese diabetic patient. *Diabetes Rev* 1999; **7**: 77-93.

UK Prospective Diabetes Study Group. Intensive blood-glucose control with sulphonylureas or insulin compared with conventional treatment and risk of complications in patients with type 2 diabetes (UKPDS 33). *Lancet* 1998; **352**: 837-53.

9. Pharmacological treatment I:

**α-glucosidase inhibitors
Sulphonylureas
Meglitinide analogues
Future therapies to improve insulin
    secretion**

When non-pharmacological treatments are
unable to achieve or maintain adequate
glycaemic control, oral antidiabetic drugs are
indicated. Several differently acting classes are
currently available, and this chapter considers
the α-glucosidase inhibitors, the sulphonylureas
and the meglitinides.

α-glucosidase inhibitors

Slowing the rate at which glucose enters the
circulation after a meal reduces the extent of
the post-prandial rise in glycaemia in type 2
diabetes. Inhibitors of intestinal α-glucosidase
enzymes slow the rate of carbohydrate digestion
and provide one means of reducing post-
prandial hyperglycaemia.

> α-glucosidase inhibitors slow the rate of
> intestinal carbohydrate digestion

Brief history

The first α-glucosidase inhibitor, acarbose, was
introduced in the early 1990s (Figure 9.1).
Recently two further α-glucosidase inhibitors,
miglitol and voglibose have been introduced in
some countries, but not the UK. To date, this
class of drugs has been used extensively in
Germany, but not much elsewhere.

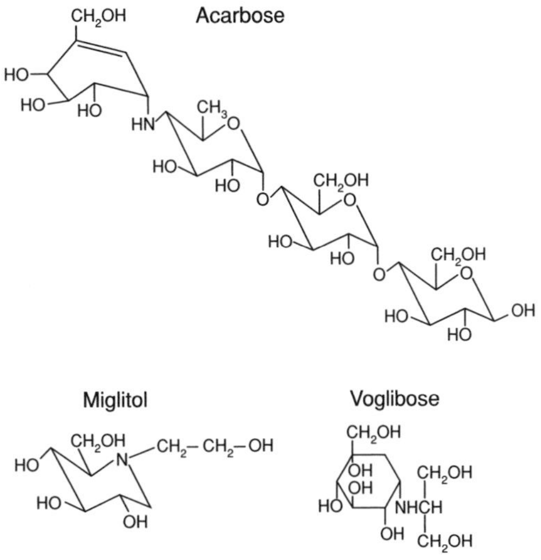

Figure 9.1
Chemical structures of the α-glucosidase inhibitors
acarbose, miglitol and voglibose.

Pharmacokinetics

Acarbose and voglibose are absorbed in trivial
amounts (acarbose <2% and voglibose <5%).
Acarbose is degraded by amylases in the small
intestine and by intestinal bacteria, and some
of the degradation products are absorbed. Most
of the acarbose and degradation products that
are absorbed are eliminated over 24 hours in
the urine. Miglitol is almost completely
absorbed and eliminated unchanged in the urine
(Table 9.1).

Mode of action

α-glucosidase inhibitors slow the process of
carbohydrate digestion by competitively
inhibiting the activity of α-glucosidase
enzymes located in the brush border of the
enterocytes lining the intestinal villi (Figure
9.2). Acarbose also causes a small reduction in
the activity of α-amylase. The main
α-glucosidases are glucoamylase, sucrase,
maltase and dextrinase, and the inhibitors bind
to these enzymes with high affinity, thus
preventing the enzymes from cleaving their

Table 9.1
Dosage and pharmacokinetic features of the α-glucosidase inhibitors.

	Dosage	Amount absorbed	Plasma protein-bound	Elimination of absorbed drug and metabolites
Acarbose	Up to 3 x 100 mg/day	<2%*	–	Urine
Miglitol	Up to 3 x 100 mg/day	>95%†	negligible	Urine
Voglibose	Up to 3 x 5 mg/day	<5%	–	Urine

* About 30% absorbed as metabolites produced by intestinal bacteria.
† Where doses are submaximal, <70% of a maximum dose is absorbed.

normal disaccharide and oligosaccharide substrates into absorbable monosaccharides. The varying affinities with which the inhibitors bind to the enzymes give the inhibitors slightly different activity profiles. Acarbose shows greatest affinity for glycoamylase, then sucrase, then maltase, and then the dextrinases, while miglitol is an especially potent inhibitor of sucrase, and voglibose is generally more potent than acarbose on other α-glucosidases.

The consequence of inhibiting α-glucosidase activity is to defer the completion of carbohydrate digestion until the substrate is further along the intestinal tract. This, in turn, delays and spreads glucose absorption over a longer period, which reduces the height of the post-prandial hyperglycaemic peak, but prolongs its duration. Thus, α-glucosidase inhibitors must be taken with meals containing digestible carbohydrate (not monosaccharides). These inhibitors do not significantly affect the absorption of glucose itself, but miglitol does interfere slightly with sodium-dependent glucose transport across the brush border.

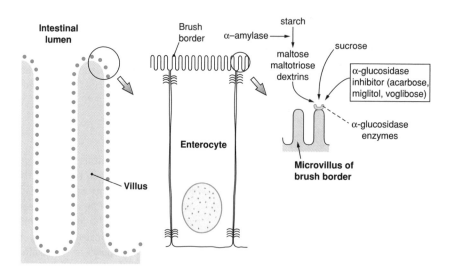

Figure 9.2
α-glucosidase inhibitors (acarbose, miglitol and voglibose) competitively inhibit the activity of α-glucosidase enzymes in the brush border of intestinal enterocytes.

Because the α-glucosidase inhibitors move glucose absorption more distally along the intestinal tract, they alter the release of intestinal hormones that are dependent on glucose absorption. Thus secretion of gastric inhibitory polypeptide (GIP), mainly from the jejunal mucosa, may be reduced by α-glucosidase inhibitors. In contrast, secretion of glucagon-like peptide-1 (7-36 amide) (GLP-1), mainly from the ileal mucosa, is increased by α-glucosidase inhibitors. Both GIP and GLP-1 enhance nutrient-induced insulin secretion, and these alterations probably balance each other out. Overall, the α-glucosidase inhibitors usually reduce post-prandial insulin concentrations because of the smaller rise in post-prandial glycaemia. Although lower concentrations of insulin and glucose during the post-prandial period imply a reduction in insulin resistance, euglycaemic hyperinsulinaemic clamp studies have demonstrated little improvement in insulin sensitivity.

Indications and contraindications

An α-glucosidase inhibitor can be used as adjunctive monotherapy for type 2 patients who are not adequately controlled by non-pharmacological measures. Because α-glucosidase inhibitors reduce post-prandial hyperglycaemia they can be a useful first-line monotherapy in patients who have only slightly raised basal glucose concentrations but more severe post-prandial hyperglycaemia. They can also be used as combination therapy in patients inadequately controlled with other classes of oral antidiabetic agent or insulin (Table 9.2).

When starting therapy with an α-glucosidase inhibitor, it is important to establish that the patient's meals are consistently rich in complex carbohydrate. The selected α-glucosidase inhibitor should always be taken with meals starting with a low dose and titrating up slowly. Monitoring of glycaemic control is recommended, although the post-prandially directed action of these agents is unlikely to induce hypoglycaemia. Thus, the α-glucosidase

Table 9.2
Clinical use of the α-glucosidase inhibitors.

Indications	Patients with type 2 diabetes inadequately controlled by non-pharmacological measures or other antidiabetic agents.
Type of therapy	Monotherapy, or in combination with any other antidiabetic agent.
Treatment schedule	Should be taken with meals rich in digestible complex carbohydrate. Dose should be titrated slowly to be compatible with meals.
Cautions and contraindications	Renal and hepatic disease; history of chronic intestinal disease.
Side-effects	Gastrointestinal disturbances (eg flatulence, abdominal discomfort and diarrhoea).
Adverse reactions	Gastrointestinal disturbances are occasionally severe. Very rarely associated with abnormal liver function.
Precautions	Serum creatinine and liver enzymes should be checked routinely if using high dosages.

inhibitors are antihyperglycaemic as opposed to hypoglycaemic agents. Limitations to their use are usually determined by tolerability to their gastrointestinal side-effects, which include flatulence. Patients who are already experiencing gastrointestinal problems – on metformin therapy, for example – are not good candidates for an additive α-glucosidase inhibitor, and treatment should not be given to patients with a history of chronic intestinal disease.

> Gastrointestinal side-effects are prominent with the α-glucosidase inhibitors

The hepatic effects of high doses of acarbose and its degradation products can occasionally increase liver enzyme concentrations, so it is recommended that alanine transaminase is checked regularly in patients receiving a maximum dose. If liver enzymes are raised, acarbose dosages should be reduced to a level at which normal enzyme concentrations are re-established. Since absorbed α-glucosidase inhibitors and their degradation products are largely eliminated in the urine, individuals with severe renal impairment are contraindicated.

Pregnancy and breast feeding are regarded as contraindications for *all* oral antidiabetic drugs, mainly due to caution and a lack of data, rather than evidence of any detrimental effect (page 50).

Efficacy

The main effect of the α-glucosidase inhibitors is to reduce post-prandial excursions of glycaemia. This, in turn, tends to smooth out the daily blood glucose profile, lowering post-prandial peaks and reducing interprandial troughs. Given as monotherapy to patients who comply appropriately with dietary advice, an α-glucosidase inhibitor will typically reduce peak post-prandial glucose concentrations by 1–3 mmol/l and occasionally by up to 4 mmol/l. The incremental area under the post-prandial plasma glucose curve can be halved in some individuals. Further, there is often a carry-over benefit of a small reduction in basal glycaemia of up to about 1 mmol/l. The accompanying decrease in HbA_{1c} is usually about 0.5%, but may be >1%, if a high dose of the drug is tolerated and dietary compliance maintained.

An α-glucosidase inhibitor can be used for additive efficacy in combination with any other class of antidiabetic agent, although there may then be a trivial reduction in the absorption of the initial drug. α-glucosidase inhibitors do not cause weight gain, can reduce post-prandial hyperinsulinaemia, and have been associated with a small lowering of triglyceride concentrations in some studies. Their ability to reduce interprandial hypoglycaemia and their generally good safety record are further advantages, but poor gastrointestinal tolerability has limited their use.

> The α-glucosidase inhibitors do not cause weight gain

Adverse effects

The most common problems experienced with the α-glucosidase inhibitors are gastrointestinal side-effects. If the dose is too high (relative to the amount of complex carbohydrate in the meal), then undigested oligosaccharides will pass into the large intestine, where they will be fermented by the resident bacteria, producing flatulence, meteorism, borborygmi, abdominal discomfort and, sometimes, diarrhoea. This is most likely to occur during the initial titration of the drug and can be minimized by slowing titration and ensuring that the patient complies with the dietary requirement of meals rich in complex carbohydrate. In some patients gastrointestinal symptoms gradually subside with time, which suggests that the gastrointestinal tract adapts.

Isolated cases of raised liver enzyme concentrations with acarbose do not seem to cause permanent abnormalities, and hypoglycaemic episodes are only likely to occur when an α-glucosidase inhibitor is used in combination with a sulphonylurea or insulin. No significant drug interactions are apparent.

> The α-glucosidase inhibitors are unlikely to cause hypoglycaemia as monotherapy

Sulphonylureas

Sulphonylureas have been the mainstay of oral treatment for type 2 diabetes for the past 40 years. This class of drug stimulates insulin secretion to lower blood glucose concentration (page 138).

> Sulphonylureas act principally by stimulating insulin secretion

Brief history

Sulphonamide antibacterial drugs were noted to cause hypoglycaemia in the early 1940s. Subsequent investigations into the chemical basis for this effect gave rise to the first sulphonylureas (carbutamide and tolbutamide) in the mid-1950s. By the 1960s, several so-called first-generation sulphonylureas as they were now known (eg acetohexamide, tolazamide and chlorpropamide) had become available, offering a range of different pharmacokinetic options. In the 1970s, however, a large multicentre trial in the US, the University Group Diabetes Program (UGDP), raised controversial questions about possible detrimental cardiovascular effects of sulphonylureas. These findings have not been confirmed by long-term clinical experience, however, and a succession of

more potent 'second-generation' sulphonylureas (eg glibenclamide – also called glyburide – gliclazide and glipizide) emerged in the 1970s and 1980s. Glimepiride was introduced in the mid-1990s and a slow-release formulation of gliclazide in 2000. Sulphonylureas currently used in the UK are illustrated in Figure 9.3.

Pharmacokinetics

The main differences between the individual sulphonylureas relate to their pharmacokinetics (Table 9.3). The duration of action varies from <12 hours (tolbutamide) to >24 hours (chlorpropamide), mainly due to differences in their rates of metabolism, metabolite activity and rates of elimination. All are well absorbed and most reach their peak plasma concentration within two to four hours. They are all

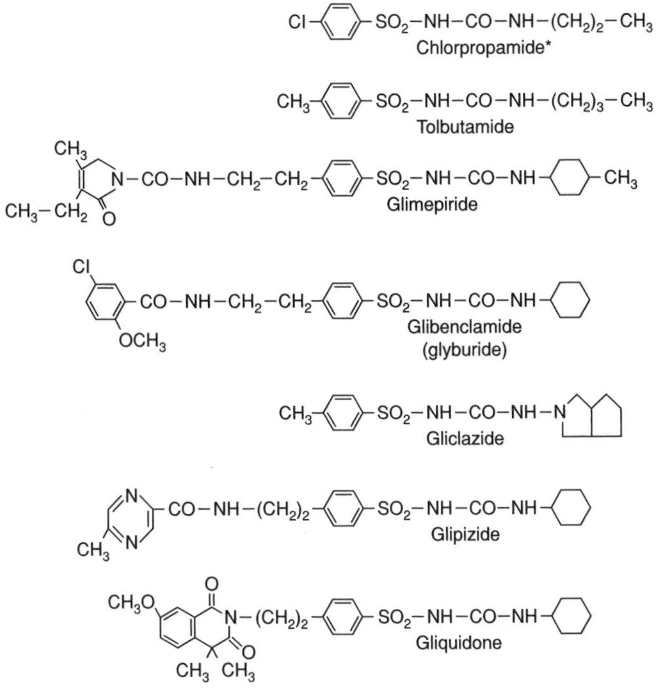

Figure 9.3
Chemical structures of the sulphonylureas chlorpropamide, tolbutamide, glimepiride, glibenclamide (glyburide), gliclazide, glipizide and gliquidone.
*Chlorpropamide is no longer recommended for new patients.

Table 9.3
Pharmacokinetic features of the sulphonylureas.

	Daily dosage (mg)[†]	Duration of action*	Activity of metabolites	Main elimination route
Chlorpropamide[1]	100–500	Long	Active	Urine >90%
Glibenclamide[§2]	2.5–15	Intermediate–long	Active	Bile >50%
Gliclazide MR[2a]	30–120	Intermediate–long	Inactive	Urine ~65%
Gliclazide[2a]	40–320	Intermediate	Inactive	Urine ~65%
Glimepiride[2]	1–6	Intermediate	Active	Urine ~60%
Glipizide[2b]	2.5–20	Short–intermediate	Inactive	Urine ~70%
Gliquidone[2]	15–180	Short–intermediate	Inactive	Bile ~95%
Tolbutamide[‡1]	500–2000	Short	Inactive	Urine ~100%

* Long = >24 hours; intermediate = 12–24 hours; short = <12 hours.
† Large dosages should be divided and related to meal pattern.
‡ Should be taken immediately before meals.
§ Glibenclamide is also known as glyburide (micronized formulation available in US).
[1] = first-generation sulphonylurea; [2] = second-generation sulphonylurea; [a] = modified-release formulation of gliclazide (Diamicron MR);
[b] = extended-release formulation (intermediate duration) of glipizide (Glucotrol XL).

metabolized by the liver, but their metabolites and routes of elimination vary considerably. Since all are highly protein-bound they can interact with other highly protein-bound drugs (eg the salicylates, sulphonamides, and warfarin), which can increase the potential for hypoglycaemia.

> Sulphonylureas are highly protein-bound in the circulation and there is increased potential for hypoglycaemia when they are administered with other protein-bound drugs

Mode of action

The sulphonylureas stimulate insulin secretion through a direct effect on the pancreatic β-cells. They bind to the sulphonylurea receptor (SUR1) on these cells, which is a component of the transmembrane complex that houses the ATP-sensitive Kir 6.2 potassium channels (K-ATP channels). Binding of the sulphonylurea closes K-ATP channels, reducing potassium efflux and favouring membrane depolarization. In turn, depolarization opens voltage-dependent calcium channels, increasing calcium influx, raising intracellular calcium concentrations and activating calcium-dependent proteins that control the release of insulin granules (Figure 9.4). In this way, the sulphonylureas lead to a prompt release of pre-formed insulin granules adjacent to the plasma membrane (first-phase insulin release). They subsequently increase the extended (second) phase of insulin release which begins about 10 minutes later as insulin granules are translocated to the membrane from deeper within the β-cell and new granules are formed. The increased release of insulin continues as long as drug stimulation continues, provided the β-cells are functionally capable. The sulphonylureas may also potentiate insulin release through SURs on insulin granules and through activation of protein kinase C. They can cause hypoglycaemia because they initiate insulin release when glucose concentrations are below the normal threshold for glucose-stimulated insulin release (about 5 mmol/l).

This class of drug also seems to exert some weak extra-pancreatic effects which suppress hepatic gluconeogenesis and potentiate insulin-mediated glucose uptake into muscle and adipose tissue. These actions generally require supra-therapeutic concentrations and are probably not clinically relevant. The sulphonylureas have been shown to transiently stimulate and then suppress glucagon secretion by isolated islets, but this effect is not considered to impact significantly on their clinical action. The hepatic extraction of insulin has been reduced by sulphonylureas in some studies, which could help to increase the systemic availability of insulin.

Indications and contraindications

Sulphonylureas have remained a popular first-line oral antidiabetic drug choice for type 2 patients who have not achieved or maintained adequate glycaemic control with non-pharmacological measures (Table 9.4). They are usually preferred for patients who are not overweight since they can cause weight gain, but the availability of sulphonylureas with

different pharmacokinetic properties has provided a choice of agent to accommodate the needs of patients with other medical conditions and contraindications or intolerance to other therapies. The sulphonylureas can be used in combination with any differently acting oral antidiabetic agent and have been used in combination with bedtime insulin in some, although this is not a widely accepted practice in the UK. Chlorpropamide is no longer recommended for new patients.

Starting sulphonylurea therapy, or indeed any other antidiabetic drug therapy, must be considered carefully within the context of the

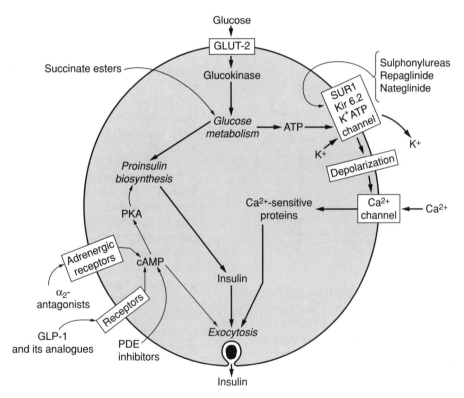

Figure 9.4
The insulin-releasing effect of sulphonylureas and other agents on the pancreatic β-cell. Sulphonylurea binds to the sulphonylurea receptor (SUR1) within the plasma membrane of the pancreatic β-cell. This binding closes the Kir 6.2 potassium channels, reducing potassium efflux, depolarizing the cell, and opening voltage-dependent calcium influx channels. Subsequently, raised levels of intracellular calcium bring about insulin release. Sulphonylureas may also enhance nutrient-stimulated insulin secretion through other actions on the β-cell. GLUT-2 = glucose transporter isoform-2; GLP-1 = glucagon-like peptide 1 (7–36 amide); PDE = phosphodiesterase; cAMP = cyclic adenosine monophosphate; PKA = protein kinase A; Kir 6.2 K+ ATP channel = adenosine triphosphate-sensitive potassium inwardly-rectifying channel.

Table 9.4
Clinical use of the sulphonylureas.

Indications	Patients with type 2 diabetes inadequately controlled by non-pharmacological measures or other types of oral antidiabetic agents.
Type of therapy	Monotherapy, or in combination with other antidiabetic agents (except other insulin-releasing agents).
Treatment schedule	A low dose to begin with, escalated slowly. Schedule should be adjusted if necessary to minimize the risk of hypoglycaemia. Maximum effect may be achieved before the maximum permitted dose is reached.
Cautions and contraindications	Should be used cautiously in patients with hepatic or renal disease (see pharmacokinetics) or porphyria.
Side-effects	Occasional, usually transient, sensitivity reactions. Chlorpropamide can lead to facial flushing after alcohol has been consumed – rarely, it causes hyponatraemia.
Adverse reactions	Risk of hypoglycaemia, especially with high doses of longer-acting preparations.
Precautions	Interactions with other protein-bound drugs such as the salicylates and sulphonamides.

overall care plan. An assessment of which agent is most likely to achieve the therapeutic goals of the care plan must be made, taking full account of the accompanying medical and lifestyle circumstances and other commitments of the patient. Once an agent has been selected, contraindications should be checked again. The duration of action and route of elimination of the particular sulphonylurea may be important considerations if the prospect of interprandial hypoglycaemia is likely, or if renal or liver disease are a concern. Shorter-acting preparations and those without active metabolites are generally preferred for

individuals at risk of hypoglycaemia and the elderly. Transient sensitivity reactions can occur.

The starting dose should always be low and blood glucose monitored in an appropriate way (chapter 5) – for example, by a member of the care team every two weeks, preferably supplemented by home self-monitoring. Dosage may be increased at two- to four-week intervals as required, until the glycaemic target is achieved. If symptomatic hypoglycaemic episodes occur, an attempt should be made to confirm blood glucose level with home self-monitoring. In such cases, and where an increase in dosage produces no further improvement in glycaemic control, patients should be returned to their previous dose. It is not uncommon for the maximum blood glucose-lowering effect to be achieved far below the maximum permitted drug dosage – probably because the drug is already producing its maximum increase in insulin secretion for the patient's prevailing β-cell capability. Long-term glycaemic control should be checked using HbA_{1c} levels (or fructosamine if HbA_{1c} is not available).

If the glycaemic target is not achieved, the addition of another class of agent should be considered, with the same evaluation and titration procedure followed. If the new combination still fails to give adequate control, some patients may benefit from the addition of a third, differently acting, oral therapy, but compliance is known to deteriorate with the number of agents taken. If adequate glycaemic control is not achieved with a combination of oral therapies, it is quite likely that the natural history of the type 2 diabetes has progressed to a state of severe β-cell failure. It is then usually advised to switch to insulin therapy (page 165).

Always start with a low dose of sulphonylurea. Monitor blood glucose by an appropriate method and increase dosages at two- to four-week intervals as necessary until the glycaemic target is achieved

Efficacy

The blood glucose-lowering efficacy of sulphonylureas has been evaluated in many retrospective and prospective studies, and from over 40 years of clinical experience. Given as monotherapy in type 2 patients who are not adequately controlled by non-pharmacological measures, sulphonylureas usually reduce fasting plasma glucose (FPG) by 2–4 mmol/l, and this is usually associated with a decrease in HbA_{1c} levels of 1–2%. Since the hypoglycaemic effect of sulphonylureas is due mainly to increased insulin secretion, the effectiveness of sulphonylureas is dependent on adequate β-cell function, and is independent of age and body weight.

The progressive β-cell failure that occurs during the natural history of type 2 diabetes may require the sulphonylurea dosage to be increased when glycaemic control deteriorates. Rapid and uncontrollable deterioration of glycaemic control during sulphonylurea therapy, sometimes termed sulphonylurea failure, occurs in 5–10% of patients each year. The inability to maintain acceptable glycaemic control is generally similar for all sulphonylureas (and other oral antidiabetic agents), and reflects an advanced extent of β-cell failure. In other words, it is mainly disease progression, rather than drug failure and the term 'sulphonylurea failure' is something of a misnomer. However, some differences have been observed between individual sulphonylureas. In the UKPDS, the 'secondary failure' rate of chlorpropamide was higher than that of glibenclamide. Further, a five-year comparative study showed a lower secondary failure rate for gliclazide than either glibenclamide (glyburide) or glipizide. Individuals who have adequate β-cell function usually respond well to the sulphonylureas, and early use of sulphonylureas as first-line monotherapy in these patients is much more successful than late intervention in patients with little or no remaining β-cell reserve. Patients who respond well to the sulphonylureas tend to have less severe fasting hyperglycaemia on presentation.

Insulin concentrations during sulphonylurea therapy do not usually extend beyond the range observed in the non-diabetic population (including those with impaired glucose tolerance), and suggestions that sulphonylurea-induced hyperinsulinaemia might increase the risk of detrimental insulin-induced effects on the cardiovascular system remain unsubstantiated. Sulphonylurea therapy generally seems to have little effect on the blood lipid profile, although some studies have noted a small decrease in plasma triglyceride level and small improvements in other lipid parameters, possibly as a result of improved glycaemic control.

When a sulphonylurea is used in combination with another type of oral antidiabetic (that is not an insulin-releaser), the glucose-lowering efficacy of the sulphonylurea is approximately additive to the effect of the other agent (dependent, of course, on adequate β-cell function). Sulphonylurea–metformin combinations are commonly used, and once-daily sulphonylureas are convenient in this respect. Early use of combination therapy is indicated when optimal titration of a single agent does not achieve adequate glycaemic control. A combination of two different types of agent is more likely to achieve the glycaemic target and will also 'buy time' during which control is better maintained. If institution of combination therapy is only undertaken as a last resort after 'failure' of a single oral agent, it is likely that β-cell failure is already advanced and combination therapy will offer limited benefit.

Adverse effects

Hypoglycaemia is the most common and serious adverse event experienced with the sulphonylureas, and patients on sulphonylurea therapy should receive instruction as to how to recognize and prevent this side-effect, and how to react when the symptoms occur. Hypoglycaemia is less likely to occur in patients on shorter-acting and slow-release formulations, and more likely with longer-acting preparations and irregular eating habits. Hypoglycaemia is also more likely to occur in patients with good control. Estimates of the incidence of mild hypoglycaemia (ie hypoglycaemia not requiring assistance from another individual) are mostly based on patient-reported symptoms and are unconfirmed by blood glucose measurements. In the UKPDS, about 20% of patients treated with a sulphonylurea reported one or more episodes of hypoglycaemia a year and similar accounts have emerged from other studies. Glibenclamide (glyburide) causes mainly interprandial hypoglycaemia, while chlorpropamide reportedly causes hypoglycaemia mostly in the early mornings before breakfast. The typical symptoms of hypoglycaemia are listed in Table 9.5.

> Hypoglycaemia is the most common and severe adverse event associated with sulphonylurea therapy

The UKPDS reported that more severe hypoglycaemia (ie that requiring the assistance of another person or medical intervention) occurred in about 1% of sulphonylurea-treated patients a year. However, much lower rates – 0.2–2.5 episodes per 1,000 patient years – have emerged from adverse-event reports to the regulatory authorities and from physician questionnaires. The mortality risk associated with sulphonylurea-induced hypoglycaemia is about 0.014–0.033 per 1,000 patient years, with the longer-acting agents carrying the greatest risk. For comparison, the incidence of insulin-induced hypoglycaemia has been estimated as high as 100 per 1,000 patient years.

> Weight gain is a recognized feature of sulphonylurea therapy

Mild hypoglycaemic reactions require a reassessment not only of the choice of agent, but the treatment schedule, any intercurrent illness, any potential drug interactions (Table 9.6), and any modifiable features of the patient's lifestyle such as diet and meal patterns. Alcohol consumption can predispose to hypoglycaemia and should be reconsidered. The possibility of an acute cerebrovascular event should be excluded. Severe hypoglycaemic episodes causing neuroglycopenic coma should be treated in a similar manner to the insulin-induced severe hypoglycaemia (discussed in chapter 11 and opposite) but excluding the use of glucagon.

> Severe sulphonylurea-induced hypoglycaemia is a medical emergency

Table 9.5
Signs and symptoms of hypoglycaemia and actions to be taken by the patient.

Symptoms	Physiological mechanism	Onset occurs when blood glucose is: (mmol/l)*	Intervention required
Hunger, sweating, tremor, palpitations	Autonomic response to subnormal glycaemia	Below ~3.5	Take glucose-rich sweets, drink, or food
Cognitive dysfunction, incoordination, atypical behaviour, speech difficulty, drowsiness, dizziness	Neuroglycopenia (brain deprived of glucose)	Below ~2.8	Take glucose-rich sweets or drink, and seek assistance
Malaise, headache, nausea, reduced consciousness	Severe neuroglycopenia	Below ~2.0	Third party intervention required+
Convulsions, coma	Severe neuroglycopenia	Below ~1.5	Medical intervention essential+

*Approximate concentration of glucose in arterialized venous blood below which symptoms are induced by insulin infusion in non-diabetic individuals. Symptoms often seem to occur at higher glucose concentrations in diabetic patients.
+Glucagon is *not* suitable for treating hypoglycaemia in type 2 patients since it stimulates insulin secretion.
Hospitalization is strongly recommended for patients with severe sulphonylurea-induced hypoglycaemia.

Table 9.6
Drugs able to potentiate the hypoglycaemic effect of sulphonylureas.

Displace them from plasma proteins:	Salicylates, sulphonamides, warfarin, phenylbutazone, fibrates
Decrease their hepatic metabolism:	Warfarin, monoamine oxidase inhibitors, chloramphenicol, phenylbutazone
Decrease their renal excretion:	Salicylates, probenecid, allopurinol
Intrinsic hypoglycaemic activity:	Salicylates, alcohol, monoamine oxidase inhibitors

Other adverse effects which can occur with sulphonylurea therapy are sensitivity reactions (usually rashes), but these are transient, reversible and rarely lead to erythema multiforme. Fever, jaundice and blood dyscrasias are very rare. Some sulphonylureas have been noted to precipitate acute porphyria. Chlorpropamide, in particular, can lead to facial flushing after alcohol consumption, and has been reported to cause photosensitivity. This drug may also increase renal sensitivity to antidiuretic hormone, which very occasionally leads to sufficient water retention to create hyponatraemia. Conversely, glibenclamide has a mild diuretic action. Weight gain is a recognized feature of sulphonylurea therapy – typically a gain of 1–4 kg which stabilizes after about six months. This is attributed to the increased insulin concentrations with their anabolic effects and reduced loss of glucose in the urine.

> Severe sulphonylurea-induced hypoglycaemia has a high case-fatality rate

Cardiac muscle and vascular smooth muscle express various isoforms of the SUR which bind sulphonylureas with much lesser affinity than the SUR1 expressed by the pancreatic β-cells. Thus, while very high concentrations of

sulphonylureas can cause contraction of these muscles, this is not considered likely to be clinically significant at therapeutic concentrations.

> Longer-acting sulphonylureas, such as chlorpropamide and glibenclamide should be avoided in the elderly

Management of sulphonylurea-induced hypoglycaemia

Recurrent symptoms suggestive of hypoglycaemia should prompt a reduction in dose or withdrawal of sulphonylurea therapy. The importance of the effects of alcohol may be underestimated in elderly patients and the potential for drug interaction must always be borne in mind. Presentation with altered conscious level or focal neurological signs may lead to an erroneous diagnosis of acute cerebrovascular event, but the possibility of hypoglycaemia should always be excluded in patients with type 2 diabetes presenting with any of these features.

> All sulphonylureas have the potential to cause severe hypoglycaemia

Patients with severe sulphonylurea-induced hypoglycaemia should be admitted to hospital quickly; relapse following initial resuscitation with oral or iv glucose is well recognized and may necessitate prolonged iv infusion of dextrose. An iv bolus of glucose leads to further release of insulin, especially in subjects whose β-cell function is relatively well preserved. This predictable consequence of treatment, combined with the long duration of action of drugs such as chlorpropamide and glibenclamide, explains the tendency for hypoglycaemia to recur.

> Relapse after resuscitation is common in severe sulphonylurea-induced hypoglycaemia

The antihypertensive agent diazoxide and the somatostatin analogue octreotide offer a more direct approach by inhibiting stimulated endogenous insulin secretion; but although these drugs have been used successfully as adjuncts to iv dextrose, neither is licensed for this indication in the UK.

- *iv dextrose* – remains the mainstay of therapy; continuous infusion of 5–10% dextrose may be required for several days.

- *Diazoxide* – antagonizes the actions of sulphonylureas by opening ATP-sensitive potassium channels in the membranes of β-cells (pages 12 and 30). However, associated adverse cardiovascular effects, including tachycardia and orthostatic hypotension, may be hazardous in elderly patients who may have compromised vasculature or impaired baroreceptor reflexes.

- *Hydrocortisone* – has been advocated, but there is scant evidence of efficacy and high doses may lead to hypokalaemia.

- *Glucagon* – stimulates endogenous insulin release and therefore cannot be recommended.

- *Mannitol* – is advocated for cerebral oedema; dexamethasone is a widely used alternative.

- *Octreotide* – has been shown to be an effective and well-tolerated inhibitor of sulphonylurea-induced hypoglycaemia under controlled experimental conditions, but clinical experience in this indication is limited.

Serum potassium should be monitored and iv supplements administered if hypokalaemia develops – high plasma insulin levels will increase potassium transport into cells. Where chlorpropamide accumulation is suspected, renal elimination may be greatly enhanced by forced alkaline diuresis. General supportive measures and correction of any underlying or contributory factors, eg acute renal impairment, are also necessary.

Meglitinide analogues

The first phase of glucose-stimulated insulin secretion is diminished or lost early in the natural history of type 2 diabetes. Consequently, the plasma insulin rise during digestion of a meal is delayed. An initial surge of insulin release is particularly important for the suppression of hepatic glucose production, and failure to accomplish this in type 2 diabetes makes a substantial contribution to post-prandial hyperglycaemia. It is difficult to organize sulphonylurea regimens that give maximum insulin release during meal consumption and minimum insulin release at other times, but a group of agents known as 'prandial' insulin releasers, has emerged to produce a rapid but short-lived stimulation of insulin secretion. These, also known as the meglitinides, can be taken immediately before a meal so that the prompt stimulation of extra insulin release reinstates an initial surge of insulin and limits the raised insulin concentrations to the period of meal digestion. Repaglinide and nateglinide are the two meglitinides available for clinical use in the UK.

> Repaglinide and nateglinide constitute a group of rapid-acting secretagogues, meglitinides, also known as 'prandial' insulin releasers.

Brief history

The non-sulphonylurea portion of glibenclamide – a benzamido compound termed meglitinide – was shown to stimulate insulin secretion in the early 1980s. Derivatives of meglitinide, such as repaglinide, and similar compounds, such as the D-phenylalanine derivative nateglinide, have been developed as rapid insulin releasers. Repaglinide was introduced in 1998 and nateglinide in 2001.

Pharmacokinetics

Benzamido prandial insulin releasers differ from sulphonylureas in their structure (Figure 9.5) and most importantly in their pharmacokinetics.

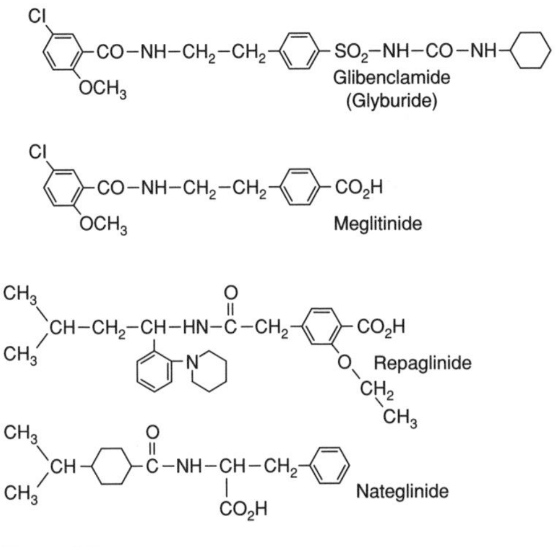

Figure 9.5
Chemical structures of meglitinide, repaglinide and nateglinide compared with glibenclamide (glyburide).

Repaglinide and nateglinide are rapidly absorbed. Absorption is almost complete for repaglinide and about 73% for nateglinide. Peak plasma concentrations are achieved within an hour, and >98% of the circulating drug is protein bound. Both agents are rapidly metabolised by the liver: repaglinide to inactive metabolites excreted mainly in the bile; nateglinide to mostly inactive metabolites eliminated in the urine. When taken about 15 min before a meal, repaglinide and nateglinide produce a prompt insulin-releasing effect. This is limited to about three hours for repaglinide or less for nateglinide, thus coinciding with the duration of meal digestion.

Mode of action

The mechanism through which benzamido prandial insulin releasers stimulate insulin secretion is essentially the same as that of the sulphonylureas. These drugs also bind to the SUR1 on the plasma membrane of the β-cell – but at a different site. This binding closes the ATP-sensitive Kir 6.2 potassium channel, leading to depolarization, voltage-dependent calcium influx, and activation of calcium-dependent proteins that control insulin release (Figure 9.4).

Repaglinide and nateglinide bind to a different site on the SUR1 to that of the sulphonylureas

Since the Kir 6.2 potassium channel is closed when either the benzamido binding site *or* the sulphonylurea binding site on the SUR1 is bound with its respective agonist, there is no additive advantage in giving a prandial insulin releaser in addition to a sulphonylurea. (The pharmacokinetic differences would enable the 'prandial' benzamido compound to bind before the sulphonylurea but this has not been translated into a clinical advantage). Due to the short half-life of the prandial insulin releasers, the insulin-releasing effect of these agents predominantly enhances the first phase and early second phase of secretion, and is not sustained as long as that of the sulphonylureas. No other actions of the benzamido compounds on the β-cell, or extra-pancreatic effects, have yet been established.

Indications and contraindications

In the USA repaglinide and nateglinide are indicated for use as monotherapy and in combination with metformin. In Europe the indication is the same for repaglinide, but nateglinide is only available for combination use with metformin. A 'prandial' insulin releaser could be appropriate for an individual with an irregular lifestyle in which meals are unpredictable and may be missed (Table 9.7). A prandial insulin releaser is also likely to benefit an individual who regularly experiences interprandial hypoglycaemia. Such cases require a reassessment of the choice of agent, taking full account of the pharmacokinetics, dosage and timing, and the potential for addition of an α-glucosidase inhibitor to help smooth out the daily glucose profile. Prandial insulin releasers can be used effectively in combination with any other differently acting oral antidiabetic (ie non insulin-releasing) agent, eg metformin. The protocol for starting repaglinide as monotherapy or either meglitinide as second-line therapy is similar to that for starting a sulphonylurea (page 139). A meglitinide should be taken 15–30

Table 9.7
Clinical use of meglitinides.

*Indications**	Patients with type 2 diabetes inadequately controlled by non-pharmacological measures or other types of oral agents that do not stimulate insulin secretion. Patients prone to interprandial hypoglycaemia on a sulphonylurea.
*Type of therapy**	Monotherapy, or in combination with other antidiabetic agents (except other insulin-releasing agents).
Treatment schedule	Take about 15 minutes before each main meal. The initial dose should be low (eg 0.5 mg repaglinide or 60 mg nateglinide) and escalated slowly to 4 mg or 180 mg, respectively before each main meal.
Cautions and contraindications	Should be used with caution in patients with hepatic or severe renal disease.
Side-effects	Occasionally sensitivity reactions, usually transient.
Adverse reactions	Risk of hypoglycaemia.
Precautions	Possible interactions with erythromycin, rifampicin, gemfibrozil and some antifungal agents.

*In the UK repaglinide is indicated for monotherapy and combination therapy; neglatinide is indicated only for combination therapy.

minutes before each main meal and begun at a low dose (eg 0.5 mg repaglinide or 60 mg nateglinide). The effect on glycaemic control should be monitored, and the dosage titrated up slowly to a maximum of 4 mg repaglinide or 180 mg nateglinide before each main meal if required. As with the sulphonylureas, if a titration step gives no further benefit or a hypoglycaemic episode occurs, the patient should return to the previous dosage, and if glycaemic targets are not met, early introduction of combination therapy should be considered. The main contraindications to meglitinides are

hepatic disease and severe renal impairment (see pharmacokinetics).

The possibility of hypoglycaemia (usually only mild) and the potential for interaction with drugs that are highly protein bound should be appreciated.

Efficacy

Clinical trials have noted that repaglinide (0.5–4 mg taken about 15–30 minutes before meals) increases insulin secretion and reduces post-prandial hyperglycaemia in a dose-related manner. A dose of 4 mg has been shown to reduce the incremental area under the post-prandial glucose curve by about one-third. With appropriate titration against the complex carbohydrate content of the diet, repaglinide's effect can be limited to the period of digestion. By timing the intake of repaglinide to about 15–30 minutes before the meal, the greatest stimulation of insulin secretion occurs during the early period (within about 30 minutes) of meal digestion, thus replacing the acute insulin response which is diminished or absent in type 2 diabetes and helping to suppress hepatic glucose production.

Chronic use of repaglinide has a carry-over effect to lower the basal glycaemia. Reductions in HbA_{1c} observed with repaglinide have been similar in magnitude to those observed with the sulphonylureas, ie 1–2%. Repaglinide usually shows a greater post-prandial glucose-lowering effect but a lesser reduction in fasting glycaemia, but has not been available long enough to enable comparisons with sulphonylureas over several years. Whether intermittent daily stimulation of β-cell function with such a prandial insulin releaser is different in the long term to more protracted daily stimulation of β-cell function remains to be seen.

Although nateglinide is not licensed as monotherapy in Europe, trials in type 2 diabetic patients have noted that nateglinide exerts a dose-related (60–180 mg) increase in insulin secretion and a reduction in post-prandial hyperglycaemia. Taken about 15 min before meals, nateglinide can reduce post-prandial hyperglycaemia similarly to repaglinide, showing a greater post-prandial glucose-lowering effect than sulphonylurea therapy but a lesser reduction in basal hyperglycaemia. Reductions in HbA_{1c} are typically about 0.5–1.0%.

Repaglinide and nateglinide have been used successfully in combination with metformin. Combination of a prandial insulin releaser with metformin or a thiazolidinedione should help to reduce the risk of severe hypoglycaemia in patients with good glycaemic control. A small increase in body weight can be expected in patients starting antidiabetic therapy with a meglitinide, but there is little change in weight among patients switched from sulphonylurea therapy. Plasma lipid profiles do not seem to be significantly affected by therapy with a meglitinide.

Adverse effects

Despite the short duration of action of the prandial insulin releasers, hypoglycaemia remains the predominant adverse effect. However its incidence is much lower than with the sulphonylureas – the number of serious events, in particular, appears to be reduced. Reassessment of opportunities to minimize the risk of hypoglycaemia is recommended in any patient experiencing such episodes (page 142). Sensitivity reactions, usually transient, have been reported with repaglinide, and the manufacturers suggest caution over possible interactions with erythromycin, rifampicin and various antifungal agents. Since meglitinides have a lower binding affinity for isoforms of the SUR in cardiac and vascular smooth muscle, the possibility of clinically significant cardiovascular effects remains similarly putative for meglitinides as for the sulphonylureas.

> Meglitinides are associated with a lower incidence of serious hypoglycaemia than some of the longer-acting sulphonylureas

Future therapies to improve insulin secretion

New sulphonylurea formulations

Changes in the formulation of some sulphonylureas have already been undertaken to modify their duration of action. For example, a micronized formulation of glibenclamide (glyburide) introduced in the US increases the rate of absorption and enables an earlier onset of action. A longer-acting ('extended release') formulation of glipizide (Glucotrol XL) has also been introduced.

A 'modified release' formulation of gliclazide (Diamicron MR) is now available. While the duration of action of gliclazide is unchanged, this new formulation uses a hydrophilic matrix to match progressive delivery of gliclazide with the hyperglycaemic profile. Improved bioavailability enables once-daily dosing, while reducing the dosage from 80 mg per tablet to 30 mg per tablet. (If blood glucose remains inadequately controlled, the dose, which is given in the morning, can be increased as required.)

> Modified-release formulations of sulphonylureas with improved bioavailability allow dose reductions

Fixed-dose combinations of metformin and glibenclamide (Glyburide) have long been available in a minority of countries. Glucovance, a new combination in the USA, combines glibenclamide (G) and metformin (M) at dosages of G1.25:M250, G2.5:M500, and G5:M500 mg. Also in the USA there is a fixed-dose combination of glipizide and metformin at dosages of 2.5:250, 2.5:500 and 5:500 mg (Metaglip). It is envisaged that fixed-dose (single tablet) combinations might simplify combination therapy for many patients. Patients with particularly marked hyperglycaemia after non-pharmacological treatment would be candidates for initiation of drug therapy with a fixed combination sulphonylurea–metformin regimen. The precautions associated with both classes of agent would apply, and any dose escalation would follow the procedure described previously (page 140).

A single-tablet combination of glimepiride plus rosiglitazone (Avandaryl) is in the advanced stages of development.

> Fixed-dose sulphonylurea–metformin combination tablets are available in some countries

Novel insulin releasers

A potential future approach to synchronizing insulin secretion with meal consumption involves analogues of the intestinal hormone glucagon-like peptide-1 (7-36 amide) (GLP-1). GLP-1 potentiates nutrient-stimulated insulin secretion via receptors in the pancreatic β-cell membrane which activate cyclic adenosine monophosphate (cAMP) and this increases the insulin response to a meal. It also enhances proinsulin biosynthesis and may additionally slow gastric emptying and induce satiety. Since GLP-1 is a rapidly degraded peptide, its therapeutic application requires injection or infusion. To obviate this problem, slow-release formulations, a sublingual preparation, and aerosol forms of GLP-1 are being evaluated. Two injectable analogues of GLP-1 are advanced in development: exendin-4 (Exenatide) – discovered in the saliva of an American lizard, and GLP-1 linked to a fatty acid (Liraglutide).

Interestingly, GLP-1 and analogues have recently been found to both stimulate division of β-cells and increase new β-cell formation from uncommitted progenitor cells in the exocrine pancreatic ducts.

It may also be possible to prolong the plasma half-life of exogenous (and endogenous) GLP-1 by administration of agents that inhibit the dipeptidyl peptidase 4 (DPP4) enzyme which degrades GLP-1. Several DPP4 inhibitors are in development.

A further novel approach to enhancing insulin secretion involves succinate esters which enhance the activity of the Krebs cycle in the β-cell. This stimulates proinsulin biosynthesis and insulin secretion. However, succinate esters can serve as a nutrient fuel in a range of tissues and provide a substrate for gluconeogenesis. Thus, this approach can only be exploited if the succinate esters are targeted predominantly at β-cells.

Imidazoline compounds can also stimulate insulin secretion, possibly both independently and through a mechanism involving closure of the Kir 6.2 potassium channels in the pancreatic β-cells. Imidazoline-binding sites have been identified in pancreatic β-cells, but are not yet fully characterized.

Pancreatic β-cells express several types of phosphodiesterase (PDE) and when some (eg type III) of these are inhibited, cAMP concentrations are increased and the initiation of insulin secretion (by other agents) is promoted. Again, specific targeting of the pancreatic β-cell would be required.

Further reading

Bailey CJ, Day C. Antidiabetic drugs. *Brit J Cardiol* 2003; **10**: 128-36.

Bailey CJ, Feher MD. *Therapies for diabetes*. Sherborne Gibbs: Birmingham, 2004.

Campbell IW. Antidiabetic drugs present and future. *Drugs* 2000; **60**: 1017-28.

Chiasson JL, Josse RG, Hunt JA et al. The efficacy of acarbose in the treatment of patients with non-insulin dependent diabetes mellitus: a multicenter controlled clinical trial. *Ann Intern Med* 1994; **121**: 928-35.

De Fronzo RA. Pharmacologic therapy for type 2 diabetes. *Ann Intern Med* 1999; **131**: 281-303.

Dornhorst A. Insulinotropic meglitinide analogues. *Lancet* 2001; **358**: 1709–16.

Groop LC. Sulphonylureas in NIDDM. *Diabetes Care* 1992; **15**: 737-54.

Harrower ADB. Comparative tolerability of sulphonylureas in diabetes mellitus. In: Krentz AJ, Ed. *Drug treatment of type 2 diabetes*. Auckland: Adis International, 2000; 77-84.

Inzucchi SE. Oral antihyperglycemic therapy for type 2 diabetes. *JAMA* 2002; **287**: 360–72.

Krentz AJ, Bailey CJ. Oral anti-diabetic agents: current role in type 2 diabetes. *Drugs* 2005; **65**: 385–411.

Krentz AJ, Ferner RE, Bailey CJ. Comparative tolerability profiles of oral antidiabetic agents. *Drug Safety* 1994; **11**: 223-41.

Lebovitz HE. α-glucosidase inhibitors as agents in the treatment of diabetes. *Diabetes Rev* 1998; **6**: 132-45.

Lebovitz HE (ed). *Therapy for diabetes mellitus and related disorders*, 4th edn. American Diabetes Association: Alexandria, USA, 2004.

Rendell M. The role of sulphonylureas in the management of type 2 diabetes mellitus. *Drugs* 2004; **64**: 1339–58.

Schernthaner G, Grimaldi A, DiMario U *et al*. GUIDE study: double-blind comparison of once-daily gliclazide MR and glimepiride in type 2 diabetic patients. *Eur J Clin Invest* 2004; **34**: 535–42.

10. Pharmacological treatment II:

Metformin
Thiazolidinediones
Future therapies to improve insulin action

Insulin resistance is an important pathogenic feature of most presentations of type 2 diabetes, and a logical therapeutic target. The biguanide metformin and the thiazolidinediones (TZDs) rosiglitazone and pioglitazone are the main agents currently available to act directly against insulin resistance.

Metformin

Brief history

Galega officinalis (goat's rue or French lilac), historically used as a traditional treatment for diabetes in Europe, was found to be rich in guanidine. In 1918 guanidine was shown to have a blood glucose-lowering effect, and several derivatives (eg galegine and synthalin A) were introduced as antidiabetic drugs in the 1920s. These were discontinued and all but forgotten as insulin became widely available, and it was not until the late 1950s that three antidiabetic biguanides were reported: metformin and phenformin in 1957, and buformin in 1958 (Figure 10.1). Phenformin was withdrawn in many countries in the 1970s due to a high incidence of lactic acidosis, and buformin receives limited use in a few countries, leaving metformin as the main biguanide. Indeed metformin is currently the most extensively used oral agent for type 2 diabetes worldwide.

Pharmacokinetics

Metformin hydrochloride is a stable hydrophilic biguanide which is quickly absorbed and quickly eliminated unchanged in the urine (Table 10.1).

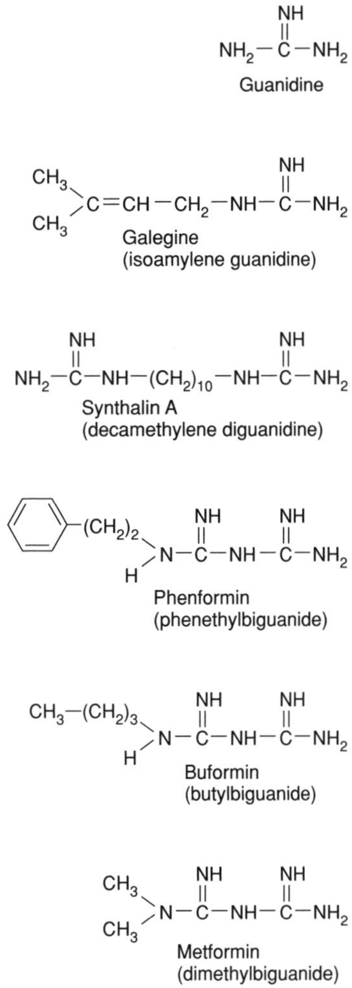

Figure 10.1
Chemical structures of guanidine, galegine, synthalin A, phenformin, buformin and metformin.

Table 10.1
Pharmacokinetic features of the biguanide metformin.

Time to peak plasma concentration	1–2 hours*
Plasma protein-bound	Negligible
Metabolism	Not metabolized
Elimination $t_{1/2}$	~6 hours
Elimination	Urine (approximately 90% eliminated in urine in 12 hours)

* 4–8 hours for prolonged-release formulation

Thus it is imperative that metformin is only prescribed to patients with sufficient renal function to avoid accumulation of the drug. Renal clearance of metformin is achieved more by tubular secretion than glomerular filtration, and the only significant interaction is competition with cimetidine which can increase plasma metformin concentration. There is little binding of metformin to plasma proteins, so metformin does not interfere with protein-bound drugs. Since it is not metabolized, it does not interfere with the metabolism of other drugs either. It is widely distributed, and high concentrations are retained in the walls of the gastrointestinal tract, providing a reservoir from which plasma concentrations are maintained. Nevertheless, peak plasma concentrations (about 2 µg/ml) are short-lived: in patients with normal renal function the plasma elimination $t_{\frac{1}{2}}$ for metformin is usually about six hours, and almost 90% of the absorbed dose is eliminated within 12 hours.

Mode of action

Metformin has a variety of metabolic effects (Table 10.2). It acts partly by improving insulin action and partly by effects that are not directly insulin-dependent. Metformin lowers blood glucose concentrations without causing overt hypoglycaemia. Its clinical efficacy requires the presence of insulin, but the drug does not stimulate insulin release and typically causes a small decrease in basal insulin concentrations in hyperinsulinaemic patients. The most evident blood glucose-lowering mechanism of metformin is its reduction of excessive hepatic glucose production (Figure 10.2). It reduces hepatic gluconeogenesis mainly by increasing sensitivity to insulin. Additionally it reduces the hepatic extraction of certain gluconeogenic substrates (such as lactate) and opposes the effects of glucagon. It decreases the rate of hepatic glycogenolysis, and the activity of hepatic glucose-6-phosphatase.

> Metformin has multiple metabolic effects; reduction of excessive hepatic glucose production is thought to be the principal mode of action

Insulin-stimulated glucose uptake and glycogen formation in skeletal muscle are enhanced by metformin. These involve increased movement of insulin-sensitive glucose transporters into the cell membrane and increased activity of glycogen synthase. Metformin also acts in an insulin-independent manner to suppress fatty acid oxidation and reduce triglyceride levels in hypertriglyceridaemic patients – this reduces the energy supply for gluconeogenesis and improves the glucose–fatty acid (Randle) cycle. Finally, preclinical studies have shown that metformin increases glucose turnover in the splanchnic bed (independently of insulin), which is likely to contribute to its blood glucose-lowering effect; it also expends extra energy to help prevent weight gain.

Table 10.2
Metabolic and other effects of metformin.

Antihyperglycaemic	Suppresses hepatic glucose output. Increases insulin-mediated glucose use. Decreases fatty acid oxidation. Increases splanchnic glucose turnover.
Weight control	Weight stabilization. Can assist weight reduction.
Improved lipid profile	Reduces hypertriglyceridaemia. Lowers NEFAs, lowers LDL-C and raises HDL-C in some patients.
Decreased hyperinsulinaemia	Decreases basal insulinaemia.
Not cause of serious hypoglycaemia	Serious hypoglycaemia very unlikely with monotherapy.
Counters insulin resistance	Decreases the endogenous/exogenous insulin requirement.
Vascular effects	Increased fibrinolysis. Decreased PAI-1.

NEFAs = non-esterified fatty acids; LDL-C = low-density lipoprotein-cholesterol; HDL-C = high-density lipoprotein-cholesterol; PAI-1 = plasminogen activator inhibitor-1.

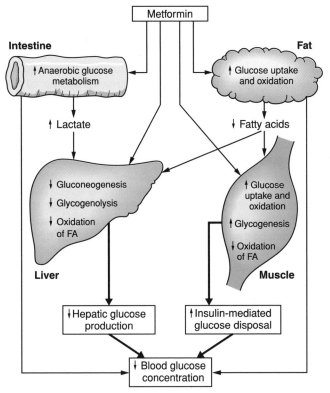

Figure 10.2
Mechanisms of action of metformin. FA = Fatty acids

At the cellular level, metformin can improve insulin sensitivity by increasing the insulin-stimulated tyrosine kinase signalling activity of the insulin receptor (page 20). Signalling is also increased through the enhanced activity of a range of post-receptor insulin-signalling pathways. Although metformin also increases insulin receptor binding when insulin receptor numbers are depleted, this is unlikely to have a significant impact on insulin action. The insulin-independent effects of metformin seem to result from changes in membrane fluidity in hyperglycaemic states and in the activities of certain metabolic enzymes. Collectively, the cellular effects of metformin counter insulin resistance and reduce glucotoxicity in type 2 diabetes.

> Metformin therapy also improves insulin action in skeletal muscle

Indications and contraindications

Metformin is customarily the therapy of choice for overweight and obese type 2 patients because it does not lead to weight gain. However, it is an equally effective antihyperglycaemic agent in normal-weight patients and is now used extensively as first-line monotherapy for type 2 diabetes inadequately controlled by diet, exercise, or lifestyle management. Metformin can be used in combination with any other class of oral antidiabetic agent or with insulin.

> Metformin does not lead to weight gain or serious hypoglycaemia

> Metformin is widely regarded as the drug of choice for overweight or obese patients with type 2 diabetes

Starting treatment with metformin should follow the same protocol as starting treatment with a sulphonylurea (page 139). The main contraindications are listed in Table 10.3. Patients are excluded if there is evidence of impaired renal function (eg serum creatinine >120–130 µmol/l or 1.4–1.5 mg/dl, dependent on lean body mass) to avoid the risk of drug accumulation. Cardiac or respiratory insufficiency, and any other condition predisposing to hypoxia or reduced perfusion (eg septicaemia) are further contraindications, as is liver disease, alcohol abuse, or a history of metabolic acidosis. Metformin can otherwise be used in the elderly, provided there is no renal insufficiency. It should be noted that the improved insulin sensitivity may cause ovulation to resume in cases of anovulatory polycystic ovary syndrome (PCOS). Indeed, metformin is often used 'off-label' in the treatment of PCOS. Under close supervision, metformin has also been used in cases of non-alcoholic steatohepatitis, although special caution is advised.

Metformin should be taken with or immediately before meals to minimize the possibility of gastrointestinal side-effects. The starting dose should be 500–850 mg/day (or 500 mg twice a day; one tablet with each of the morning and evening meals). Blood glucose concentration should be monitored and the dosage increased slowly (one tablet at a time), at intervals of about two weeks, until the glycaemic target is attained. As with the other oral agents outlined (chapter 9), if the target is not attained and a higher dosage produces no greater effect, the dosage should be stepped down, and combination therapy considered (eg addition of a sulphonylurea, prandial insulin releaser or thiazolidinedione). The most effective dose is usually about 2000 mg/day in divided doses with meals, but the absolute maximum allowed is 2550–3000 mg, dependent on country. A prolonged-release formulation of metformin (Glucophage XR in the USA, Glucophage SR in the UK) offers the opportunity for once-daily administration, and this may reduce gastrointestinal side-effects. Fixed-dose combinations of metformin plus a sulphonylurea are now available in some countries (page 148). There is also a fixed-dose combination of metformin plus rosiglitazone (Avandamet) (page 161).

Abdominal discomfort and other gastrointestinal side-effects are not uncommon during the introduction of metformin. Symptoms usually remit if the dose is reduced and re-titrated slowly, and only about 5–10% of patients cannot tolerate any dose at all. Unexplained diarrhoea in diabetic patients is sometimes linked to metformin. During long-term treatment, it is advisable to recheck

Table 10.3
Clinical use of metformin.

Indications	Patients with type 2 diabetes inadequately controlled by non-pharmacological measures or other oral antidiabetic agents.
Type of therapy	Monotherapy, or in combination with any other antidiabetic agent.
Treatment schedule	Metformin should be taken with meals and dose escalated slowly to a maximum of 2550 (or 3000*) mg/day.
Cautions and contraindications	Renal and hepatic disease; cardiac or respiratory disease or any other hypoxic condition; severe infection; alcohol abuse; history of acidosis; intravenous radiographic contrast media.
Side-effects	Gastrointestinal symptoms (eg diarrhoea); metallic taste; possibly reduced absorption of vitamin B_{12} and folic acid; ovulation in polycystic ovarian syndrome.
Adverse reactions	Risk of lactic acidosis if contraindications breached: risk of hypoglycaemia with combination therapy.
Precautions	Contraindications should be observed, especially renal function (eg creatinine level): interacts with cimetidine.

*Maximum dose varies between countries.

yearly for contraindications, particularly a raised serum creatinine level. In patients with poor diet, metformin can reduce absorption of vitamin B_{12} and a haemoglobin measurement is also advised. Deficiency of vitamin B_{12} sufficient to cause megaloblastic anaemia is, however, very unusual. Treatment should be temporarily stopped during use of iv radiographic contrast media, surgery and any other situation in which the exclusion criteria could be invoked. Substitution with insulin may then be appropriate.

About 5% of patients cannot tolerate any dose of metformin due to gastrointestinal side-effects

The contraindications to metformin must be observed

Standard monitoring of glycaemic control by home blood glucose measurement, or measurement of fasting or random plasma glucose or HbA_{1c} at clinic visits is recommended with all diabetes treatment programmes. Since type 2 diabetes is a progressive disease, it may be necessary to increase the drug dosages or move to another stage in the treatment algorithm at any time. Metformin alone is unlikely to cause serious hypoglycaemia, but hypoglycaemia becomes an issue when metformin is used in combination with an insulin-releasing agent or insulin.

Efficacy

The long-term blood glucose-lowering efficacy of metformin is similar to that of the sulphonylureas, but the mechanism of action is different. Optimally titrated metformin monotherapy typically reduces fasting plasma glucose (FPG) by 2–4 mmol/l in type 2 patients inadequately controlled on non-pharmacological therapy, which corresponds to a decrease in HbA_{1c} of 1–2%. While metformin's effect is dependent on the presence of some endogenous β-cell function, it is independent of weight, age and duration of diabetes. (As the United

Kingdom Prospective Diabetes Study illustrated, diabetes is characterized by a progressive increase in hyperglycaemia with time, principally due to deterioration of β-cell function, irrespective of the therapies used.)

Monotherapy with metformin offers several advantages. Its mechanism of action (it does not stimulate insulin secretion) means that it is unlikely to cause severe hypoglycaemia. Indeed, the reduction in insulin concentration, notably in hyperinsulinaemic patients, should actually improve insulin sensitivity by relieving the insulin-induced down-regulation of insulin receptors and suppression of post-receptor insulin pathways. Body weight tends to stabilize or decrease slightly during metformin therapy, and small improvements in the blood lipid profile may be observed in hyperlipidaemic patients. Thus, plasma concentrations of triglyceride, free fatty acids and low-density lipoprotein (LDL)-cholesterol tend to fall, while high-density lipoprotein (HDL)-cholesterol tends to rise. These effects appear to be independent of the antihyperglycaemic effect, although a lowering of triglyceride and free fatty acid levels is likely to improve insulin sensitivity and benefit the glucose–fatty acid cycle. In the United Kingdom Prospective Diabetes Study, patients who started oral antidiabetic therapy with metformin showed a reduced risk of myocardial infarction of 39% after 10 years. In addition to effects on body weight and lipid profile, several other potentially vasoprotective effects, including increased fibrinolysis and a reduced plasminogen activator inhibitor-1 (PAI-1) concentration, have been reported.

Metformin significantly reduced the risk of myocardial infarction in the United Kingdom Prospective Diabetes Study

Combination of metformin with a sulphonylurea, meglitinide, acarbose or a thiazolidinedione produces an additive blood glucose-lowering effect, provided that the combination is instituted before severe β-cell failure. Although there is an increased risk of hypoglycaemia, the other effects of the two agents in combination are generally intermediate – the weight gain seen with a sulphonylurea is reduced in combination with metformin, for example, while the insulin reduction and improved lipid profile seen with metformin monotherapy are lessened in combination. Consistent with its ability to improve insulin sensitivity, when metformin is added to patients on insulin therapy, a reduction in insulin dosage is usually required. At the same time, most patients also show an improvement in glycaemic control. Metformin reduces the weight gain associated with insulin therapy, and decreasing the insulin dosage in itself decreases the risk of hypoglycaemic episodes. The regimen usually involves once-daily long-acting insulin analogue or bedtime NPH or twice-daily NPH with metformin at mealtimes.

> Metformin may be usefully combined with the sulphonylureas, meglitinides, thiazolidinediones and insulin

Adverse effects

The most serious adverse event associated with metformin is lactic acidosis. The incidence is rare (about 0.03 cases per 1000 patient-years), but the associated mortality rate is about 50%. Since the background incidence of lactic acidosis among type 2 patients has not yet been established, it is likely that a proportion of cases are falsely attributed to the drug. Most cases in patients receiving metformin are due to malprescription. A commonly overlooked contraindication is renal insufficiency, which results in metformin accumulation. Excessive concentrations of metformin increase glycolysis to lactate, particularly in the splanchnic bed. The situation is aggravated by any co-existing hypoxic condition or impaired liver function. Although hyperlactataemia also occurs in cardiogenic shock and other illnesses that decrease tissue perfusion, metformin is usually

an incidental factor in such cases. Metformin should be stopped in all cases of suspected or proven lactic acidosis, however, regardless of cause.

Severe lactic acidosis is typically characterized by a raised blood lactate concentration (eg >5 mmol/l), decreased pH (eg <7.25), and increased anion gap (eg $[Na^+] - [Cl^- + HCO_3^-]$ >15 mmol/l). Presenting symptoms are usually non-specific but often include hyperventilation, malaise and abdominal discomfort. Patients with suspected metformin-associated lactic acidosis should be admitted to hospital promptly and treatment with iv bicarbonate commenced immediately, regardless of cause. If a raised plasma metformin concentration (eg >5 µg/ml) is found, circulating metformin can be removed by haemodialysis. Supportive measures to address any co-existing hypoxaemia or hypotension should also be initiated.

> Lactic acidosis is a rare but potentially lethal side-effect of biguanide treatment

Thiazolidinediones

The thiazolidinediones (TZDs) are agents which improve insulin sensitivity by stimulating a nuclear receptor known as the peroxisome proliferator-activated receptor-gamma (PPARγ). The TZDs are also referred to as PPARγ agonists, glitazones, insulin sensitizers and enhancers of insulin action.

> The thiazolidinediones are insulin-sensitizing drugs that stimulate PPARγ

Brief history

The antidiabetic activity of TZDs was described in the early 1980s and the first to become available for clinical use was troglitazone (Figure 10.3). Troglitazone was introduced in Japan and the US in 1997, but withdrawn in 2000 due to reports of fatal idiosyncratic

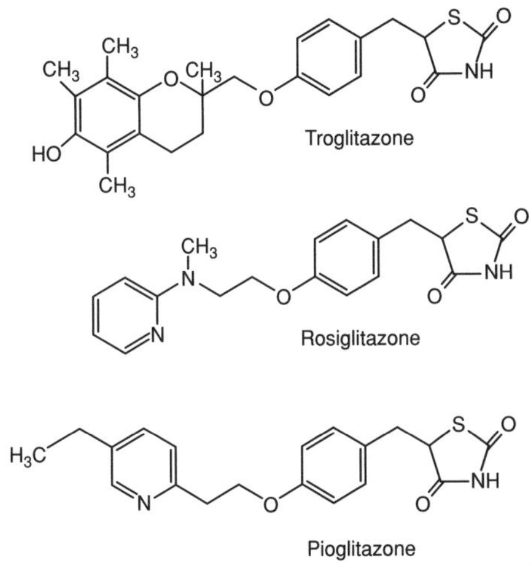

Figure 10.3
Chemical structures of the thiazolidinediones, troglitazone, rosiglitazone and pioglitazone.

hepatotoxicity. The drug was withdrawn by the UK distributor just weeks after its introduction in late 1997. Two other TZDs, rosiglitazone and pioglitazone, that have not been associated with this severe side-effect, were introduced in Japan and the US in 1999 and in Europe in 2000.

Pharmacokinetics

Rosiglitazone and pioglitazone are quickly and almost completely absorbed (peak concentration reached within one to two hours, slightly longer when taken with food) (Table 10.4). Both agents are extensively metabolized by the liver, rosiglitazone mainly to weakly active metabolites excreted more in urine than bile, pioglitazone to more active metabolites excreted mostly in bile. Rosiglitazone metabolism is undertaken mainly by CYP2C8, an isoform of cytochrome P450 which is not widely activated. Thus rosiglitazone interacts with few other drugs (paclitaxel, gemfibrozil and rifampicin). Pioglitazone is metabolized partly by CYP2C8, CYP3A4 and other isoforms of P450, and could potentially interfere with the metabolism of oral contraceptives, nifedipine and some other agents. However, to date, no significant drug interactions have been reported. Although both TZDs are almost completely bound to plasma proteins, their concentrations are generally low and they have not been reported to interfere with other protein-bound drugs.

Mode of action

Stimulation of PPARγ appears to be the principal mechanism through which TZDs enhance insulin sensitivity. PPARγ is mostly (and strongly) expressed in adipose tissue where it operates in association with the retinoid X receptor (RXR) to increase transcription of certain insulin-sensitive genes (Figure 10.4). These genes include lipoprotein lipase (LPL), the fatty acid transporter protein (FATP), the adipocyte fatty acid-binding protein (aP2), fatty acyl-CoA synthase and the insulin-sensitive glucose transporter, GLUT-4. Stimulation of PPARγ by a TZD will promote adipocyte differentiation and lipogenesis, and increase the local effects of insulin.

Table 10.4
Pharmacokinetic features of the thiazolidinediones rosiglitazone and pioglitazone.

	Rosiglitazone	Pioglitazone
Time to peak plasma concentration	Approximately 1 hour	<2 hours
Plasma protein-bound	>99%	>99%
Hepatic metabolism	Mainly by CYP2C8 to several weakly active metabolites	Mainly by CYP2C8 and CYP3A4 to active metabolites
Elimination $t_{1/2}$	Approximately 3.5 (100–150)* hours	3–7 (16–24)* hours
Elimination	Mainly urine (>60%)	Mainly bile (>60%)

* values in parentheses include metabolites.

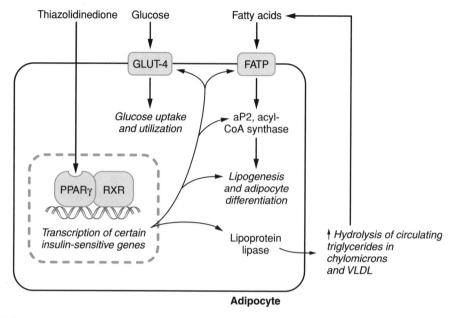

Figure 10.4
Mechanism of action of a thiazolidinedione on an adipocyte PPARγ receptor (peroxisome proliferator-activated receptor gamma). RXR = retinoid X receptor; GLUT-4 = glucose transporter isoform 4; FATP = fatty acid transporter protein; aP2 = adipocyte fatty acid-binding protein; VLDL = very low density lipoproteins.

> Activation of PPARγ seems to be the principal mechanism through which the thiazolidinediones promote insulin action

Stimulation of adipogenesis via PPARγ encourages differentiation of new small insulin-sensitive adipocytes, mainly in subcutaneous depots. Stimulation of lipogenesis via PPARγ reduces circulating non-esterified fatty acid (NEFA) concentrations which facilitates glucose uptake by muscle and insulin-sensitive adipocytes, and reduces gluconeogenesis in the liver by correcting the glucose–fatty acid cycle. TZDs can also reduce adipocyte production of cytokine tumour necrosis factor-α (TNFα) and the hormone resistin, which have been implicated in the development of insulin resistance (page 21). Also TZDs increase production of the adipocyte hormone adiponectin, which improves many of the metabolic and other actions of insulin. The lowering of insulin concentrations in hyperinsulinaemic patients, and the lowering of circulating triglyceride levels in some patients are further mechanisms which may help to improve insulin sensitivity.

PPARγ is weakly expressed in skeletal muscle and liver where it also appears to enhance certain insulin actions (Table 10.5). TZDs are reported to increase glucose uptake via GLUT-4 in muscle, and decrease gluconeogenesis in the liver, possibly by reducing expression of phosphoenolpyruvate carboxykinase and increasing expression of glucokinase.

TZDs, like metformin, are antihyperglycaemic, rather than hypoglycaemic, agents and require the presence of insulin to generate significant blood glucose-lowering effects. Their clinical efficacy is dependent on insulin levels sufficient to activate the genes listed above. They are not a substitute for the absence of insulin and they *selectively* enhance some effects of insulin on

Table 10.5
Metabolic effects of the thiazolidinediones.

Adipose tissue	Muscle	Liver
↑ Glucose uptake	↑ Glucose uptake	↓ Gluconeogenesis
↑ Fatty acid uptake	↑ Glycolysis	↓ Glycogenolysis
↑ Lipogenesis	↑ Glucose oxidation	↑ Lipogenesis
↑ Differentiation	↑ Glycogenesis*	↑ Glucose uptake*

* = an inconsistent finding.

cellular metabolism and differentiation: they do not enhance all insulin effects. Thus TZDs act co-operatively with insulin to create an insulin-sparing and glucose-lowering effect linked to their lipogenic activity. Interestingly, the glucose-lowering activity of TZDs remains evident in animals devoid of adipose tissue, demonstrating the importance of the less prominent effects of the TZDs on other tissues.

Indications and contraindications

Rosiglitazone and pioglitazone are available for use as monotherapy in non-obese and obese patients with type 2 diabetes inadequately controlled by non-pharmacological measures. In Europe TZDs are only indicated for monotherapy

when metformin is not appropriate. TZDs can also be used in combination with other oral antidiabetic drugs in patients inadequately controlled by monotherapy. In Europe (but not the USA) TZDs are not presently indicated for use with insulin.

The general principles for initiating treatment with a TZD are essentially the same as those for initiating sulphonylurea or metformin treatment. The main cautions are listed in Table 10.6. Rosiglitazone and pioglitazone can lead to fluid retention with increased plasma volume, reduced haematocrit and a decrease in haemoglobin. The risk of oedema and anaemia should be appreciated, and patients with any evidence of congestive heart disease

Table 10.6
Clinical use of the thiazolidinediones.

Indications	Type 2 diabetic patients inadequately controlled by non-pharmacological measures or other oral antidiabetic agents.
Type of therapy	Monotherapy, or in combination with any other antidiabetic agents.*
Treatment schedule	Pioglitazone (15 or 30 mg/day); rosiglitazone (2 or 4 mg/day). Dose should be escalated gradually up to a typical maximum of 45 mg/day for pioglitazone† and 8 mg/day for rosiglitazone.
Cautions and contraindications	Congestive heart disease; heart failure‡; oedema; anaemia; impaired liver function.
Side-effects	Fluid retention; increased plasma volume; reduced haematocrit; decreased haemoglobin; ovulation in polycystic ovarian syndrome.
Adverse reactions	Risk of oedema and anaemia: risk of hypoglycaemia with combination therapy.
Precautions	Check for contraindications; monitor liver enzymes (eg alanine transaminase) periodically; potential effect on oral contraceptive activity (pioglitazone).

*In Europe, monotherapy only when metformin not appropriate. Insulin combination not available in Europe. Also, only combination with metformin or a sulphonylurea indicated in Europe. Please refer to the product labelling sheet for specific indications in different countries.
†Maximum recommended daily dosage in combination therapy may vary between countries.
‡Definition of heart failure in the product label varies between countries.

or heart failure are contraindicated (although precisely whom to exclude on the basis of cardiac status currently varies according to the different product labelling sheets in Europe and the US).

Haemoglobin should be checked before starting a TZD, bearing in mind that reductions of up to 1 g/dl may occur during therapy. No adverse effects on blood pressure have been noted, despite the increase in plasma volume. Liver function should also be checked – by measuring serum alanine transaminase (ALT) level – both before starting therapy and periodically thereafter based on clinical judgement. Pre-existing liver disease or the development of elevated ALT levels are contraindications, although hepatotoxicity has not been a major concern with either rosiglitazone or pioglitazone. Precautionary checks of liver function remain because of the cases of fatal idiosyncratic hepatotoxicity seen with troglitazone.

> Liver function should be checked before and periodically during treatment with the thiazolidinediones

The starting dose should always be low – 2 mg rosiglitazone once or twice a day or 15 mg pioglitazone once a day. Glucose monitoring and dosage titration are important, particularly bearing in mind that the TZDs exert a slowly generated antihyperglycaemic effect. In fact, full expression of the appropriate dosage may not occur until two to three months after first administration – rosiglitazone 8 mg/day and pioglitazone 30 or 45 mg/day are commonly used dosages. If no effect is observed after three months, it is appropriate to consider the patient a non-responder.

Rosiglitazone and pioglitazone can be used in the elderly, provided there are no contraindications. In women with anovulatory polycystic ovary syndrome (PCOS) the improvement in insulin sensitivity may cause ovulation to resume.

Efficacy

The slowly generated blood glucose-lowering effect of TZDs in type 2 diabetes is explained by the substantial contribution of the nuclear effect, altering the expression of certain insulin-sensitive genes (Figure 10.4). Hence, maximal effect may take two to three months to occur, much longer than for other oral antidiabetic agents. It should be noted that not all patients respond to TZDs, and that the efficacy of this class of drug is highly dependent on adequate insulin concentrations being present.

> The thiazolidinediones require the presence of adequate quantities of insulin to exert their metabolic effects

Monotherapy with a TZD is likely to reduce fasting plasma glucose (FPG) by about 2–3 mmol/l and HbA_{1c} by 1–1.5%. Greater reductions may occur in patients presenting with marked hyperglycaemia but substantial insulin reserve. A similar glucose-lowering effect is often seen when these drugs are combined with those from another class (Table 10.7). Estimates of insulin sensitivity and endogenous β-cell function (based on analysis of basal glucose and insulin concentrations) have indicated that TZD addition improves both these parameters.

If switching oral combinations to include a TZD, triple oral therapy (eg metformin, sulphonylurea or meglitinide and TZD) is often used during the change-over period while the TZD is titrated up and one of the other agents titrated down. Permanent triple therapy has been shown to be effective in some studies and this is licensed for rosiglitazone in Europe.

In addition to improved glycaemic control, TZDs influence other aspects of metabolism. They invariably reduce circulating NEFA concentrations, one of the mechanisms, in fact, through which they can improve glycaemic control (page 158). Rosiglitazone seems to cause a small rise in total

Table 10.7

Blood glucose-lowering effects of rosiglitazone and pioglitazone in type 2
diabetic patients. Data from published controlled studies ≥4 months.

	Dose (mg/day)	↓ HbA$_{1c}$* (%)
Monotherapy		
Rosiglitazone	8	0.6–1.5
Pioglitazone	30	0.6–1.5
Combination with sulphonylurea[†]		
Rosiglitazone	4	0.9–1.1
Pioglitazone	30	1.2–1.3
Combination with metformin[†]		
Rosiglitazone	8	0.8–1.5
Pioglitazone	30	0.6–0.8
Combination with insulin		
Rosiglitazone	8	1.2[a]
Pioglitazone	30	1.2[b]

* = decrease from baseline; [†] = patients poorly controlled on existing treatment before
rosiglitazone or pioglitazone added in; [a] = average decrease in insulin dose of 9 units/day;
[b] = 16% of patients reduced their insulin dose by >25%.

cholesterol levels, but this stabilizes within three to six months. This increase is accounted for by a rise in both the LDL-cholesterol and the HDL-cholesterol levels, which leaves the LDL:HDL and the total:HDL ratios little changed or slightly higher. HDL-cholesterol levels may continue to rise after six months. Pioglitazone appears to have little effect on total cholesterol, but has been shown to reduce triglyceride concentrations in most studies. Both TZDs reduce the proportion of small dense (more atherogenic) LDL-cholesterol.

> Rosiglitazone and pioglitazone have some different effects on plasma lipids

Weight gain has been observed during TZD therapy, similar in magnitude to that seen during sulphonylurea therapy – typically 1–4 kg and stabilizing over six to 12 months. There is preliminary evidence that the distribution of body fat is also altered: visceral adipose depots may be reduced while subcutaneous adipose depots increase.

> Weight gain and oedema are prominent side-effects of the thiazolidinediones

There are data to suggest that the TZDs exert a range of effects on vascular function which might reduce cardiovascular risk. They have been reported to down-regulate plasminogen activator inhibitor-1 (PAI-1) and to decrease urinary albumin excretion to a greater extent than would be expected by the improvement in glycaemic control. TZDs can also increase vascular reactivity and reduce C-reactive protein (CRP) concentrations and carotid intimal-medial thickness. Preclinical studies have noted that chronic treatment of diabetic and glucose-intolerant animals with a TZD can preserve β-cell granulation and reduce β-cell failure.

A fixed-dose combination of metformin (M) plus rosiglitazone (R) (Avandamet) is available in the USA and Europe. Tablet strengths (mg) include M500:R1, M500:R2, M500:R4, M1000:R2 and M1000:R4, but not all of them are available in all countries. The combination reduces the tablet burden for those patients taking it. Precautions for both agents must be observed.

Adverse effects

Rosiglitazone and pioglitazone have shown encouraging tolerability. The precautions related to heart disease, oedema, anaemia and liver function include intermittent monitoring in accordance with package labelling. Pioglitazone has rarely been associated with an elevation in creatine kinase concentration and myalgia. More than mild hypoglycaemia may occur when the TZDs are used in combination with other antidiabetic agents. If contraindications arise during treatment, monitoring should be intensified and then, if necessary, treatment discontinued.

PPARγ is expressed by many tissues: activation of PPARγ in macrophages can reduce the production of some inflammatory cytokines and might affect atherogenesis. Stimulation of PPARγ in colon cells has been variously reported to increase and decrease cell division and differentiation in different animal and cell models.

Future therapies to improve insulin action

Other PPARγ agonists

Several novel TZDs and other types of PPARγ agonists have been shown to improve insulin action and glycaemic control during preliminary clinical trials in type 2 patients, and we expect these to be developed further. Several agonists of both PPARα and γ (so-called dual PPARs or PPARα/γ agonists) are under investigation. They have both glucose-lowering and triglyceride-lowering activity.

Vanadium salts

Early clinical studies have confirmed that vanadium salts improve glycaemic control in type 2 patients. They act within two to three weeks by reducing hepatic glucose production and enhancing insulin-mediated glucose use in muscle. These effects occur in part by an inhibitory effect on the phosphatases that dephosphorylate and deactivate the insulin receptor. Other cellular actions which could increase and mimic the effects of insulin have also been noted. Concern over the toxic effects of vanadium accumulation are a current challenge.

Insulin receptor-signalling enhancers

Other substances have been reported to enhance insulin receptor signalling by phosphatase inhibition or direct interaction with the insulin receptor, and compounds have been described that increase insulin action independently of the insulin signalling pathway, eg by affecting translocation of GLUT-4 glucose transporters or the activity of enzymes of glycogenesis, glycolysis and glucose oxidation directly. Few of these options have proved suitable for clinical evaluation. Lipoic acid, which has recently been tested for the treatment of diabetic neuropathy, has been reported to improve both insulin sensitivity and glycaemic control in clinical trials.

Other agents

Deficiencies in certain minerals, notably chromium and magnesium, are associated with decreased insulin sensitivity, and patients with these deficiencies have shown improved glycaemic control after supplementation with magnesium salts or trivalent chromium. Extra intake of the antioxidant vitamins C and E continues to produce equivocal effects on glycaemic control in the trials to date. Agents designed to inhibit fatty acid oxidation, inhibit glucose-6-phosphatase, or suppress the secretion or action of counter-regulatory hormones such as glucagon have been described, but have not yet given rise to viable treatments. The amylin analogue pramlintide is an injectable peptide that has been shown to improve glycaemic control through several neurally mediated effects, including delayed gastric emptying, decreased glucagon secretion and a satiety action. Pramlintide reduces weight gain and is currently being considered as an adjunct to insulin therapy.

Further reading

Bailey CJ, Day C. Antidiabetic drugs. *Br J Cardiol* 2003; **10**: 128–36.

Bailey CJ, Day C. Thiazolidinediones. *Br J Diabetes Vasc Dis* 2001; **1**: 7-13.

Bailey CJ, Feher MD. *Therapies for diabetes*. Sherborne Gibbs: Birmingham, 2004.

Bailey CJ. Potential new treatments for type 2 diabetes. *TIPS* 2000; **21**: 259-65.

Bailey CJ, Turner RC. Metformin. *N Engl J Med* 1996; **334**: 574-9.

Cusi K, DeFronzo RA. Metformin: a review of its metabolic effects. *Diabetes Rev* 1998; **6**: 89-131.

Evans AJ, Krentz AJ. Recent developments and emerging therapies for type 2 diabetes mellitus. In: Krentz AJ, Ed. *Drug treatment of type 2 diabetes*. Auckland: Adis International, 2000; 1-22.

Howlett HCS, Bailey CJ. A risk-benefit assessment of metformin in type 2 diabetes mellitus. In: Krentz AJ, Ed. *Drug treatment of type 2 diabetes*. Auckland: Adis International, 2000; 61-76.

Inzucchi SE. Oral antihyperglycemic therapy for type 2 diabetes. *JAMA* 2002; **287**: 360–72.

Krentz AJ, Bailey CJ. Oral anti-diabetic agents: current role in type 2 diabetes. *Drugs* 2005; **65**: 385–411.

Lebovitz HE (ed). *Therapy for diabetes mellitus and related disorders*, 4th edn. American Diabetes Association: Alexandria, USA, 2004.

Yki-Jarvinen H. Thiazolidinediones. *N Eng J Med* 2004; **351**: 1106–18.

11. Pharmacological treatment III: insulin

Insulin preparations
Insulin species
Duration of insulin action
Starting insulin therapy
Insulin delivery systems
Unwanted effects of insulin therapy
Special situations
Patient acceptability
Combination therapy with oral agents
Discontinuation of insulin therapy

Insulin is life-sustaining in patients with type 1 diabetes because of the absence of endogenous insulin production due to near-complete β-cell destruction. Insulin is often used to improve metabolic control in patients with type 2 diabetes. The United Kingdom Prospective Diabetes Study (page 59) highlighted the progressive nature of type 2 diabetes, showing that a substantial proportion of patients will eventually require insulin to achieve and maintain their glycaemic target (Figure 11.1). Others will be treated with insulin rather than oral antidiabetic agents because complications such as advanced diabetic nephropathy make insulin the safest option (page 89). Clinical trial data have suggested that insulin may decrease mortality after acute myocardial infarction (page 99) and insulin is often required temporarily in type 2 patients during other severe acute illnesses such as major sepsis, and surgery. Insulin is also regarded as the treatment of choice for gestational diabetes when dietary measures prove insufficient.

In the UK, about 20–25% of type 2 diabetic patients are estimated to require insulin within 10 years of diagnosis, although a greater proportion of patients, namely those who are inadequately controlled on other therapies, would probably benefit. In the US, >30% of type 2 patients are currently receiving insulin, partly because there was previously a smaller range of oral agents available in the US, but also because the US has a greater proportion of

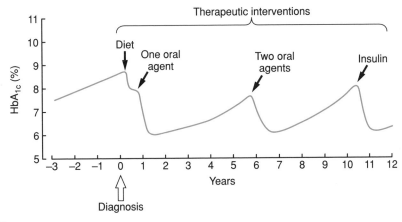

Figure 11.1
Typical changes in HbA$_{1c}$ values during treatment of a patient with type 2 diabetes requiring diet, then one oral antidiabetic agent, then two differently acting oral antidiabetic agents, and eventually insulin therapy, to control the progressive natural history of the disease.

severely obese type 2 patients whose condition cannot be controlled with oral agents.

In recent decades, developments in insulin manufacture have led to successive refinements, initially with improvements in purity, and then with the mass production of human sequence insulin. These advances have been coupled with advances in injection devices, making the practicalities much less daunting and more comfortable. Even after decades of experience, however, the optimal use of insulin and avoidance of its major unwanted side-effect – hypoglycaemia – remain elusive targets. The reality is that subcutaneous insulin injection can only ever approximate to the exquisitely sensitive response of normal islet β-cells to glucose and other endogenous regulators (chapter 2). Further, there are fundamental problems with exogenous insulin use:

- Delivery into the systemic rather than portal circulation causes plasma insulin concentrations to be equally high in both circulation systems (in the physiological situation, portal levels are much higher), so that hyperinsulinaemia is a common occurrence.
- Systemic delivery delays the onset of action, and results in a relatively prolonged effect, compared with endogenously secreted insulin; there is suboptimal matching of delivery peak and decline of insulin concentrations relative to meals. In particular, it is difficult to mimic the endogenous surge of insulin into the portal circulation at the beginning of a meal, which normally promptly suppresses hepatic glucose production.
- There is no scope for reducing plasma insulin levels in response to fasting or exercise once an injection has been given.
- It is difficult to control the fasting plasma glucose concentration (by suppressing hepatic glucose production) without inducing hypoglycaemia during the night.
- There is day-to-day variability in the absorption of intermediate-duration

insulin in individual patients – more than is generally appreciated.
- There is an accompanying need for dietary restriction, including consuming an approximately similar quantity of carbohydrate at a set (meal) time each day and the need for between-meal snacks to prevent interprandial hypoglycaemia in some patients.

Certain clinical situations present further considerations:

- Obese patients with inadequately controlled type 2 diabetes (common) and those with additional causes for insulin resistance (page 22) have higher insulin requirements.
- Insulin clearance is impaired by complications such as renal impairment (relatively common) or the presence of hepatic cirrhosis.

A selection of rapid-, short-, intermediate- and long-acting insulins, as well as mixtures of rapid–intermediate and short–intermediate insulins are available (Table 11.1). Finer needles, pen injector devices, new types of power injectors and mini-pumps now facilitate insulin administration.

Most patients will be started on insulin under the guidance of the local hospital diabetes resource centre or clinic. Some – the elderly, senile or infirm, for example – may be unable to self-administer insulin, in which case a responsible relative or district nurse is called in. Insulin therapy should always be accompanied by self-monitoring of capillary blood glucose by the patient where possible (page 65).

Insulin preparations
The variety of insulin preparations is daunting, but the types and methods of delivery can be summarized quite succinctly. Insulins are usually classified according to their onset and duration of action (Figure 11.2).

Table 11.1
Synopsis of insulin preparations

Category	Generic type	Examples	Onset of action (minutes)*	Duration of action (hours)*
Rapid	–	Aspart, Lispro	10–20	3–4
Rapid–intermediate	–	Novomix, Humalog	10	10–20
Short	Regular, neutral†	Actrapid, Humulin S, Insuman rapid	15–60	4–8
Short–intermediate	Regular–isophane (NPH) mixtures	Mixtard, Humulin M3, Insuman combo	15–60	12–20
Intermediate	Isophane (NPH)	Insulatard, Humulin I	60–120	12–20
Long	Crystalline zinc suspensions, 'Lente'	Ultratard	120–240	18–24+
	Long-acting analogues	Lantus (glargine) Levemir (detemir)	60–120	18–24+

*Times of onset and duration of action are approximate ranges that vary between individuals depending on dose and site of subcutaneous injection and pathophysiological state.
†Regular (neutral) insulin was previously termed 'soluble', but the term 'soluble' is no longer exclusively applicable to short-acting insulins.
+ indicates duration of action may exceed 24 hours.
NPH = neutral protamine Hagedorn.

With increasing use of more intensive (basal-bolus) insulin treatment regimens, it is becoming pragmatic to categorize insulins according to the timing and purpose of administration:

- basal (maintenance, background), eg intermediate, long-acting
- bolus (meal, prandial), eg rapid-acting, short-acting
- biphasic (mixed, premixed), eg rapid-acting + isophane (NPH), short-acting + isophane (NPH).

Insulins also vary in terms of:

- species and method of manufacture (animal-derived, semi-synthetic or synthetic)
- modifications which prolong duration of action
- designated mode of delivery (syringe, pen injector, or infusion device, for example)

- strength – in the UK, all insulin preparations contain 100 units/ml (U100). Other strengths (U40, U80 and U500) are available in some other countries (or can be obtained by special request to the manufacturer).

Insulin species

Therapeutic insulin is derived from three sources:

Bovine

Bovine insulin is extracted from cattle pancreas. It is effectively obsolete but still available for patients who have been using it for many years. Long-term use is often associated with the presence of anti-insulin antibodies. Bovine insulin differs from human insulin (Figure 2.1) in three amino acids: A8 alanine, A10 valine and B30 alanine.

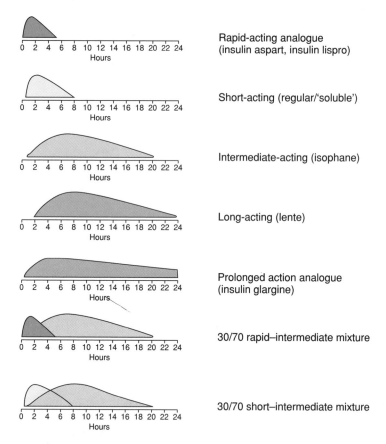

Figure 11.2
Approximate times of onset and durations of action of various insulins following subcutaneous injection.

Porcine

Porcine insulin differs from human insulin in a single amino-acid (alanine replaces threonine at B30). It is reserved mainly for patients with type 1 diabetes who have experienced a decrease in the warning symptoms for hypoglycaemia with human insulin.

Human

Human insulin is most commonly used and now manufactured predominantly using recombinant DNA technology. Chemical (enzymatic) modification of porcine insulin (emp) is still employed by one major manufacturer (Novo Nordisk) in the production of so-called 'semi-synthetic' insulin. The method of manufacture is always stated on the bottle:

- *prb* – produced from the precursor molecule proinsulin and synthesized using recombinant DNA by bacteria containing the human proinsulin gene
- *pyr* – produced recombinantly from a precursor synthesized by yeast
- *ge* – genetically engineered – a more generic label.

Animal-derived insulins are unacceptable to devout followers of Islam and Judaism and to strict vegans.

Analogues

Recently introduced insulin analogues (rapid-acting lispro and aspart, long-acting detemir, and prolonged duration insulin glargine) are genetically engineered:

Lispro differs from human insulin by the transposition of two amino acids on the B chain; from B28 proline and B29 lysine to B28 lysine and B29 proline (lys–pro becoming 'lispro'). In *aspart*, aspartate replaces proline at position B28.

For *glargine* two additional arginine molecules (B31 arginine and B32 arginine) are located at the C-terminus of the B-chain, conferring additional positive charges and thereby altering the isoelectric point. In addition, asparagine is replaced by arginine at A21, to confer stability.

For *detemir*, the B29 lysine is acylated with a C14 fatty acid side chain (myristic acid) and the B30 threonine has been deleted.

Duration of insulin action

Short-acting insulins

Short-acting insulins are also known as regular, neutral and unmodified insulins. The term 'soluble' was previously used to describe short-acting insulins, but this is no longer exclusively applicable to short-acting insulins. Short-acting insulins differ slightly in their pharmacokinetics according to species. Onset of action following subcutaneous injection is fastest for human, followed by porcine, then bovine insulin.

> Human sequence short-acting insulins have a slightly faster onset and shorter duration of action than animal insulins

These differences, which may reflect lipophilic properties, are minor. For insulin to exert its effects in target tissues it must be absorbed from the subcutaneous injection site and diffuse from the interstitial space into the circulation. The rate at which this occurs is the principal determinant of the speed of onset of action, but other factors that influence pharmacokinetics include:

- site of injection – absorption from abdominal wall is faster than from thigh
- volume injected – smaller volumes are more quickly absorbed
- local mechanical factors – massage of injection site or exercise of local muscles will increase absorption rate.

Insulin can become denatured and lose efficacy if exposed to extremes of high or low temperature; storage at 4°C in a domestic refrigerator is usually recommended, freezing is not. Following subcutaneous injection of a human short-acting insulin preparation, the action profile is likely to be:

- onset around 30 minutes
- peak at one to three hours
- duration of four to eight hours.

When injected intravenously, the plasma half-life of a short-acting insulin is less than five minutes; continuous infusion is therefore required to maintain plasma levels. The only notable exceptions are when an iv bolus is required in a diagnostic endocrine test (eg the insulin tolerance test), when possible severe insulin resistance is being assessed, or for research purposes. Short-acting and rapid-acting insulins are the only preparations suitable for iv administration – other insulins must be injected subcutaneously.

> Rapid-acting and short-acting insulins are suitable for iv use

Pharmacokinetic properties dictate the timing of injections of short-acting insulin. Ideally, subcutaneous injections should take place 30–45 minutes before meals, in order to match peak action to glucose absorption from the gastrointestinal tract – but this is not always practical. A delayed meal carries the risk of hypoglycaemia. For an elderly patient, possibly senile, or reliant on a third party for insulin administration, it may be safer to ensure that the meal has been eaten first (tight glycaemic control is not usually an objective of treatment for such patients, and pharmacokinetic considerations are less of a concern). In contrast, patients using pen injection devices may prefer to take their insulin as the meal is served – although this applies more to rapid-acting insulins.

Rapid-acting insulins

The amino acid substitutions within these insulin molecules (page 169) reduce the tendency of the molecules to self-associate (as dimers and hexamers). This results in more rapid absorption into the bloodstream after subcutaneous injection (Figure 11.3). Compared with human short-acting insulin, rapid-acting insulins (eg aspart and lispro) are characterized by an earlier peak and reduced duration of action:

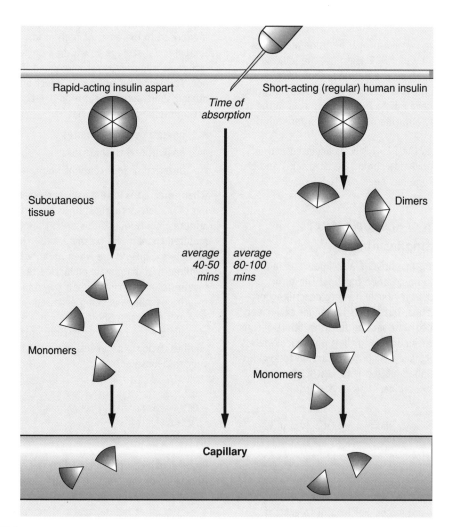

Figure 11.3
Rapid-acting insulin aspart dissociates into monomers more quickly than regular short-acting insulin. Adapted from Heller S. *Prescriber* 2000; **11**: 47-53.

- onset at 10–20 minutes
- peak at 40–60 minutes
- duration of three to four hours.

The rapid-acting analogues are an alternative to short-acting insulin, designed for use immediately before (or even just after) meals (Figure 11.4). Compared with human short-acting insulin, they produce an additional reduction in post-prandial peak glucose concentration of about 1–2 mmol/l. In patients with type 2 diabetes, they are conveniently administered as pre-mixed (biphasic) preparations suitable for twice-daily use.

Twice-daily mixtures

Short-acting insulins may be mixed in the syringe with longer-acting preparations (isophane or, less commonly, lente). If insulins are mixed at home or in the surgery, the short-acting preparation *must* be drawn into the syringe before the longer-acting preparation to avoid contaminating the short-acting vial with protamine or zinc. Fixed, premixed combinations are also available: 30/70, eg Humulin M3, Human Mixtard 30 are 30:70 ratios of short to isophane. This book uses the European nomenclature, which states the percentage of the shorter-acting insulin before the percentage of the longer-acting

component. A 30/70 mixture twice daily is often favoured in the UK (Figure 11.5). If the glucose profile suggests it might be advantageous, it is acceptable to use a different preparation for the morning and evening injection.

Pre-mixed preparations comprising a mixture of rapid-acting analogues and protamine have been designed for administration immediately before (or in some circumstances just after) meals. Examples are Humalog Mix 25 comprising lispro and neutral protamine-lispro (25% and 75% respectively), or Novomix 30 comprising aspart and protamine-aspart (30% and 70% respectively).

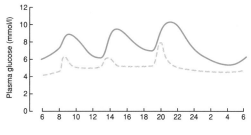

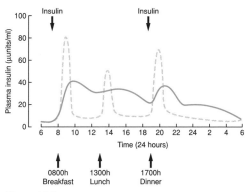

Figure 11.5
Daily plasma glucose and insulin profiles of a non-diabetic individual (- - - -) and a patient with type 2 diabetes (———). The type 2 diabetic patient was treated twice daily with a mixture of short- and intermediate-acting insulin. A slightly larger dose of both was given in the morning before breakfast than in the evening before dinner.

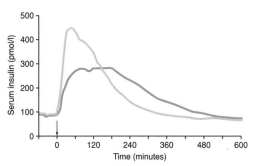

Figure 11.4
Serum insulin levels rise and fall rapidly with insulin aspart. Reproduced with permission from Heller S. *Prescriber* 2000; **11**: 47-53. - - - - = insulin aspart; ——— = short-acting insulin.

The nomenclature for premixed insulins varies from country to country.

In Europe the percentage of the shorter-acting insulin ingredient is stated first; in the US the percentage of the longer-acting ingredient is stated first

Multiple daily ('basal–bolus') injections

Another approach is to administer a longer-acting *'basal'* insulin at bedtime (around 2200 hours) to provide control until the morning, then to administer short-acting insulin injections ('bolus') approximately 30 minutes before breakfast, lunch and dinner. Coupled with frequent blood glucose testing, this regimen forms the basis for so-called intensified insulin therapy (or 'basal–bolus' regimen) in pursuit of a near-normal daily glucose profile, and is encouraged, where appropriate, in type 1 patients (see Figure 11.6). It may also be useful in some type 2 patients, particularly those who require insulin during pregnancy (once-daily injection of a medium- or long-acting insulin is rarely sufficient). Multiple injections may be unsuitable for elderly or infirm patients, in whom excellent glycaemic control is not the

primary objective. Increasing insulin dose to reduce fasting hyperglycaemia increases the risk of hypoglycaemia during interprandial periods, especially at night. A general guide is that if the patient requires a total daily dose of ≥30–40 units, this is split into two or more injections. The exception is when insulin is administered solely at bedtime to type 2 patients whose principal aim is to control a severely raised fasting plasma glucose concentration. Insulin glargine appears to be especially useful to such patients, by stabilizing insulin throughout a 24-hour period and reducing the risk of hypoglycaemia (page 173).

Intermediate-duration insulins; isophane

Insulin is complexed with the fish sperm protein protamine to produce an isophane preparation. Isophane preparations have a slower onset and longer duration of action than unmodified short-acting insulins and are known generically as isophane or neutral protamine Hagedorn (NPH). They are well-established and widely used and have the following action profile:

- onset at about one to two hours
- peak at four to eight hours
- duration of 12–18 hours.

Once-daily NPH or lente insulin regimens seldom provide adequate glycaemic control: twice-daily regimens are more effective

Such preparations (eg Humulin I, Human Insulatard) may be used twice daily as monotherapy. In type 2 patients who have been inadequately controlled with oral agents, a single morning dose is seldom enough. More commonly, morning and evening administration is required. The morning dose is often given in conjunction with a short-acting insulin and pre-mixed preparations, often termed *'biphasic'* or 'short–intermediate', are usually preferred in this respect. A twice-daily short–intermediate or rapid–intermediate pre-mixed 'biphasic' regimen

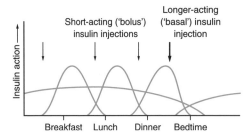

Figure 11.6
Typical intensive multiple daily ('basal–bolus') insulin regimen. A subcutaneous injection of a longer-acting ('basal') insulin is usually given at bedtime; glargine can, in principle, be administered at any set time. Short-acting or rapid-acting ('bolus') insulin injections are given before or with each of the main meals. Arrows show times of injections. → = longer-acting insulin; → = short-acting insulin.

may be used in which the pre-mix is given before or with the morning and evening meals.

A further alternative approach is to give an intermediate-acting insulin as monotherapy at bedtime, and to supplement it with an oral agent during the day. The principal aim of this type of regimen is to control pre-breakfast hyperglycaemia by suppressing overnight hepatic glucose production. The insulin-mediated suppression of fatty acid release from adipocytes may help to reduce glucose output from the liver by reducing the energy source for gluconeogenesis. However, waning of insulin action in the pre-breakfast period, possibly coupled with an intrinsic tendency for fasting plasma glucose concentrations to creep up at this time (the so-called 'dawn phenomenon') are factors that may detract from successful control. Because increasing the insulin dose carries a risk of night-time hypoglycaemia, a second injection pre-breakfast is often required. Increasingly, a single bedtime dose of isophane (NPH) or long-acting analogue is used in combination with daytime oral agents (page 186).

Long-acting insulins; PZI and lente preparations

Protamine zinc insulin (Hypurin bovine PZI, CP Pharmaceuticals) is not used much nowadays, although some patients have been successfully maintained on it for many years. It is a long-acting (>24 hours) insulin, but presents problems if mixed with short-acting analogues (excess protamine will tend to convert some of the short-acting into longer-acting insulin). Patients need not be transferred if this does not present a problem, but increasing the zinc content of the insulin preparation will result in amorphous (micro-crystalline) and crystalline insulins with prolonged action:

- onset at two to four hours
- peak at six to 18 hours
- duration of 18–>24 hours (amorphous, 18 hours; semilente, ie 30% amorphous, 70% crystalline, 18–24 hours; crystalline, ≥24 hours.

Lente insulin, such as Human Monotard (Novo Nordisk), is best used twice daily. Lente insulins contain an excess of zinc which can modify the action of a short-acting insulin if mixed in the same syringe. Although this should, in theory, delay the rise in plasma insulin concentration, in practice it seems to be of minor clinical significance as long as the mixture is prepared and injected without delay. Combinations of lente and short-acting insulins are not suitable for pre-mixed biphasic (short–intermediate mixed) preparations. Lente insulins have become less popular with the emergence of the biphasics.

Prolonged-action soluble insulins

The first example of a prolonged-action soluble insulin analogue, insulin glargine (Lantus, Sanofi-Aventis) became available in 2000. This analogue was designed to avoid the peak insulin concentration typically observed with conventional longer-acting insulins such as lente. Insulin glargine shows the following action profile (Figure 11.7):

- onset at about 90 minutes
- prolonged plateau, rather than peak
- duration of about 24 hours or longer.

While insulin glargine is soluble at acid pH in the vial, when injected subcutaneously it forms a microprecipitate at the injection site (because the latter is at a slightly alkaline, physiological pH). The stability of this microprecipitate slows absorption of insulin into the circulation, which means that a single daily injection can provide a fairly stable level of insulin for most of a 24-hour period, more closely mimicking the basal component of insulin secretion in healthy subjects. 'Basal' insulin secretion accounts for about half of all daily insulin secretion, the rest being secreted in response to meals. In principle glargine could be administered at any set time, although pre-breakfast or evening are usually preferred. The peakless action of glargine has been associated with a reduced incidence of hypoglycaemia (especially nocturnal episodes).

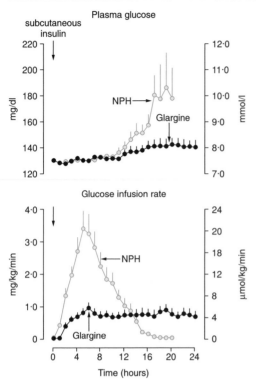

Figure 11.7
Plasma glucose and rates of glucose infusion required to maintain plasma glucose concentration at the target of 7.2 mmol/l in 20 patients with type 1 diabetes following injection of either 0.3 units/kg insulin glargine or NPH
Reproduced with permission from Bolli GB, Owens DR. *Lancet* 2000; **356**: 443-4.

> Insulin glargine is a clear solution – the era when all clear preparations were short-acting insulins has passed

Another clear insulin preparation with a long action is detemir, (Levemir, Novo Nordisk), introduced in the UK in 2004. Detemir has a fatty acyl group attached to the B chain (B29 lysine) of the insulin molecule which binds to albumin in the circulation. Detemir may not be quite as long-acting as glargine or as peakless, but it has been reported to produce very predictable effects on glycaemic control, with little day-to-day variability. There have also been accounts of fewer episodes of hypoglycaemia and less weight gain with detemir.

Starting insulin therapy

Indications

Insulin treatment should be considered for patients in whom glycaemic control has remained unsatisfactory with non-pharmacological measures and a combination of differently acting, optimally titrated, oral agents. It should also be considered for symptomatic patients with serious co-morbidity and for patients contraindicated for, or intolerant of, other oral therapies.

Procedure

The insulin starting dose is dependent on the extent of existing hyperglycaemia, whether or not the patient is obese, concomitant therapies and co-morbidity. If the HbA_{1c} is >8% on current therapy:

- consider starting at 10 units/day
- monitor fasting plasma glucose (eg by self-monitoring)
- titrate up by two units/day to achieve target control
- if patient is obese, consider adding one unit/day to starting dose for each BMI unit >30
- if there is renal or hepatic impairment consider starting at a lower insulin dose.

If the HbA_{1c} is <8% on current therapy, consider starting at six units/day and then monitor, titrate and adjust as above.

Selection of regimen

The insulin regimen should be tailored to the individual patient's circumstances. Twice-daily isophane (NPH) is a popular choice. The total daily dose is divided: about two-thirds is given before breakfast and one-third before dinner/at bedtime. Alternatively, a mixture of short-acting and intermediate-acting insulins, eg 'biphasic' pre-mixed 30/70 might be appropriate or a pre-mixed rapid–intermediate preparation.

More complicated regimens should only be used if necessary. These might include:

- bedtime intermediate-acting or longer-acting insulin with pre-meal supplements of rapid-acting or short-acting insulin ('basal–bolus')
- bedtime intermediate-acting or longer-acting insulin with day-time oral agents
- pre-meal supplements of rapid-acting or short-acting insulin plus an oral insulin action enhancer such as metformin (or a thiazolidinedione) at bedtime and in the morning if required.

Note that a combination of insulin with a thiazolidinedione is not presently permitted in Europe. Other regimens are discussed elsewhere in this chapter.

Insulin delivery systems

Subcutaneous injections

Self-administered subcutaneous injection using a syringe has traditionally been the mainstay of insulin therapy. Injections have been made more convenient and less unpleasant by features such as disposable plastic syringes and ultrafine, lubricated needles. Technical problems with modern syringes are now very uncommon.

> Disposable plastic insulin syringes may be used several times (by the same individual)

It is no longer considered necessary to clean the injection site with alcohol before injecting (although the site should be clean), or to draw back on the plunger (to check that a vein hasn't been entered), or to compress the preferred site routinely. Too shallow an injection will be delivered intradermally, which can be painful and may cause local atrophy (evident as pitting), while too deep an injection may be delivered intramuscularly. The recommended procedure for subcutaneous insulin injection is outlined in Table 11.2.

Table 11.2
Recommended procedure for insulin injection.

1. Shake vial gently and invert.
2. Draw air (equivalent to injection volume) into syringe.
3. Pierce vial cap.
4. Expel air and draw insulin into syringe up to required mark on syringe.
5. Inject syringe contents at 90° to skin surface.

Anatomical injection sites

Traditionally, patients are advised to vary the location of their injection site (Figure 11.8). This helps to avoid local reactions to insulin, although these are now infrequently encountered in patients with type 2 diabetes.

Allergy

Local allergic reactions are uncommon with modern insulin preparations; transient tender nodules developing at the injection site are suggestive, but generalized allergic reactions are rare.

Lipohypertrophy

Localized areas of lipohypertrophy, although comfortable for injections, are thought to cause erratic absorption of insulin at the site. The hypertrophy is attributed to the trophic effects of insulin on fat metabolism. Avoidance of the area may lead to regression; liposuction has also been used.

Lipoatrophy

Lipoatrophy has been rare since the introduction of highly purified insulins and human insulins. Its incidence may be reduced by injection of highly purified short-acting insulin around the edge of the lesion.

Patients may occasionally complain of recurrent minor local bleeding or bruising, but this rarely presents any cause for serious concern.

Pen injector devices

These continue to increase in popularity and are suitable for most insulin-treated patients. So-

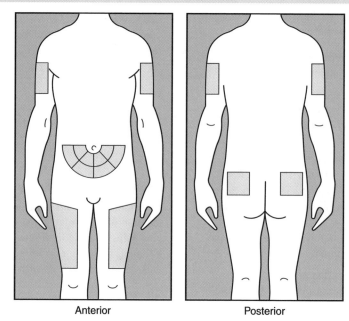

Anterior   Posterior

Figure 11.8

Recommended sites for subcutaneous insulin injection. Reproduced with permission from Krentz AJ. *Churchill's Pocketbook of Diabetes*. Edinburgh: Churchill Livingstone, 2000.

called pen injectors are self-contained devices which obviate the need to draw insulin into a syringe from the vial. They use replaceable insulin cartridges and the mechanized dosage selection facilitates more accurate dispensing of injection volumes. Errors arising from air bubbles are also eliminated if the needle is cleared by expelling two to four units before use. The required dose is dialled and then injected by depressing a plunger. Pens can be very useful for the visually impaired (magnifiers are available) and patients with arthritis or other physical problems interfering with their manual dexterity. They can also improve compliance – particularly in children and adolescents. In fact, few patients now elect to use a conventional syringe.

A selection of pen designs incorporating different features to appeal to different patients is available (no extra charge) and patients should be allowed to choose the one that suits them best. Options include preloaded, entirely

disposable one-piece pens containing 3 ml of 100-unit insulin and an integral needle, and reusable pens which can take cartridges containing either 1.5 ml or 3 ml of 100-unit insulin. The latter require disposable needles. The maximum single dose delivered by the current pen injectors ranges from 36 to 100 units. Pens may be used to give boluses of short- or rapid-acting insulin more conveniently before meals (this is more common among type 1 patients) or to deliver premixed ('biphasic') insulins – used by about 75% of type 2 patients in the UK – more conveniently twice-daily. The Autopen will accept animal insulin cartridges. While, overall, glycaemic control is not necessarily improved with pen injector use, these tools have several definite advantages over conventional syringes:

- more accurate dosing
- portability
- ease of use (especially with impaired dexterity or vision)
- more convenient.

Other modes of delivery

Other modes of insulin delivery, either infrequently used or currently at an experimental stage, include the following:

Continuous subcutaneous infusion

Continuous subcutaneous insulin infusion (CSII) is a specialized insulin delivery technique suitable for intensive therapy but offered by relatively few centres; it currently has a limited role for patients with type 2 diabetes. Type 2 patients wanting excellent glycaemic control during pregnancy are potential candidates. The apparatus now comprises convenient, miniature, programmable pumps (produced by Minimed, Disetronic and Deltec).

Pulmonary insulin

Several pulmonary delivery devices using different insulin preparations are advanced in clinical trials, eg Exubera Inhale (Pfizer, Aventis) and AERX Aradigm (Novo Nordisk, iDMS). The lungs have a large surface area, making them an attractive site for insulin delivery by aerosol. The current devices are likely to suit preprandial dosing with a bolus of rapid- or short-acting insulin. Combined with a long-acting basal insulin or with oral antidiabetic agents, this approach is attractive for selected patients with type 2 diabetes. However, bioavailability is low, making this a potentially expensive option, and long-term safety data are awaited.

Jet injectors

Jet injectors are designed to eject a gaseous stream at high pressure. The stream contains tiny particles of insulin which penetrate the skin. The procedure may be uncomfortable and insulin delivery erratic, and the principal indication, true needle-phobia, is rare.

Oral and nasal insulin

Oral and nasal insulin delivery are still at the experimental stage. Bioavailability via each of these routes seems low. Nasal absorption is rapid, but the use of absorption enhancers may damage the nasal mucosa. Orally active preparations may prove difficult for accurate and repeatable dosing.

Unwanted effects of insulin therapy

A significant proportion of patients with type 2 diabetes require insulin therapy in the long-term because oral agents are unable to provide adequate glycaemic control – so-called 'secondary failure', usually due to disease progression (chapter 9). Reservations about insulin therapy in patients with type 2 diabetes, particularly elderly patients, have focused on the risks of hypoglycaemia and weight gain. Theoretical concerns about promotion of atherosclerosis have also exercised clinicians for decades, but without any definitive outcome.

Weight gain

Weight gain is a common consequence of initiating insulin (and sulphonylurea) treatment in patients with type 2 diabetes. Over the course of the United Kingdom Prospective Diabetes Study, the gain in weight (beyond that observed in patients treated with diet alone) was more than doubled in the insulin-treated group compared with the glibenclamide group (4.0 *vs* 1.7 kg). Reduced urinary glucose loss is a likely explanation, coupled with the general anabolic effects of insulin. Dietary counter-measures may be partially effective, particularly when combined with an exercise programme, and weight gain is not inevitable, but certainly can detract from the sense of achievement for some patients; it is almost universally cited as undesirable. Also, greater obesity exacerbates insulin resistance and certain cardiovascular risk factors. Weight gain tends to plateau after a few months, however, and there is evidence that combination therapy with insulin and metformin can limit weight gain (page 186).

Hypoglycaemia

Hypoglycaemia occurs with considerably lower frequency in type 2 diabetes than in type 1, but may be of paramount importance in the elderly, socially isolated, demented or otherwise infirm type 2 patient. The United Kingdom Prospective Diabetes Study associated insulin treatment with an average of 1.8 episodes of severe hypoglycaemia per year (severe hypoglycaemia being defined as hypoglycaemia requiring the assistance of another person or medical attention). Increased duration of insulin therapy increases the risk of hypoglycaemia. Concomitant use of oral antidiabetic agents and near-normal glycaemia control may increase the risk of hypoglycaemia.

> Severe hypoglycaemia is relatively uncommon in insulin-treated patients with type 2 diabetes compared to those with type 1 diabetes

Causes of iatrogenic hypoglycaemia

Iatrogenic hypoglycaemia either results from a mismatch between the supply of glucose for metabolic requirements (eg due to a missed meal) and the rate of glucose use (eg an increase during or following physical exercise), or a relative excess of insulin leading to a fall in the circulating glucose concentration. There are other causes in insulin-treated patients, but their influence varies from patient to patient and most are considered uncommon or rare in patients with type 2 disease. Some may, however, assume greater importance with the increasing incidence of type 2 diabetes in the young. These include:

- *Changes in insulin pharmacokinetics* – Pharmacokinetics are commonly affected by exercise, which enhances insulin absorption in the exercising limb, and renal impairment, which is also relatively common in type 2 patients (chapter 6). Less significant influences are a change in insulin species from, for example, bovine to human (this is more of a problem in type 1 patients) and a change in anatomical injection site (which is rarely clinically significant).
- *Changes in insulin sensitivity* – Insulin sensitivity will increase with marked weight loss and the withdrawal of certain drugs that induce insulin resistance (eg the corticosteroids). It will also increase with

hypopituitarism or Addison's disease, but both conditions are rare. Hypothyroidism is a more common condition, but a rare cause of hypoglycaemia in insulin-treated patients.

Much more rarely (especially in type 2 diabetes), malabsorption syndromes, gastroparesis due to autonomic neuropathy, and eating disorders such as anorexia and bulimia, have all been associated with the development of hypoglycaemia in insulin-treated patients.

Relative severity of iatrogenic hypoglycaemia

Cerebral function is critically dependent on an adequate supply of glucose from the circulation. Glucose is transported into the brain across the blood–brain barrier by a facilitative glucose transporter protein. The most serious consequence of acute hypoglycaemia is cerebral dysfunction with the risk of:

- injury (to self or others)
- generalized epileptic seizures
- coma.

Cognitive impairment progresses to loss of consciousness as plasma glucose levels fall. Seizures and transient focal neurological deficits may occur with severe neuroglycopenia. Prolonged severe hypoglycaemic coma, often exacerbated by excessive alcohol consumption, may lead to cerebral oedema and permanent brain damage. The effects of recurrent hypoglycaemia on cerebral function in middle-aged and elderly patients are not particularly well documented.

Clinically, hypoglycaemia induced by exogenous insulin is similar to sulphonylurea-induced hypoglycaemia (page 142) and may be graded as follows:

- *Grade 1* – biochemical hypoglycaemia (eg plasma glucose <3.0 mmol/l [54 mg/dl]) in the absence of symptoms
- *Grade 2* – mildly symptomatic (successfully treated by the patient)

- *Grade 3* – severe (the assistance of another person is required)
- *Grade 4* – very severe (causing coma or convulsions).

Note that biochemical definitions of hypoglycaemia may differ according to the circumstances of the patient and may be modulated by previous episodes of hypoglycaemia. The physiological response to acute hypoglycaemia comprises:

- suppression of endogenous insulin secretion
- activation of a hierarchy of counter-regulatory hormone responses.

Counter-regulatory hormone responses to hypoglycaemia

Most of the data concerning counter-regulatory hormone responses to acute hypoglycaemia have been derived from healthy subjects and patients with type 1 diabetes; more studies are required in patients with type 2 diabetes. However, long-duration insulin therapy in patients with type 2 disease is associated with an increased risk of hypoglycaemia; progressive insulin deficiency is thought to result in a situation similar to that in patients with type 1 diabetes, where the counter-regulatory hormone responses to hypoglycaemia are impaired. Patients with type 2 diabetes who progress rapidly to a need for insulin are more likely to be affected. As the plasma glucose concentration falls below certain thresholds, hormones which antagonize insulin's actions are secreted in the following sequence: glucagon and catecholamines, then cortisol and growth hormone.

Catecholamine secretion occurs in the setting of generalized sympathetic nervous system activation. Glucagon and catecholamines are the principal hormones protecting against acute hypoglycaemia. They stimulate glycogenolysis and gluconeogenesis, thereby increasing hepatic glucose production (chapter 2); enhanced hormone-stimulated lipolysis may also contribute

to recovery from hypoglycaemia by facilitating gluconeogenesis. If healthy subjects are given carefully controlled doses of insulin, increased secretion of these two hormones occurs at arterial plasma glucose levels of approximately 3.8 mmol/l; cortisol secretion occurs at lower glucose levels. If the response of either glucagon or catecholamines is inadequate, the other will usually compensate. Deficiency of both hormones will result in severe hypoglycaemia.

> Failure of counter-regulatory hormone responses predisposes to severe recurrent hypoglycaemia

Cortisol and growth hormone play a less important role during acute hypoglycaemia, and are more important in the later recovery of glucose levels.

Antecedent hypoglycaemia can alter the glycaemic threshold for counter-regulatory hormone secretion; scrupulous avoidance of hypoglycaemia may restore symptoms. Clinical studies have shown that intensive insulin therapy leads to symptoms which develop at lower plasma glucose levels, resulting in less time between the onset of symptoms and the development of severe neuroglycopenia. Biochemical evidence of recurrent hypoglycaemia, if well documented, is therefore a contraindication to intensive insulin therapy and a dose reduction should be considered. Non-diabetic patients with chronic recurrent hypoglycaemia due to insulinomas may also lose the typical symptoms and signs of hypoglycaemia.

Warning symptoms of hypoglycaemia

The symptoms and signs of acute hypoglycaemia are conveniently divided into two main categories (Table 11.3): autonomic (or adrenergic) if they arise from activation of the sympathoadrenal system; and neuroglycopenic if they result from inadequate cerebral glucose delivery. Under experimental conditions, adrenergic activation occurs at a higher plasma glucose concentration than that at which cerebral function becomes impaired (about

Table 11.3

Autonomic, neuroglycopenic and non-specific symptoms and signs in acute hypoglycaemia. Sourced from Hepburn DA *et al. Diabetes Care* 1991; **14**: 949-57.

Autonomic (adrenergic)	Neuroglycopenic	Non-specific
Tremor	Impaired concentration	Hunger
Sweating	Confusion	Weakness
Anxiety	Irrational, uncharacteristic or inappropriate behaviour	Blurred vision
Pallor	Difficulty in speaking	
Nausea	Non-co-operation or aggression	
Tachycardia	Drowsiness, progressing to coma	
Palpitations	Focal neurological signs including transient hemiplegia	
Shivering	Focal or generalized convulsions	
Increased pulse pressure	Permanent neurological damage if prolonged, severe hypoglycaemia	

2.7 mmol/l). Thus, the patient is alerted to the falling plasma glucose concentration by adrenergic activation and is usually able to take corrective action. If the warning symptoms are deficient or their perception is impaired, eg by certain drugs or alcohol, then the patient may become irrational and aggressive due to the onset of neuroglycopenia. Prompt assistance from another party may then be required to avert loss of consciousness and more serious sequelae.

> Severe hypoglycaemia carries risk of coma, convulsions, injury and (albeit rarely) even death

Risk factors for severe hypoglycaemia

Insulin treatment of long duration (ie five years or more) is often associated with defective glucagon responses to hypoglycaemia in patients with type 1 diabetes. In addition, intensive insulin therapy (aiming for sustained near-normoglycaemia) can lead to the loss of the normal autonomic hypoglycaemia warning symptoms, giving rise to a high risk of recurrent severe hypoglycaemia. Factors predisposing to severe hypoglycaemia include:

- a history of severe hypoglycaemia
- a history of symptomatic unawareness of hypoglycaemia

- intensive insulin therapy regimens aiming for near-normoglycaemia (eg during pregnancy)
- glycated haemoglobin within the non-diabetic range
- long-duration insulin treatment
- excessive or inappropriate alcohol consumption.

(It should be noted that this list is derived mainly from studies in type 1 patients.)

Driving and insulin treatment

Patients who have lost their warning symptoms for hypoglycaemia should not drive motor vehicles. The fact that hypoglycaemia while driving could have serious consequences should be explained to the patient, preferably in writing. This advice should also be recorded in the patient's case notes; fatalities have occurred. In the UK, patients should be reminded that it is their legal responsibility to inform the driving licensing authority if:

- treatment with hypoglycaemic potential, including insulin, is commenced (patients should be advised not to drive until their glycaemic control is acceptable)
- significant tissue complications – eg acute or chronic visual impairment, severe peripheral neuropathy, ischaemic heart

disease, cerebrovascular disease – develop. Expert advice is required if night vision is affected by extensive retinal photocoagulation (chapter 6).

- hypoglycaemia unawareness occurs.

In these circumstances, a report from the responsible clinician will usually be requested by the licensing authority. If a patient is involved in a road traffic accident in which hypoglycaemia is thought to have been contributory, the police will usually notify the licensing authority and the patient's licence (usually renewed every three years if insulin-treated) is likely to be withdrawn until there is convincing evidence that the risks have become acceptable. General precautions for driving on insulin treatment are listed in Table 11.4. The regulations concerning public service and heavy goods vehicles differ, of course, and vary from country to country. In the UK, taxi licences are granted by the local authority, and insulin treatment not necessarily disallowed, as long as glycaemic control is deemed satisfactory. Certain professions, such as the armed forces, often exclude insulin-treated patients, however, which can lead to conflicts of interest and encourage some patients to avoid insulin treatment longer than is advisable. The regulations are flexible in many cases, though, subject to regular, satisfactory medical reports. A commitment to frequent self-monitoring is required.

> Patients who have lost their hypoglycaemic warning symptoms must not drive motor vehicles

Recreational implications for insulin treatment

Certain sports, such as scuba diving, carry predictable risks for patients at risk of hypoglycaemia. It is important to note that post-exercise hypoglycaemia can occur several hours after the event, which can lead to diagnostic difficulties if appropriate enquiries

Table 11.4
Advice for insulin-treated diabetic drivers.

- A supply of readily accessible glucose tablets (or a suitable alternative) must always be carried in the car
- Plan each journey
- Make provisions for unexpected delays
- Check blood glucose before, and periodically during, long journeys
- Take regular breaks on long journeys and avoid fatigue
- Have regular meals and snacks at the designated times
- If hypoglycaemia develops, stop the car at the earliest safe opportunity, switch off the engine, remove the ignition key and vacate the driver's seat (take care on busy roads)
- Always carry an identity card or bracelet confirming your diagnosis
- Never drink alcohol before driving

are not made. Patients may find that they have to reduce their insulin dose substantially before rigorous exercise; this should always be planned. Conversely, patients with minimal endogenous insulin secretion may need to consume additional carbohydrate both before and during exercise. Insulin sensitivity tends to improve rapidly with aerobic exercise (page 128), but the effect is lost rapidly if the exercise programme is interrupted for more than a few days.

Long-haul travel

Adjustment of insulin dosing during long-distance travel is often relatively easy for patients with type 2 diabetes, particularly if a twice-daily regimen is applied and some endogenous insulin secretion present. Plans should be discussed with the diabetes care team ahead of travel, and the relevant airline informed. Insulin should not be stowed in the hold (freezing will denature it), nor should it be exposed to extreme heat, such as direct sunlight.

Insulin treatment has implications for driving, certain occupations and some recreational activities

Meticulous glucose control

Meticulous avoidance of low glucose levels – ie those <4.0 mmol/l – may restore the warning symptoms of hypoglycaemia in some insulin-treated patients. The use of rapid-acting insulin analogues is being explored, but it is often difficult to decide whether improvements in glycaemic control are attributable to altered pharmacokinetics or education and greater input from the diabetes care team. Although the loss of warning symptoms has been described as a form of acquired autonomic dysfunction, it is generally accepted that classic diabetic autonomic neuropathy *per se* is not responsible in most cases.

Nocturnal hypoglycaemia

The frequent occurrence of nocturnal hypoglycaemia – which may affect more than 50% of patients and often goes unrecognized – is an important cause of hypoglycaemic unawareness. Conventional strategies to minimize nocturnal hypoglycaemia include:

- reducing the dose of evening intermediate insulin
- moving the time of the evening injection of intermediate insulin to 2200 hours
- eating a snack containing 10–20 g carbohydrate before bed
- avoiding excessive alcohol consumption.

The contribution of the evening dose of short-acting insulin to the problem of hypoglycaemia at 0200–0300 hours may well have been underestimated in the past and recent evidence points to a lower rate of nocturnal hypoglycaemia when the insulin analogues lispro or insulin aspart are used in place of conventional short-acting preparation. Since lispro and aspart have a shorter duration of action their effects will dissipate earlier in the evening, resulting in lower plasma insulin concentrations in the early hours of sleep.

In addition, studies in children have shown that the physiological responses to hypoglycaemia are impaired during stages 3–4 (the slow-wave) of sleep.

Evening doses of conventional short-acting insulins may contribute to nocturnal hypoglycaemia in some patients

Insulin species and hypoglycaemia risk

In the UK there has been intense debate about the effect of insulin species on the warning symptoms of hypoglycaemia. A minority of patients with type 1 diabetes complained that their symptoms reduced in intensity when they changed from animal to human sequence insulin. It is recognized that a change in species may necessitate changes in dosage, and minor differences in pharmacokinetics and, in some patients with diabetes of long duration, the presence of high titres of anti-insulin antibodies is thought to be responsible. This is particularly true for patients changing from bovine to the less immunogenic porcine or human insulin preparations. Whether there is any effect of species *per se* on the symptom complex of hypoglycaemia remains less certain, with most studies showing no appreciable difference. Alternative causes of hypoglycaemia must always be excluded (page 178) and the great majority of patients in the UK and elsewhere are now treated with human sequence insulin.

Treatment of insulin-induced hypoglycaemia

Insulin-treated patients are advised to carry dextrose tablets at all times, but surveys indicate that a high proportion do not comply; periodic reiteration of the advice is required. At the onset of symptoms patients should take either:

- two to four dextrose tablets

- two teaspoonfuls (10 g) of sugar, honey or jam (ideally in water)
- a small glass of a carbonated, sugar-containing soft drink.

If there is no improvement within five to 10 minutes, the treatment should be repeated. If the next meal is not imminent, a snack (eg biscuit, sandwich, piece of fruit) should be eaten to maintain blood glucose levels. Over-treatment ('emptying the fridge') should be avoided if possible.

Where the hypoglycaemia is more severe (grade 3 or 4; page 178), a friend, colleague or relative may notice its development before the patients themselves. A subtle change in appearance or behaviour may prompt another person to encourage oral carbohydrate consumption. Unfortunately, cognitive dysfunction may lead to a negative or even hostile response. As the level of consciousness falls, it becomes hazardous to try to forcibly administer carbohydrate by mouth. Alternatives then include:

- *Buccal glucose gel* – proprietary thick glucose gels (eg Hypostop), or honey, can be smeared on the buccal mucosa; efficacy is variable.
- *iv glucose* – 25 ml of 50% dextrose or 100 ml of 20% dextrose may be administered into a large vein, ideally after cannulation. Paramedical expertise is required – extravasation of hypertonic 50% dextrose can cause tissue necrosis and thrombophlebitis may also complicate iv delivery – but this technique will usually lead to restoration of consciousness within a few minutes.
- *Glucagon* – parenteral glucagon is not recommended for type 2 patients because there may be sufficient remaining β-cells to respond with increased insulin secretion.

Recovery from hypoglycaemia may be delayed if:

- the hypoglycaemia has been very prolonged or severe

- an alternative cause for impairment of consciousness (eg stroke, drug overdose) co-exists (the hypoglycaemia may cause falls and head injury)
- the patient is post-ictal (convulsion caused by severe hypoglycaemia).

If cerebral oedema is suspected, adjunctive treatment, ie iv dexamethasone (4–6 mg, six-hourly) or mannitol, is usually administered in an intensive care setting. However, evidence for the efficacy of these drugs, or for other measures such as controlled hyperventilation, is scarce. Cranial CT imaging should be performed.

> Hypertonic 50% dextrose must be administered into a large vein in order to avoid extravasation

Special situations
Surgery

Insulin-treated patients require careful monitoring to avoid hypo- and hyperglycaemia during surgery or other invasive procedures that have required them to be 'nil-by-mouth'. An iv infusion with dextrose is usually recommended. Subcutaneous insulin is recommenced with the first meal after the procedure. Some patients treated with oral antidiabetic drugs (especially long-acting sulphonylureas and metformin) are best converted to insulin temporarily ahead of major surgery. This is usually done as part of inpatient treatment (Table 11.5). The management of type 2 diabetes during surgery is outlined in Table 11.6. Note that patients with type 2 disease are more likely to require surgery than non-diabetic individuals – for diabetic foot complications, for example. They may also have complications (eg nephropathy, autonomic neuropathy) which can adversely affect outcome. Poor metabolic control impedes wound healing in general and exacerbates plasma electrolyte disturbances, and the hormonal response to surgical stress can lead to major metabolic decompensation.

Table 11.5
Dextrose and insulin infusions* for control of perioperative diabetes.

- Glucose is administered via a drip counter at a rate of 100 ml/hour of 10% dextrose (containing an appropriate amount of potassium).

- Short-acting (regular, 'soluble') insulin (50 units) is added to 50 ml saline (0.9%) in a 50 ml syringe and delivered via a variable rate electromechanical pump (with built-in battery supply).

- Insulin (approximately 1 unit/ml) is co-infused via a Y-connector at a variable rate, with the aim of maintaining blood glucose concentrations at approximately 5–10 mmol/l.

Sample regimen:

Infusion rate (units/hour)	Blood glucose (mmol/l)
0	0–3.9[†]
1	4.0–6.9
2	7.0–9.9
3	10.0–14.9
4	≥15.0[†]

[†]Call medical staff to review. Recheck blood glucose and treat hypoglycaemia if necessary.

- Starting infusion rate is 2 units/hour. Rate is then increased or reduced on the basis of hourly blood glucose measurements.

- Advantage = Adjustable ratio of insulin to glucose.

- Disadvantage = Risk of both hypo- and hyperglycaemia if infusion rate incorrect or delivery interrupted.

*Note that insulin requirements are variable and that the infusion rates suggested are just a guide.

Hormonal stress response to intercurrent illness

Transient insulin resistance may arise in the course of intercurrent illnesses, such as severe sepsis. Temporary increases in insulin dosage, sometimes necessitating a change to iv or multiple subcutaneous doses, are required. Insulin may also become temporarily necessary during illness in patients previously well-controlled by oral antidiabetic agents; re-introduction of oral therapy may be possible following recovery.

Anti-insulin antibodies

The role of acquired anti-insulin antibodies, once thought to be an important mechanism of insulin resistance, has faded with the introduction of modern, less antigenic insulin preparations.

Renal failure

Care is required with insulin treatment in patients with progressive renal impairment. Decreased insulin degradation by the failing kidneys, reduced renal gluconeogenesis, and anorexia with decreased calorie intake may all contribute. Reductions in insulin dosage, sometimes substantial, may be required.

> Progressive renal failure may necessitate a reduction in insulin dose

Some patients with end-stage renal failure on continuous ambulatory peritoneal dialysis (page 92) inject their insulin into the dialysate bags to deliver it intraperitoneally. Insulin requirements vary widely from patient to patient, partly dependent on the strength of the dialysate used; hypertonic solutions can contain high concentrations of glucose.

Transient deterioration of retinopathy

Transient deterioration in pre-existing retinopathy may follow rapid improvement in glycaemic control, for example when insulin treatment is commenced. This phenomenon has mainly been observed in trials in patients with type 1 diabetes, but may also occur in some type 2 patients. Careful surveillance and explanation of this apparent paradox is required. The long-term prognosis is generally much better with improved glycaemic control.

Insulin neuritis

An analogous complication is so-called insulin neuritis in which acute symptomatic neuropathy develops following the institution of insulin treatment; this condition is uncommon.

Patient acceptability

Clinical studies suggest that insulin therapy can be successful if patients are selected appropriately and prepared carefully. Twice-daily isophane or pre-mixed ('biphasic') insulins are used routinely in many centres; pen injectors are suitable for most patients and may increase acceptability by increasing convenience. Morbidly obese patients inadequately controlled with oral agents remain a particularly difficult therapeutic problem. Some centres use a combination of oral antidiabetic agents and bedtime insulin. Patient acceptance of insulin

---

Table 11.6
Management of diabetes during surgery and other invasive procedures.

Measures are required to (a) avoid hypoglycaemia and (b) maintain good metabolic control:

● Liaison with the anaesthetist is recommended.

● Metabolic control should be optimized in good time if possible (this may require temporary insulin treatment for some patients otherwise not on insulin).

● The patient should be placed near the start of a morning list on the day of operation, if possible.

● During emergency surgery, any major metabolic disturbance should be corrected as far as possible. The effects of previously administered antidiabetic therapy necessitate even more frequent monitoring and use of dextrose and insulin as indicated.

● Electrolyte disturbances should be corrected before surgery wherever possible.

Diet- or tablet-treated diabetes:
In well-controlled patients undergoing minor procedures such as endoscopy, avoidance of glucose- and lactate-containing iv fluids, and missing out their short-acting sulphonylurea (or meglitinide) dose on the morning of surgery may be sufficient. In any case:

● Blood glucose levels should be monitored every one to two hours pre- and postoperatively.

● Longer-acting sulphonylureas (eg chlorpropamide, glibenclamide) should be discontinued several days before surgery since they may cause serious and prolonged postoperative hypoglycaemia; these should be temporarily replaced by insulin or short-acting agents (eg tolbutamide).

● Metformin should also be avoided perioperatively and at the time of radiological contrast investigations because of the risk of lactic acidosis. If renal function is normal (metformin is contraindicated if renal impairment is present), then discontinuation of the drug on the evening before the procedure should allow sufficient elimination. Thiazolidinediones should also be discontinued perioperatively and any insulin replacement started at about half the usual rate.

● Management of major surgery should follow that for insulin-treated patients.

Insulin-treated patients:

● For all but the most trivial procedures, patients should be stabilized pre-operatively with iv dextrose and insulin infusion as outlined in Table 11.5.

● Plasma electrolytes should be checked frequently and the amount of potassium adjusted accordingly.

● Subcutaneous insulin should be restarted with an appropriate meal. When it is reinstated, the initial injection should include a short-acting insulin and the iv infusion should be terminated 30–60 minutes later to minimize the risk of transient insulinopenia.

● Other special situations include acute myocardial infarction (chapter 7), open heart surgery with cardiopulmonary bypass (which requires considerably more insulin to compensate for the glucose-containing fluids used in the procedure), and labour (which should be managed with dextrose–insulin infusion in insulin-treated patients). Insulin requirements fall rapidly back to pre-pregnancy levels after placenta delivery and insulin may no longer be required in women with gestational diabetes or diabetes previously managed with diet or oral agents. NB Dexamethasone and β-agonists may cause metabolic decompensation.

---

can be facilitated by a positive attitude from the diabetes care team and discussion of the possibility of subsequent insulin treatment early in the course of the disease. Some studies suggest that quality of life is not necessarily impaired by the additional complexity of insulin treatment. Indeed, the sense of wellbeing experienced by patients who improve on insulin after months or years of hyperglycaemia can be rewarding for both patients and healthcare professionals alike. Adequate support from a multidisciplinary diabetes care team is an important component of safe and effective insulin therapy.

Combination therapy with oral agents

Sulphonylureas with insulin

No clear long-term benefits of such combined therapy have yet emerged, but this approach has enthusiastic support and is gaining popularity. Several studies (generally relatively small-scale and of limited duration) have suggested that concomitant treatment with insulin and a sulphonylurea may allow a reduction in insulin dose of up to 50%. Typically, isophane insulin is administered at bedtime, with sulphonylureas taken during the day. The aim is to control fasting plasma glucose concentration with the bedtime insulin by suppressing hepatic glucose production. Clearly, given the mode of action of sulphonylureas (page 138), this approach is dependent on partial residual β-cell function and its use in the longer term is not yet clear. Since β-cell function seems to deteriorate inexorably in most patients with type 2 diabetes, it is likely that the sulphonylureas will eventually lose their effect; full replacement therapy with insulin would then be required.

Metformin with insulin

There is increasing evidence that metformin may help to avert weight gain when patients with type 2 diabetes are transferred to insulin. A recent randomized trial showed that metformin and insulin (at bedtime) were associated with better glycaemic control and the lowest risk of hypoglycaemia during the first year of therapy than other regimens, including twice-daily insulin. Patients assigned to this combination used more insulin to attain fasting blood glucose targets, possibly gaining the confidence to increase insulin dose due to the low risk of hypoglycaemia. Some centres now routinely continue metformin in overweight patients when insulin is introduced, but further studies are required.

> Metformin may help to limit the weight gain associated with insulin treatment in some patients with type 2 diabetes

Thiazolidinediones with insulin

There is evidence that these insulin-sensitizing drugs may allow the insulin dose to be reduced (often >20%) and improve glycaemic control in insulin-treated type 2 patients. In Europe concerns about cardiovascular side-effects (especially increased oedema) have prevented the licensing of thiazolidinediones for use in combination with insulin. Weight gain (part of which is likely to be fluid retention) is not eliminated by combining insulin with a thiazolidinedione; both drugs have the potential to cause weight gain as monotherapy.

> Combination therapy with insulin and a thiazolidinedione may allow the insulin dose to be reduced (not licensed in Europe)

Discontinuation of insulin therapy

In some situations it may be appropriate to discontinue insulin treatment. Certain elderly or infirm patients, once-obese patients who have slimmed through dietary and exercise measures, and patients who took insulin because of a concurrent condition that has subsequently resolved, may all benefit from discontinuation. The essential criterion is that the patient has endogenous insulin secretion sufficient to permit control with oral agents or even diet alone, but certain other criteria should also be satisfied:

- There should be no history of ketosis. An exception is ketosis that was clearly associated with a severe acute illness such as major sepsis (which can sometimes precipitate ketosis in patients with type 2 diabetes).
- The patient should not have been underweight at diagnosis (this usually indicates marked insulin deficiency).
- Serum markers of autoimmune type 1 diabetes (eg islet cell antibodies) should be absent.

Patients with secondary forms of diabetes (chapter 3) represent a heterogeneous group. A history of diabetes complicating chronic pancreatitis will point to the need for insulin treatment due to severe β-cell destruction, for example. On the other hand, temporary steroid-induced diabetes may not require insulin, provided the steroid dose can be lowered sufficiently.

Demonstration of the previous inadequacy of oral agents (so-called primary or secondary failure) usually means that insulin treatment should continue. The need for small doses of insulin (eg <20 units/day) is not always a reliable guide to the success of oral agents because insulin requirements vary considerably between patients. In any case, very careful expert supervision is needed when insulin is withdrawn.

> Insulin dose cannot be reliably equated with need for insulin treatment

Transfer back to oral agents requires reconsideration of the potential risks and benefits. Measurement of plasma (or urinary) C-peptide, which is co-secreted with insulin on an equimolar basis, provides a measure of endogenous insulin reserve. Stimulation tests (eg peak C-peptide response six minutes after a 1 mg iv injection of glucagon) have been used in clinical trials to improve the accuracy of classification. These are rarely used in routine clinical practice, where the decision to use insulin treatment rests principally on clinical judgement.

Further reading

Cryer PE. Diverse causes of hypoglycaemia-associated autonomic failure in diabetes. *N Engl J Med* 2004; **350**: 2272-9.

Evans A, Krentz AJ. Benefits and risks of transfer from oral agents to insulin in type 2 diabetes. In: Krentz AJ (Ed). *Drug treatment of type 2 diabetes*. Auckland, ADIS International 2000; 85-101.

Edelman SV, Henry RR. Insulin therapy for normalizing glycosylated hemoglobin in type II diabetes. Application, benefits and risks. *Diabetes Rev* 1995; **3**: 308-34.

Galloway JA. Treatment of NIDDM with insulin agonists or substitutes. *Diabetes Care* 1990; **13**: 1209-39.

Hayward RA, Manning WG, Kaplan SH *et al*. Starting insulin therapy in patients with type 2 diabetes. *JAMA* 1997; **278**: 1663-9.

Hermann LS. Optimising therapy for insulin-treated type 2 diabetes mellitus. *Drugs Aging* 2000; **17**: 283-94.

Hirsch IB. Insulin analogues. *N Engl J Med* 2005; **352**: 174–83.

Selam JL. Implantable insulin pumps. *Lancet* 1999; **354**: 178-9.

Turner RC, Cull CA, Frighi V *et al*. Glycemic control with diet, sulphonylurea, metformin, or insulin in patients with type 2 diabetes mellitus (UKPDS 49). *JAMA* 1999; **281**: 2005-12.

United Kingdom Prospective Diabetes Study Group. United Kingdom Prospective Diabetes Study (UKPDS) 13: relative efficacy of randomly allocated diet, sulphonylurea, insulin, or metformin in patients with newly diagnosed non-insulin dependent diabetes followed for three years. *Br Med J* 1995; **310**: 83-8.

Yki-Jarvinen H. Combination therapies with insulin in type 2 diabetes. *Diabetes Care* 2001; **24**: 758-67.

Yki-Jarvinen H, Ryysy L, Nikkila K *et al*. Comparison of bedtime insulin regimens in patients with type 2 diabetes mellitus. A randomized controlled trial. *Ann Intern Med* 1999; **130**: 389-96.

1) Identifying individuals at increased risk of type 2 diabetes

Type 2 diabetes should be suspected in individuals with:

Obesity
Abdominal obesity
First-degree relative with type 2 diabetes
History of gestational diabetes and/or large babies
Previous glucose intolerance and/or hyperinsulinaemia
Ethnic predisposition
Dyslipidaemia
Hypertension
Low birth weight
Microalbuminuria
Atherothrombotic symptoms
High parity
Diabetogenic drug therapy
Recurrent infections
Old age

2) Diagnosis of type 2 diabetes*

A) With symptoms**
i)   random venous plasma glucose ≥11.1 mmol/l (≥200 mg/dl)
     or
ii) fasting *plasma* glucose ≥7.0 mmol/l (≥126 mg/dl)
     or
iii) 75 g OGTT[†], two-hour *plasma* glucose ≥11.1 mmol/l (≥200mg/dl)

B) Without symptoms
Measurement of i), ii), or iii) (above) on two separate occasions. If fasting or random values are equivocal, a two-hour value after a 75 g OGTT[†] should be used

*Diagnosis is normally based on two separate measurements of plasma or blood glucose. It should normally be confirmed by at least one plasma or blood glucose measurement made by a recognized clinical chemistry laboratory
**Polyuria or polydipsia, plus visual disturbance, fatigue, unexplained weight loss, recurrent infection, macrovascular complications, retinopathy, nephropathy, or neuropathy
[†]OGTT = oral glucose tolerance test

3) Diagnostic glucose concentrations for type 2 diabetes, impaired glucose tolerance and impaired fasting glucose

	Glucose concentration, mmol/l (mg/dl)			
	Whole blood		Plasma	
	Venous	Capillary	**Venous**	Capillary
Diabetes mellitus				
Fasting	≥6.1 (≥110)	≥6.1 (≥110)	**≥7.0 (≥126)**	≥7.0 (≥126)
Two hours post-glucose load*	≥10.0 (≥180)	≥11.1 (≥200)	**≥11.1 (≥200)**	≥12.2 (≥220)
Impaired glucose tolerance (IGT)				
Two hours post- glucose load*	≥6.7 (≥120) and <10.0 (<180)	≥7.8 (≥140) and <11.1 (<200)	**≥7.8 (≥140) and <11.1 (<200)**	≥8.9 (≥160) and <12.2 (<220)
Impaired fasting glucose (IFG)				
Fasting			**≥5.6 (≥100) and <7.0 (<126)**	≥6.1 (≥110) and <7.0 (<126)

*Two hours after a 75 g oral glucose load, conducted after an overnight fast

4) 75 g oral glucose tolerance test

Procedure

- Patient asked to withhold food after last meal of previous day (nothing to eat or drink from midnight, except water, until test).

- Morning medications should be deferred until after test.

- Patient should arrive at least 30 minutes in advance of test, preferably by transport (ie with minimal physical exertion).

- Start test at 0800–0900 hours.

- Insert venous line (unless capillary test, eg finger prick, is to be performed).

- Take pre-test blood sample (approximately 15–30 minutes before test; this sample is not usually used for measurement, but serves to verify that patient was stable when compared with next 'time zero' sample). Collect blood into fluoride-oxalate tube (unless immediate capillary measurement being performed).

- Take 'time zero' blood sample.

- Within about five minutes, patient consumes 75 g anhydrous D-glucose dissolved in about 300 ml water.

- Take blood samples at ½, 1, 1½ and 2 hours.

- Remove venous line.

- A simplified approach involves the measurement of glucose in the fasting state (time zero) and two hours after the glucose challenge (since these are the values used for diagnostic purposes).

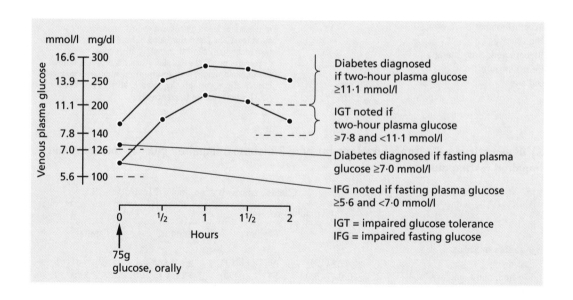

5) HbA$_{1c}$

HbA$_{1c}$ (glycated haemoglobin A$_{1c}$) is a measure of the non-enzymatic attachment of *glucose* to the terminal valine of the β chain of haemoglobin. HbA$_{1c}$ is expressed as a percentage of the haemoglobin that is glycated (normally about 4–6%). HbA$_{1c}$ has largely replaced HbA$_1$, which is a measure of *all sugars* attached to the terminal β chain of haemoglobin. HbA$_{1c}$ is the largest component (60–80%) of HbA$_1$. Values for HbA$_{1c}$ are therefore about 1–2% (absolute units) lower than HbA$_1$. Since the lifespan of an erythrocyte is about 120 days, HbA$_{1c}$ gives an indication of average glycaemia over half of this period, ie over 60 days. However, more recent changes in glycaemia will have a slightly greater impact on the extent of glycation, so HbA$_{1c}$ provides a more useful indication of glycaemia over the 40–60 days (six to eight weeks) preceding the assay.

Guidelines for optimal glycaemic control suggest aiming for an HbA$_{1c}$ value of ≤ 6.5% (European Policy Group), or <7% (American Diabetes Association), based on a non-diabetic reference range of 4–6%.

6) Ideal targets for metabolic control

	European Diabetes Policy Group	American Diabetes Association
HbA$_{1c}$ %	≤6.5	<7.0
Fasting plasma glucose		
mmol/l	≤6.0	–
mg/dl	<110	–
Preprandial plasma glucose		
mmol/l	–	5.0–7.2
mg/dl	–	90–130
Fasting total cholesterol		
mmol/l	<4.8	–
mg/dl	<185	–
Fasting LDL-cholesterol		
mmol/l	<3.0	<2.6
mg/dl	<115	<100
Fasting HDL-cholesterol		
mmol/l	>1.2	>1.1 (Men), >1.29 (Women)
mg/dl	>46	>40 (Men), >50 (Women)
Fasting triglycerides		
mmol/l	<1.7	<1.7
mg/dl	<150	<150
Blood pressure		
mmHg	<130/80*	<130/80*
Body mass index		
kg/m²	18.5–25	
Waist circumference cm (inches)	Men <102 (<40)† Women <88 (<35)†	
Waist:hip ratio	Men <0.95 Women <0.80	

European Diabetes Policy Group 1999
American Diabetes Association Position Statement 2004
* British and European Hypertension Societies guidelines 2003/4
† Metabolic Syndrome: National Cholesterol Education Program (Adult Treatment Panel III) 2001

7) Starting therapy with oral antidiabetic agents

Agent	Recommended daily dose (mg)*	Duration of action†	Starting dose (mg)‡	Exclusions and contraindications	Side-effects and adverse events	Precautions§
α-glucosidase inhibitors (slow rate of carbohydrate digestion[a])						
Acarbose	150–300	Short	50 td; with main meals	Intestinal diseases, severe kidney disease	Gastrointestinal intolerance	Check LFT for high dose ? check creatinine
Miglitol[f]	75–300	Short	25 }			
Sulphonylureas[b] (increase insulin secretion)						
Chlorpropamide	100–500	Long	100 od	Choice of agent restricted by severe liver or kidney disease, or porphyria	Hypoglycaemic episodes, sensitivity reactions, weight gain	Interactions with other protein-bound drugs
Glibenclamide[c]	2.5–15	Intermediate-long	2.5 od			
Gliclazide[d]	40–320	Intermediate	40 od[d]			
Glimepiride	1–6	Intermediate	1 od			
Glipizide[e]	2.5–20	Short-intermediate[e]	2.5 od or bd			
Gliquidone	15–180	Short-intermediate	15 od or bd			
Tolbutamide	500–2000	Short	500 od or bd			
Meglitinide non-sulphonylurea 'prandial' insulin releasers (increase insulin secretion)						
Repaglinide	1–16	Very short	0.5 bd or td, before main meals	Liver or severe kidney disease	As for sulphonylureas but less severe hypoglycaemia	Drug interactions
Nateglinide	180–540	Very short	60 td before main meals			
Biguanides (counter insulin resistance)						
Metformin	500–3000	Short-intermediate	500 od or bd, 850 od, with meals	Kidney, liver, cardiac or any hypoxic disease	Gastrointestinal, risk of lactic acidosis	Check creatinine; vitamin B_{12} or Hb
Thiazolidinediones (improve insulin sensitivity)						
Rosiglitazone	2–8	Intermediate	2 od or bd	Cardiac failure, oedema, anaemia, liver disease	Oedema, anaemia, weight gain	Check LFT, Hb
Pioglitazone	15–45	Intermediate	15 bd			
Metformin–rosiglitazone fixed dose combinations (counter insulin resistance)						
Metformin–rosiglitazone	500:1–1000:4	Intermediate	500:1 od or bd before or with meals	As for metformin and rosiglitazone	As for metformin and rosiglitazone	As for metformin and rosiglitazone
Sulphonylurea–metformin fixed dose combinations (increase insulin secretion and counter insulin resistance)[f]						
Glibenclamide–metformin	1.25:250–10:2000	Intermediate	1.25:250 od or bd before or with meals	As for sulphonylureas and metformin	As for sulphonylureas and metformin	As for sulphonylureas and metformin

* Maximum recommended daily dose can vary between countries; † long = >24 hours; intermediate = 12–24 hours; short = <12 hours; very short = < 5 hours; ‡ od = once daily; bd = twice daily; td = three times daily; titrate up dosage slowly; § glycaemic control should be monitored throughout and rigorously during titration phase with all antidiabetic drugs; thiazolidinediones, nateglinide and sulphonylurea-metformin fixed dose combinations are not indicated for initial oral antidiabetic therapy in Europe; prescribing information varies between countries. a meals should be rich in complex carbohydrate; b take with first main meal; large doses of intermediate-acting agents can usually be divided and taken before each of the two main meals, preferably breakfast and lunch; c glibenclamide = glyburide; maximum dose 20 mg in some countries; d modified-release formulation of gliclazide (Diamicron MR) – daily dose 30–120 mg; e extended-release formulation of glipizide (Glucotrol XL) – intermediate duration; f Not UK; LFT = liver function test, eg alanine transaminase; Hb = haemoglobin.

8) Insulins available in the UK

Name	Manufacturer	Species	Vial or cartridge	Onset, peak and duration of action (hours)
Rapid-acting insulins (bolus)				
NovoRapid (aspart)	Novo Nordisk	Analogue	Vial, cartridge, preloaded pen	
Humalog (lispro)	Lilly	Analogue	Vial, cartridge, preloaded pen	
Short-acting insulins (bolus)				
Actrapid	Novo Nordisk	Human	Vial, cartridge, preloaded pen	
Velosulin	Novo Nordisk	emp, Human	Vial	
Humulin S	Lilly	Human	Vial, cartridge, preloaded pen	
Hypurin Bovine Neutral	CP Pharmaceuticals	Beef	Vial and cartridge	
Hypurin Porcine Neutral	CP Pharmaceuticals	Pork	Vial and cartridge	
Insuman rapid	Aventis Pharma	Human	Cartridge, preloaded pen	
Pork Actrapid	Novo Nordisk	Pork	Vial	
Intermediate- and long-acting insulins (basal)				
Insulatard	Novo Nordisk	Human	Vial, cartridge, preloaded pen	
Humulin I	Lilly	Human	Vial, cartridge, preloaded pen	
Hypurin Bovine Isophane	CP Pharmaceuticals	Beef	Vial and cartridge	
Hypurin Bovine Lente	CP Pharmaceuticals	Beef	Vial	
Hypurin Bovine PZI	CP Pharmaceuticals	Beef	Vial	
Hypurin Porcine Isophane	CP Pharmaceuticals	Pork	Vial and cartridge	
Insuman Basal	Aventis Pharma	Human	Vial, cartridge, preloaded pen	
Monotard	Novo Nordisk	Human	Vial	
Pork Insulatard	Novo Nordisk	Pork	Vial	
Ultratard	Novo Nordisk	Human	Vial	
Lantus (glargine)	Aventis Pharma	Analogue	Vial, cartridge, preloaded pen	
Levemir (detemir)	Novo Nordisk	Analogue*	Vial, cartridge, preloaded pen	
Pre-mixed insulins (biphasic)				
NovoMix 30	Novo Nordisk	Analogue	Cartridge, preloaded pen	
Humalog Mix 25/50	Lilly	Analogue	Cartridge (not 50), preloaded pen	
Mixtard 30	Novo Nordisk	Human	Vial	
Mixtard 10–50	Novo Nordisk	Human	Cartridge, preloaded pen	
Humulin M3	Lilly	Human	Vial, cartridge, preloaded pen	
Hypurin Porcine 30/70 mix	CP Pharmaceuticals	Pork	Vial and cartridge	
Insuman Comb 15–50	Aventis Pharma	Human	Vial, cartridge, preloaded pen	
Pork Mixtard 30	Novo Nordisk	Pork	Vial	

Chart axis: 0 2 4 6 8 10 12 14 16 18 20 22 24 26 28 30 32 34

Times shown for onset and duration are approximate and may vary from person to person. Onset = the time taken for the insulin to start having an effect. Modified from the July/August 2004 *Balance*, with permission from Diabetes UK, the charity for people with diabetes (www.diabetes.org.uk). emp = enzyme modified pork.

* Human B29 tetradecanyl, des B30.

† Humulin M1 and M4 are to be withdrawn, as are the 1.5ml cartridges of Humulin I, Humulin S, Humulin M3 and Humulin M5.

9) Synopsis of antidiabetic agents

	Insulin	Sulphonylureas and meglitinides	Metformin	α-glucosidase inhibitors	Thiazolidinediones
Basal glucose	↓↓	↓	↓	– or ↓	↓[a]
Postprandial glucose	↓↓	↓↓	↓	↓	↓[a]
Insulin concentration	↑↑	↑	– or ↓	– or ↓	– or ↓
Body weight	↑	↑	– or ↓	–	– or ↑
Free fatty acids	↓	– or ↓	– or ↓	–	↓
Triglyceride	–	–	– or ↓	–	– or ↓
Total cholesterol	–	–	– or ↓	–	– or ↑
Safety risks	Hypo[b]	Hypo[b]	LA[c]	–	?[d]
Tolerability	Inject	–	GI[e]	GI[e]	–
Exclude/caution	–	Liver/renal[f]	Renal/liver/hypoxia[c]	GI[g]	Cardiac/liver[d]
Monitor[h]	–	–[f]	Creatinine, B_{12}, Hb[i]	LFT[j]	LFT, Hb[k]

↑ = increase; ↓ = decrease; – = no significant change

[a] Blood glucose-lowering efficacy may be slightly less than sulphonylurea or metformin in the shorter-term and similar in the longer-term and in combination therapy

[b] Hypoglycaemia, less severe with meglitinides ('prandial' insulin releasers).

[c] Lactic acidosis is a rare risk: patients with impaired renal or liver function or predisposition to hypoxia are excluded

[d] Safety issues may include fluid retention, haemodilution, anaemia and oedema. Patients with cardiac and liver disease are excluded

[e] Gastrointestinal disturbances, especially if dosage is increased too rapidly

[f] If liver or renal disease, select agent with appropriate pharmacokinetics and monitor accordingly

[g] Exclude patients with established gastrointestinal diseases

[h] Monitor glycaemic control for all antidiabetic drug treatments

[i] Monitor creatinine and vitamin B_{12} or haemoglobin

[j] Monitor liver function test, eg alanine transaminase, with high-dose acabose

[k] Initial rigorous monitoring of liver function test and check haemoglobin

[l] Basal blood glucose-lowering effect of meglitinides is less than sulphonylureas, but postprandial effect may be greater

10) Body mass index (BMI) kg/m²

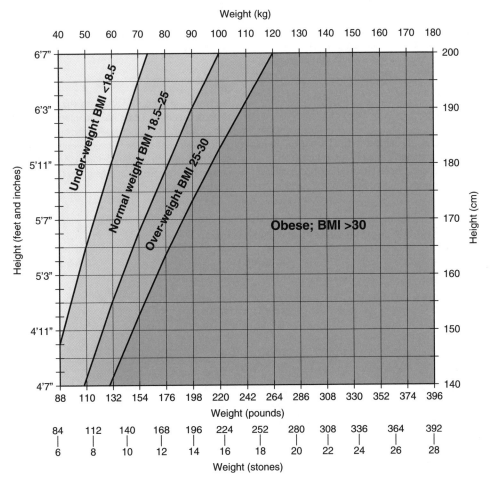

Weight (kg)

Obese; BMI >30

Under-weight BMI <18.5

Normal weight BMI 18.5–25

Over-weight BMI 25–30

Height (feet and inches)

Height (cm)

Weight (pounds)

Weight (stones)

BMI = kg/m²

11) Hypoglycaemic emergency

Sulphonylurea- or meglitinide-induced:
If mild, oral carbohydrate, such as two to four dextrose tablets, or two teaspoons of sucrose in water or milk.
If severe (ie coma), *admit to hospital as an emergency*.
NB – chlorpropamide and glibenclamide carry the highest risks of severe hypoglycaemia (although all secretagogues have this potential).
See page 143.

Insulin-induced:
If mild, as above.
If no improvement, repeat in five to 10 minutes.
Severe hypoglycaemia may require iv dextrose (25 ml 50% into a large vein). Intramuscular (im) glucagon may be given by relatives or paramedics to type 1 patients.

Failure to respond necessitates emergency hospital admission.
Alternative causes for coma, such as stroke or drug overdose, should be considered.
See page 182.

Note:
Metformin, acarbose, miglitol and the thiazolidinediones (rosiglitazone, pioglitazone) do not usually cause hypoglycaemia as monotherapy.
If acarbose contributes to hypoglycaemia (eg in combination with a sulphonylurea), oral dextrose, rather than sucrose, should be given (because of delayed intestinal digestion).

12) Laboratory data: normal values* and conversions

Measurement	Value units	Other value units
Haematology		
Erythrocyte count		
male	4.5–6.5 million/cu mm	$(x10^{12}/l)$
female	3.9–5.6 million/cu mm	$(x\ 10^{12}/l)$
Haematocrit		
male	40–54% (ml/dl)	
female	37–47% (ml/dl)	
Haemoglobin		
male	13.5–18.0 g/dl	2.09–2.79 mmol/l
female	11.5–16.0 g/dl	1.78–2.48 mmol/l
Mean corpuscular volume (MCV)	80–100 cu μm	
Mean corpuscular haemoglobin (MCH)	27–32 pg	
Mean corpuscular haemoglobin concentration (MCHC)	32–36 g/dl	
Platelets	150–500 x 10^9/l	
Reticulocyte count	0.1–2.0/100 erythrocytes	
White cell count	4.0–11.0 x 10^9/l	
Cerebrospinal fluid		
Cells	0–5 white cells/cu mm	
Glucose	2.8–4.4 mmol/l	50–80 mg/dl
Protein	0.15–0.45 g/l	
Urine		
Microalbuminuria	30–300 mg/day	
Proteinuria	>300 mg/day	
Albumin:creatinine ratio	male <2.5 mg/mmol	
	female <3.5 mg/mmol	

* Values commonly recognized as being within a 'normal range' – consult your local laboratory for precise reference ranges.

12) Laboratory data: normal values* and conversions (contd.)

Measurement	Value units	(Conversion)	Other value units
Blood			
Albumin	35–50 g/l	(÷10)	3.5–5.0 g/dl
Amylase	90–300 units/l		
Anion gap [Na^+] – [Cl^- + HCO_3^-]	7–15 mmol/l		
Aspartate transaminase (AST, SGOT)	5–35 units/l[a] (at 37°C)		
Alanine transaminase (ALT, SGPT)	5–35 units/l[a] (at 37°C)		
Bicarbonate	24–30 mmol/l		
Bilirubin – total	5–19 µmol/l	(x0.06)	0.3–1.1 mg/dl
– conjugated	1.7–6.8 µmol/l	(x0.06)	0.1–0.4 mg/dl
C-peptide (fasting)	0.2–0.8 nmol/l	(÷0.33)	0.6–2.4 ng/ml
Chloride	95–105 mmol/l		
Calcium	2.25–2.75 mmol/l	(x4)	9–11 mg/dl
Cholesterol	3.1–5.7 mmol/l	(x39)	120–220 mg/dl
Creatinine	60–133 µmol/l	(÷88.4)	0.67–1.5 mg/dl
Cortisol (morning)	150–700 nmol/l	(÷27.6)	5–25 µg/dl
Catecholamines – total	<7000 pmol/l	(÷5.9)	<1100 ng/l
– adrenaline (epinephrine)	<1300 pmol/l	(÷5.4)	<200 ng/l
– noradrenaline (norepinephrine)	<5700 pmol/l	(÷5.9)	<900 ng/l
Fatty acids (non-esterified)	0.3–0.6 mmol/l		
Glucose (fasting venous plasma)	3–6 mmol/l	(x18)	54–108 mg/dl
Glucagon (fasting)	<50 pmol/l	(x3.4)	<170 pg/ml
Glycated haemoglobin A_{1c} (HbA_{1c})	4–6 %		
Gases – pO_2	10–13.3 kPa		75–100 mmHg
– pCO_2	4.7–6.0 kPa		35–45 mmHg
Insulin (fasting)	15–130 pmol/l	(÷6.6)	2–20 µunit/ml
Lactate (fasting)	0.5–2.0 mmol/l	(x9)	4.5–18 mg/dl
Magnesium	0.7–1.1 mmol/l	(x2.6)	1.8–3.0 mg/dl
Ketones (β-hydroxybutyrate, acetoacetate, acetone)	0.05–0.2 mmol/l		
Globulin	20–35 g/l	(÷10)	2.0–3.5 mg/dl
Growth hormone (morning)	<2.0 munits/l	(x2.5)	<5.0 ng/ml
Lipoproteins – LDL-cholesterol	1.5–4 mmol/l	(x39)	60–155 mg/dl
– HDL-cholesterol	1–2 mmol/l	(x39)	40–80 mg/dl
Osmolarity	280–305 mOsmol/l		
Oestradiol (luteal)	150–1100 pmol/l	(÷3.67)	40–300 pg/ml
Oestrone (luteal)	90–460 pmol/l	(÷3.69)	25–125 pg/ml
Phosphate	0.8–1.5 mmol/l	(x3)	2.5–4.5 mg/dl
Potassium	3.5–5.0 mmol/l		
Progesterone (luteal)	15–80 nmol/l	(÷3.18)	5–25 ng/ml
Proinsulin (fasting)	<30 pmol/l	(x9)	<300 pg/ml
Prolactin (female)	<500 munits/l	(÷20)	<25 ng/ml
Protein (total)	60–80 g/l	(÷10)	6–8 g/dl
Pyruvate (fasting)	0.03–0.1 mmol/l	(÷1.13)	0.3–0.9 mg/dl
Sodium	135–145 mmol/l		
Testosterone (male)	10–42 nmol/l	(÷3.5)	3–12 ng/ml
Testosterone (female)	0.5–2.5 nmol/l	(÷3.5)	0.2–0.5 ng/ml
Thyroglobulin	<30 pmol/l		

* Values commonly recognized as being within a 'normal range' – consult your local laboratory for precise reference ranges.
a There are substantial variations in normal ranges between laboratories.

12) Laboratory data: normal values* and conversions (contd.)

Measurement	Value units	(Conversion)	Other value units
Thyroid stimulating hormone	0.5–6.0 munits/l		
Thyroxine (T_4)	70–140 nmol/l	(÷12.9)	5–10 µg/dl
Thyroxine (free)	10–25 pmol/l	(÷12.9)	0.7–2.0 ng/dl
Triiodothyronine (T_3)	1–3 nmol/l	(÷0.015)	65–200 ng/dl
Triiodothyronine (free)	3–9 pmol/l		
Triglyceride (fasting)	0.4–1.7 mmol/l	(x89)	35–150 mg/dl
Urea nitrogen	2.9–8.2 mmol/l	(x2.8)	8–23 mg/dl
Uric acid	0.18–0.48 mmol/l	(x17)	3–8 mg/dl

* Values commonly recognized as being within a 'normal range' – consult your local laboratory for precise reference ranges.
[a] There are substantial variations in normal ranges between laboratories.

Index

Page numbers in *italics* refer to *tables* and *figures*.